Acupuncture, Trigger Points and Musculoskeletal Pain

To Oina, my wife, for her patience and
forbearance during the writing of this book.

The phenomena of pain belong to that borderland
between the body and soul about which it is so
delightful to speculate from the comfort of an
armchair but which offers such formidable
obstacles to scientific inquiry.

J. H. Kellgren (1948)

Central cover illustration reproduced with permission of
D.G. Simons and J.G. Travell from Wall P.D. and Melzack R.
(eds) 1984 *Textbook of Pain*

For Churchill Livingstone
Publisher: Mary Law
Project Editor: Inta Ozols
Production Controller: Mark Sanderson
Design: Design Resources Unit
Sales Promotion Executive: Hilary Brown

Acupuncture, Trigger Points and Musculoskeletal Pain

A scientific approach to acupuncture for use by doctors and physiotherapists in the diagnosis and management of myofascial trigger point pain

P. E. Baldry MB BS FRCP

Emeritus Consultant Physician and Postgraduate Clinical Tutor, Ashford Hospital, Middlesex
Past Chairman, British Medical Acupuncture Society
President, Acupuncture Association of Chartered Physiotherapists

Foreword by

John W. Thompson PhD MB BS FRCP

Professor of Pharmacology and Head of Department of
Pharmacological Sciences, University of Newcastle upon Tyne
Consultant Clinical Pharmacologist and Consultant
in Administrative Charge, Pain Relief Clinic, Royal Victoria
Infirmary, Newcastle upon Tyne

SECOND EDITION

CHURCHILL LIVINGSTONE
EDINBURGH LONDON MADRID MELBOURNE NEW YORK AND TOKYO 1993

CHURCHILL LIVINGSTONE
Medical Division of Longman Group UK Limited

Distributed in the United States of America by Redwing
Book Company, 44 Linden Street, Brookline, MA 02146.

First edition 1989
Second edition 1993

ISBN 0-443-04580-1

British Library Cataloguing in Publication Data
A catalogue record for this book is available from the British
Library.

Library of Congress Cataloging-in-Publication Data
Baldry, Peter.
    Acupuncture, trigger points, and musculoskeletal pain:
a scientific approach to acupuncture for use by doctors and
physiotherapists in the diagnosis and management of
myofascial trigger point pain/P.E. Baldry; foreword by
John W. Thompson.—2nd ed.
        p.   cm.
    Includes bibliographical references and index.
    ISBN 0-443-04580-1: £35.00
    1. Musculoskeletal system—Acupuncture. 2. Myalgia—
Treatment. I. Title.
    [DNLM: 1. Acupuncture. 2. Fibromyalgia—diagnosis.
3. Fibromyalgia—therapy. 4. Myofascial Pain Syndromes—
diagnosis. 5. Myofascial Pain Syndromes—therapy.
WB 369 B178a]
RC925.5.B36 1993
615.8′92—dc20
DNLM/DLC
for Library of Congress   92-17401
                                               CIP

The
publisher's
policy is to use
**paper manufactured
from sustainable forests**

Produced by Longman Singapore Publishers Pte Ltd
Printed in Singapore

Foreword

Quod est ante pedes nemo spectat: coeli Scrutantur plagas.
(What is before one's feet no one looks at; they gaze at
the regions of heaven.)
                    Ennius, quoted by Cicero, *De Divinat.*, 2, 13.

This is an important and valuable book that
needed to be written. Musculoskeletal or myofascial pain is an all too common and extraordinarily neglected subject of medicine; it is
barely mentioned in many textbooks of medicine.
In reality it is a ubiquitous condition that causes
a great deal of pain and suffering and one which
unfortunately either slips by unrecognized or is
passed off as trivial or untreatable. In this book
Dr Peter Baldry has shown how musculoskeletal
pain can be simply and effectively treated by
acupuncture. But this book is much more than
that because it is really three books in one.

The first part presents an interesting historical
background to Chinese acupuncture and its
spread to the outside world, particularly to the
West. The second part deals with the principles
of trigger point acupuncture wherein, over the
course of six chapters, the reader is presented
with a detailed and critical account of the
evidence for and the nature of trigger points and
the way in which acupuncture can be used to
deactivate them. Dr Baldry spares no effort to
provide the reader with an up-to-date and
accurate account of the neurophysiology of pain
and the possible ways in which acupuncture can
be used to control it. He also grasps the difficult
and important nettle concerning the scientific
evaluation of acupuncture. The results of properly controlled experiments and trials demonstrating the efficacy of acupuncture are slowly but
surely accumulating and Dr Baldry discusses
these critically and points the way to the further
rigorous studies that are urgently needed. The
third part of the book gives a detailed and
splendidly practical account of the many different
forms of musculoskeletal pain and the way that
these can be treated with acupuncture.

Even for the reader who does not intend to use
acupuncture, this book still serves a most
valuable purpose by drawing attention to the very
large number of common musculoskeletal pain
conditions which are all too commonly overlooked. A particularly helpful feature of Dr
Baldry's book is the rich admixture of case
histories of his own patients, from which the
medical reader can learn the correct way to
diagnose and subsequently to treat these painful
conditions.

There seems little doubt that, through
unfamiliarity with this condition, much time and
effort are often expended unnecessarily both by
the medical profession and by patients seeking
the cause and treatment of pain problems which
are, in fact, musculoskeletal in origin. Dr Baldry
has performed a most valuable service in writing
this eminently readable book and I wish it the
very considerable success that it richly deserves.

John W. Thompson

Contents

Preface

The aims of this book

It is because traditional Chinese acupuncture is perforce inextricably bound up with archaic concepts concerning the structure and function of the body that most members of the medical profession in the Western world view it with suspicion and scepticism and assign it, together with various other seemingly esoteric forms of therapy, to what it has become fashionable to call alternative medicine. Moreover, it is evident that attempts during the past 40 years to place Chinese acupuncture on a more rational and scientific basis have done little to dispel this attitude.

The main purpose of this book is to bring to the attention of doctors and physiotherapists a 20th-century-evolved scientific approach to acupuncture for the relief of pain arising from myofascial trigger points, and to take acupuncture (so far as the alleviation of this type of pain is concerned) out of the category of alternative medicine by describing a method of employing it which has been developed as a result of observations made by physicians in the Western world in recent years and which therefore may readily be incorporated within the framework of present-day orthodox Western medical practice.

In this second edition, several chapters in Part Two have been considerably extended in order to incorporate recent advances in knowledge concerning the neurophysiology of pain, to describe more fully the methods employed in the diagnosis of myofascial trigger point pain, and to provide an up-to-date account of the endogenous pain modulating mechanisms involved in relieving this type of pain with acupuncture.

In addition it has been found necessary to include an entirely new chapter in view of the recently recognized diagnostic and therapeutic importance of distinguishing between the localized primary myofascial pain syndromes and the generalized fibromyalgia syndrome.

It is hoped that as a result of reading this book many more neurologists, rheumatologists, orthopaedic specialists, anaesthetists, general physicians, general practitioners and physiotherapists than at present may be led to search for trigger points in their routine clinical investigation of pain, and may be persuaded to include the type of acupuncture described in this book in their therapeutic armamentarium for cases in which there is referral of pain from these trigger points. It is hoped that this in turn may lead to the setting up of much larger-scale, statistically-controlled trials than heretofore so that the indications for and the effectiveness of this particular form of therapy may become more clearly defined.

Case histories

I offer no apology for having included case histories in this book. They are of course by their very nature essentially anecdotal and certainly no inference is meant to be drawn from them concerning the effectiveness of trigger point acupuncture, for any conclusions about that can only come from clinical trials. The sole purpose of including these vignettes is to provide illustrations from everyday clinical practice that serve to highlight certain important principles underlying the diagnosis and management of various painful musculoskeletal disorders.

Acknowledgements

My very sincere thanks are due to Professor John Thompson for the meticulous manner in which he read the manuscript of this book and then gave me much valuable advice and constructive criticism besides kindly writing a foreword.

I wish to express my gratitude to Dr Alexander Macdonald for it was he who, some years ago, first drew my attention to the aetiological importance of trigger points in the pathogenesis of musculoskeletal pain and introduced me to trigger point acupuncture as a method of alleviating it.

I thank Dr Felix Mann for having initially brought to my notice the close relationship between trigger points and traditional Chinese acupuncture points.

I wish to thank Drs Janet Travell and David Simons for the very considerable contribution they have made to my knowledge of specific patterns of myofascial trigger point pain referral. It has largely been from studying their descriptions and illustrations of these patterns in various publications referred to later in this book that I am now able to recognize them in my own patients.

I also wish to acknowledge my indebtedness to Dr David Bowsher, for it is from him in particular that I have learnt so much about what is currently known concerning the mechanisms responsible for the pain-relieving effect of acupuncture.

I am very grateful to Mr Robert Britton for having so skilfully converted my rough sketches of pain patterns into artistically executed drawings; and also to Miss Barbara Careless for her enthusiastic and careful typing of the manuscript.

I have to thank Professors Peter Williams and Roger Warwick, the editors of *Gray's Anatomy* (36th edition 1980) and its publishers Churchill Livingstone for giving me permission to reproduce Figs 12.1, 12.5, 12.9, 12.14, 13.12, 15.1, 15.2, 15.17, 15.23*, 16.8, 16.9, 16.10, 17.1, 18.1*, 18.6, 18.7*, 18.9*, 18.11*, 20.1, 20.2, 20.5*, 20.6. The illustrations from *Gray's Anatomy* marked with an asterisk originally appeared in *Quain's Anatomy* 11th edition.

Finally, I have to thank the following: Dr J. H. Kellgren and the editor of *Clinical Science* for permission to publish Figs 4.1 and 4.2; Dr Kellgren and the editor of the *British Medical Journal* for permission to publish Fig. 4.3; Dr Howard Fields and McGraw Hill, New York for permission to reproduce Figs 6.1, 6.2, 6.3 and 7.3 from *Pain* 1987; Dr David Bowsher and the editor of *Acupuncture in Medicine – The Journal of the British Medical Acupuncture Society* for permission to reproduce Figs 6.6 and 8.1; Dr Alexander Macdonald and George Allen & Unwin, London for permission to reproduce Figs 7.1 and 7.2 from *Acupuncture — from Ancient Art to Modern Medicine* 1982; Mr R. J. D'Souza for providing me with Fig. 7.3; Dr David Simons and Churchill Livingstone, Edinburgh for permission to reproduce Fig. 16.6. from *Textbook of Pain* (Wall P, Melzack R, eds) 2nd edition 1989; Professor R. W. Porter and Churchill Livingstone, Edinburgh for permission to reproduce Figs 17.1 and 17.2 from *The Lumbar Spine and Back Pain* (Jason M I V, ed) 3rd edition 1987.

Fladbury, Pershore,
Worcs WR10 2QX, 1993   P. E. B.

Introduction

For reasons to be explained later in this book, the early 1970s saw the dawn of an era when people in the Western world began taking an increasing interest in the ancient oriental mode of therapy known as acupuncture, with lay practitioners of it leading the public to believe that it has such wide ranging healing properties as to be an effective alternative to orthodox medicine in the treatment of a large number of diseases.

There is clearly no justification for such extravagant claims and it has to be said that, at the onset of this era, the medical profession in Europe and America viewed this form of therapy with considerable suspicion and continued to do so for so long as explanations as to how it might work remained inextricably bound up with abstruse concepts formulated by the Chinese 3000 years previously. This reluctance to believe in these long-established but somewhat esoteric concepts was, of course, because they had been conceived at a time when ideas concerning the structure and function of the body together with those concerning the nature of disease belonged more to the realms of fantasy than fact, and for this reason it was difficult to reconcile them with the principles upon which the present-day Western system of medical practice is based.

By chance, however, the past 15–20 years have also seen a considerable increase in knowledge concerning the neurophysiology of pain and because of this there is now a scientific explanation for acupuncture's ability to alleviate pain. It is now apparent that this technique, which involves the use of dry needles (*acus* (Latin), needle) for the purpose of stimulating peripheral nerve endings, achieves its pain-relieving effect by virtue of the fact that stimulation of this type is capable of evoking activity in pain-modulating mechanisms situated in the central nervous system.

In the light of this, the medical profession in the West has therefore had to revise its attitudes towards acupuncture so far as pain relief is concerned, for, as pointed out in the recent report on alternative therapies by the British Medical Association's Board of Science and Education (1986), its analgesic properties can now be explained on a scientific basis, and, in addition, controlled trials have provided acceptable evidence as to its usefulness in combating pain and in particular that occurring in association with certain musculoskeletal disorders.

The purpose of this book is to discuss the scientific aspects of acupuncture and to show how this type of therapy can be used in a rational manner for the relief of musculoskeletal pain by the application of a method recently developed in the Western world and based on principles that form an integral part of the system of medicine practised there.

For those trained in the Western system of medicine there are obvious advantages in using this particular method rather than the traditional Chinese one but clearly these advantages cannot be fully appreciated without knowing something about the latter. This book is therefore divided into three parts with Part One containing a brief account of traditional Chinese acupuncture. It also gives reasons as to why doctors in Europe on first learning about this type of treatment in the 17th century rejected it, and describes how certain 19th-century European and American doctors, having put on one side what they considered to be unacceptable Chinese concepts concerning this mode of therapy, devised a method of practising it principally for the relief of musculoskeletal pain that may be considered to be a forerunner of the somewhat more sophisticated one developed in recent years and described in this book. It is also pointed out that, although physicians who advocated the use of acupuncture during the last century wrote enthusiastically about it, it was never widely practised by their contemporaries, mainly it would seem because at that time there was no satisfactory explanation as to the manner in which it might work.

Part Two describes how it was fundamental laboratory investigations into the phenomenon of referred pain from musculoskeletal structures carried out by J. H. Kellgren at University College Hospital, London, in the late 1930s that prompted many physicians during the 1940s, including in particular Janet Travell in America, to study the clinical manifestations of this particular type of pain. And how, as a result of this, the latter came to recognize the importance of what she termed trigger points as being the source of pain in many commonly occurring musculoskeletal disorders.

Also, once it had been shown that it is possible to alleviate such pain by injecting trigger points with a local anaesthetic or with one or other of a variety of different irritant substances, it was discovered that this could be accomplished even more simply, as well as more safely and equally effectively, by deactivating these structures with dry needles, or in other words by performing acupuncture.

Part Two also contains a brief account of advances in knowledge concerning the neurophysiology of pain during the 1960s and 1970s and describes the various pain-modulating mechanisms now considered to be involved in the production of acupuncture analgesia. In addition it includes a discussion of some of the difficulties so far encountered in scientifically evaluating the pain relieving efficacy of acupuncture and in determining its place relative to other types of treatment in the alleviation of musculoskeletal pain.

Part Three is devoted to the practical applications of trigger point acupuncture.

REFERENCE

British Medical Association 1986 Alternative therapy. Report of the Board of Science and Education

PART ONE

Acupuncture — a historical review

1. Traditional Chinese acupuncture

The Chinese first carried our acupuncture, that seemingly strange practice whereby needles are inserted into people for therapeutic purposes, at least 3000 years ago. News of this, however, did not reach the Western world until about 300 years ago when European medical officers employed by the Dutch East Indies Trading Company in and around Java saw it being used there by the Japanese, and when at about the same time Jesuit missionaries came across it whilst endeavouring to convert the Chinese to Christianity.

From their writings it is clear that both these groups found the concepts upon which the Chinese based their curious practice difficult to comprehend, due to the fact that these appeared to be completely at variance with what Europeans by that time had come to know about the anatomy and physiology of the human body. And it has been this inability to reconcile the theoretical concepts put forward by the Chinese in support of acupuncture with those upon which modern scientific medicine is based that has for so long been the cause of such little interest being taken in it in the Western world. During the past 30 years, however, attitudes towards acupuncture in the West have been changing since research into the mechanisms of pain has provided a certain amount of insight as to how possibly it achieves its effect on pain. These, as might be expected, are entirely different from those originally put forward by the Chinese.

The prime purpose of this book is to describe a recently developed method of practising acupuncture in which dry needles are inserted into the tissues overlying what have come to be known as trigger points as a means of alleviating musculoskeletal pain. Before turning to this, however, it is necessary to give a brief account of the discovery and development of the traditional practice of Chinese acupuncture as it is only by having a proper understanding of this that the merits of the trigger point approach to acupuncture can be fully appreciated. For an explanation as to how the Chinese came to discover the therapeutic properties of acupuncture in the first place it is helpful to turn to an early Chinese medical book entitled *Huang Ti Nei Ching* and known in the English-speaking world as *The Yellow Emperor's Manual of Corporeal Medicine*. This is a most unusual textbook of medicine as it is written in the form of a dialogue between the Emperor Huang Ti and his minister Chhi-Po. It is a work which incorporates much concerning the philosophical thoughts of the ancient Chinese, their religious beliefs with particular reference to Taoism, their observations concerning the workings of the universe in general, and the application of all this to their practice of medicine.

The Western world is much indebted to the American scholar, Ilza Veith, who, in February 1945 at the Institute of the History of Medicine at Johns Hopkins University, undertook the extremely difficult task of translating this important treatise into English. This translation together with her own invaluable introductory analysis of the work was first published in 1949. Also, for those who wish to read a detailed account of how the Chinese practice of acupuncture has gradually evolved over the centuries, there is much of considerable interest in *Celestial Lancets*, an erudite study of the subject written by the two distinguished Cambridge historians, Lu Gwei-Djen and Joseph Needham (1980).

It is by no means certain that Huang Ti ever lived, with the general consensus of opinion being that he is a legendary figure, but nevertheless he is to this day worshipped as the father of Chinese medicine. It is very difficult to determine with any degree of accuracy the date the *Nei Ching* first appeared, but it seems likely that Part I, the *Su Wên* (Questions and Answers), originated in the 2nd century BC and that Part II *Chen Ching* (Needle Manual) first appeared in the 1st century BC. However not only was the latter re-named the *Ling Shu* (Vital Axis) in about AD 762 but both parts have been repeatedly revised with the addition each time of extensive commentaries by a variety of different people. This prompted Ilza Veith to say:

It is obvious that any work that has undergone the fate of the *Yellow Emperor's Canon of Internal Medicine* contains but little of its authentic original text; it is also clear that its various commentators have frequently obscured rather than elucidated its meaning. It seems impossible to determine now how much of the original text remains; especially since in former times it was difficult to distinguish text from commentary.

Nevertheless in spite of all these difficulties it is generally agreed that from a study of this work it is possible to gain a clear idea as to how the practice of acupuncture had developed in China by the 2nd century BC.

Acupuncture and a related form of heat therapy and counter-irritation known as moxibustion almost certainly had their origins long before this, as may be seen from recently discovered medical manuscripts written on sheets of silk in the tomb of the son of the Lord of Tai, a young man who died in 168 BC. As Lu Gwei-Djen & Joseph Needham point out 'the style and contents of the texts is similar to that of the *Nei Ching* but more archaic, so that they present a picture of Chinese medical thought during the two or three centuries preceding the compilation of that great classic'.

It is interesting to observe that these manuscripts, whilst certainly referring to the practice of acupuncture with needles made of stone, discuss moxibustion in even greater detail and there are reasons for believing that that technique may have been introduced even longer ago than acupuncture itself.

Moxibustion is a process by which heat is applied to the body by the burning of Artemisia leaves that have been dried to a tinder. This Artemisia tinder has come to be known in the West as moxa — a word of Japanese derivation (*mogusa*, herb for burning) because it was from Japan that the Western world first heard about this technique in the 17th century.

The classical method of performing moxibustion is to make the tinder into a cone and apply it to the skin at points identical to those used for acupuncture. Sometimes it is used as a counter-irritant by being allowed to blister and scar the skin. At other times it is used as a milder form of heat treatment, by applying it to the skin with a layer of vegetable material interposed between this and the cone in order to protect the former from damage. Yet another method is to combine moxibustion with acupuncture by placing a piece of moxa on top of a needle inserted into the body, and igniting it, when the heat from the moxa is conducted down the needle to the surrounding tissues.

Acupuncture. The concepts which prompted the ancient Chinese to use acupuncture for therapeutic purposes were complex and to the modern Western mind difficult to comprehend. They were intricately bound up with their views concerning all aspects of the living world, including in particular their belief in the existence of two cosmic regulators known as Yin and Yang.

The supremacy of power and influence accorded to these two forces in the creation of the world is well illustrated by the following quotations from the *Nei Ching*.

The principle of Yin and Yang is the basis of the entire universe. It is the principle of everything in creation. It brings about the transformation to parenthood; it is the root and source of life and death . . .

Heaven was created by an accumulation of Yang; the Earth was created by an accumulation of Yin.

The ways of Yin and Yang are to the left and to the right. Water and fire are the symbols of Yin and Yang. Yin and Yang are the source of power and the beginning of everything in creation.

Yang ascends to Heaven; Yin descends to Earth. Hence the universe (Heaven and Earth) represents motion and rest, controlled by the wisdom of nature. Nature grants the power to beget and to grow, to harvest and to store, to finish and to begin anew.

Further, the Chinese considered that, following the creation of the world, Yin and Yang continued to exert a considerable influence, and that indeed the preservation of order in all natural phenomena, both celestial and terrestrial, was dependent on the maintenance of a correct balance between them. It should be noted in this connection that neither of these two opposing forces were ever envisaged as existing in pure form but rather that each contained a modicum of the other. And moreover, there was the belief that all events both in nature and in the human body were influenced by a constantly changing relationship between them.

Yin and Yang were thus said to be ubiquitous essential components of all things, with in some cases Yang being predominant and in others Yin. In the universe for example, phenomena such as the sun, heaven, day, fire, heat and light were all considered to be predominantly Yang in nature, whereas their opposites, the moon, earth, night, water, cold and darkness were considered to be predominantly Yin. The individual structures of the body were also thought to have either Yang or Yin qualities. For example, five hollow viscera — the stomach, small intestine, large intestine, bladder and gall bladder — were said to be Yang organs because lying near to the surface on opening the body they get exposed to light. In contrast, five solid viscera — the heart, lungs, kidneys, spleen and liver — were said to be Yin organs due to their being in the dark recesses of the body.

The conclusion reached by the Chinese that five organs had Yang and five had Yin characteristics was apparently not a fortuitous one but seemingly because five was considered to be a dominant number in their conception of the universe. This stemmed from their fundamental belief in the theory of the five elements, which stated that Yin and Yang consist of five elements, namely water, fire, metal, wood and earth, and that man and indeed all natural phenomena are products of an interaction between these two opposing forces.

The theory of the five elements was extremely complicated and there is little to be gained by going into it in detail except to say, in view of its relevance to the traditional practice of Chinese acupuncture, that in its application to the organs of the body the *Nei Ching* teaches that:

The heart is connected with the pulse and rules over the kidneys. The lungs are connected with the skin and rule over the heart. The liver is connected with the muscles and rules over the lungs. The spleen is connected with the flesh and rules over the lungs. The kidneys are connected with the bones and rule over the spleen.

With this background it is now possible to see how these various considerations concerning Yin and Yang came to be applied to matters concerning the maintenance of health and the development of disease. It was considered that in order to be healthy these two opposing forces have to be in a correct state of balance (crasis) and that it is when this is not so that disease occurs (dyscrasia).

Further, it was considered that this health-giving balance between Yin and Yang only exists when a special form of energy, known as chhi, flows freely through a system of tracts. And, as a corollary to this, that disease develops when a collection of 'evil air' in one or other of the tracts obstructs the flow of chhi through it as this leads to an imbalance between Yin and Yang. It was in attempting to dispel this 'evil air' or wind that the Chinese were first led to insert needles into these tracts, and then from this, over the course of centuries, to develop a somewhat complex system of therapy now known to the Western world as acupuncture (from the Latin *acus*, a needle; and *punctura*, a prick).

As it is only possible to understand how the Chinese developed their system of acupuncture by having some knowledge of their original, somewhat primitive ideas concerning the anatomy and physiology of the body, these will now be discussed.

The knowledge of anatomy and physiology possessed by the Chinese when they first started to practise acupuncture was obviously both scanty and inaccurate. It is therefore surprising to find that from an early date and certainly by the time the *Su Wên* was compiled in the 2nd century BC they had with considerable perspicacity come to realize that blood circulates continuously around the body. For in this manuscript Chhi-Po says:

The flow (of blood) . . . runs on and on, and never stops; a ceaseless movement in an annular circuit.

Chhi-Po is here showing remarkable intuition especially when it is remembered that it was another 1700 years before the Western world came round to this view. This tardy realization of the true state of affairs in the West was of course because Galen, that remarkably influential early Greek physician, had categorically stated that the movement of blood in the vessels of the body is by means of a tidal ebb and flow. This remained the official view for centuries and anyone who dared to question it was considered a blasphemous heretic. Indeed it was not until 1628 that William Harvey with considerable courage published his proof that blood moves around the body in a continuous circle in his *Exercitatio Anatomica de Motu Cordis et Sanguinis in Animalibus*.

The ancient Chinese admittedly had no scientific evidence to support their belief in the circulation of the blood but because of their inherent conviction that the workings of the body are a microcosmic representation of those to be found in the macrocosm or universe itself, they may have come to this conclusion from observing the meteorological water-cycle that occurs in nature.

It should be noted that the Chinese at an early date not only correctly concluded that blood circulates around the body but also that this is effected by a pumping action of the heart, for in the *Su Wên* it says 'the heart presides over the circulation of the blood and juices and the paths in which they travel'. Moreover, they were quick to appreciate that the action of the heart is reflected in movements of the pulse felt at the wrist, and were able to measure the pulse rate by using an instrument capable of measuring time by a regulated flow of water, an apparatus similar to that used by the ancient Greeks for timing speeches in their law courts and called by them a clepsydra.

The ancient Chinese also with much ingenuity attempted to estimate the time it takes for blood to circulate around the body and to assist with this calculation measured the approximate total length of the great blood vessels. Although their conclusion that the circulation time is 28.8 minutes was about 60 times too slow, modern methods

having now shown it to be only 30 seconds, it was nevertheless a praiseworthy effort, especially when it is remembered that even William Harvey several hundred years later got the calculation wrong!

The Chinese whilst realizing that blood circulates around the body in specially designed vessels also believed, as did the ancient Greeks, that there is a separate substance very difficult to define in modern terms but which could perhaps best be described as a vital force or special form of energy, that also circulates around the body.

The Greeks referred to it as pneuma and considered it to be present with the blood in arteries. The Chinese called a substance of similar nature chhi, with part of it having Yang properties and the other part Yin properties. Following the appearance of the *Ling Shu* in about 762 AD it has always been said that the Yin chhi circulates around the body in the blood vessels, whilst the Yang chhi travels outside them in a completely separate system of channels or tracts.

This system of tracts, which anatomically is not demonstrable, has nevertheless always been very real to the Chinese who from the beginning believed it to consist of an intricate network of main channels, connecting channels and tributaries similar to the rivers, tributaries and canals which together make up the waterways of the earth. The idea is to be found clearly expressed in a book entitled the *Kuan Tzu* written about the late 4th century BC where it says 'one can say water is the blood and the chhi of the earth, because it flows and penetrates everywhere in the same manner as the circulation . . . in the tract and blood vessel systems'.

A belief in the existence of such tracts was vital to the Chinese in developing their practice of acupuncture and it is because of the essential part these channels play in this that they are specifically known as acu-tracts. Nonetheless it must be emphasized that it is the lack of any tangible proof of their existence that has been one of the main reasons why the Western world has viewed the traditional Chinese method of practising acupuncture with such considerable suspicion since first hearing about it 300 years ago.

The Chinese have always visualized and described these tracts in a three-dimensional form and considered them to be at variable depths along their individual courses. Clear descriptions of this are given in their writings, although their illustrations merely give the impression that the tracts run in a relatively straight line along the surface of the body. It should be noted that modern Western writers often refer to the Chinese acu-tracts as meridians but this is better avoided because as Lu Gwei-Djen & Joseph Needham in the *Celestial Lancets* point out 'the analogy with astronomical hour-circles or terrestial longitude is so far-fetched that we do not adopt the term'.

The Chinese described 12 main acu-tracts corresponding in number with the months of the year with each one being considered to have a connection with and taking its name from an organ of the body. However, as already stated, the Chinese were of the opinion that there were only ten principal organs, five with Yin characteristics and five with Yang characteristics. Therefore in order that the 12 tracts could be linked with 12 organs they found it necessary to include the pericardium amongst the Yin organs, and to invent a structure with no known equivalent in modern anatomy, which they called the san chiao (triple warmer) and included this amongst the Yang organs.

It is of interest to note that because the brain was considered to be nothing more than some form of storage organ it was not included amongst the principal organs. The *Nei Ching* in fact states that it is the liver which 'is the dwelling place of the soul or spiritual part of man that ascends to heaven'.

Those who pioneered the development of acupuncture in ancient China believed that acu-tracts for most of their course are situated in the depths of the body's tissues, but that at certain points, now known in the West as acu-points, they come to lie immediately under the skin surface where needles can readily be inserted into them.

It will be remembered that, according to traditional Chinese teaching, the purpose of inserting needles into acu-points in disease is to release noxious air or 'wind' (malignant chhi) that impedes the free flow of chhi in acu-tracts and thereby disturbs the balance between Yin and Yang.

It is possible to gain some idea as to how the Chinese have always thought about acu-points by studying the various names they use to describe them in their writings. One of the commonest of these being chhi hsüeh — hsüeh being a word meaning a hole or minute cavity or crevice; in the *Su Wên*, chhi hsüeh are described as pores or interstices in the flesh that are connected to the naturally occurring Yin and Yang forms of chhi in the acu-tract and blood vessel systems. It is also said that these 'holes' in the flesh are open to invasion by malignant chhi from outside the body but that if and when this onslaught occurs it is readily repelled by acupuncture!

The *Nei Ching* in several places says that there are 365 acu-points. A figure no doubt arrived at because of its symbolic association with the number of degrees in the celestial circle, the number of days in the year and the number of bones in the human body. This however was only the number of points supposed to be present in theory for even in the *Nei Ching* itself only 160 points actually receive names, and with the passage of time even fewer have remained in regular use.

The Chinese have given each of their acu-points a specific name and just as they have named acu-tracts after various rivers so they have incorporated into the names of acu-points references to such parts of nature's waterway system as tanks, pools and reservoirs. Also, during the course of time, acu-points along the length of each tract have been individually numbered, and, as every tract bears the name of the organ to which it is supposed to be linked, it necessarily follows that each point may be identified by reference to the name of the tract along which it is situated and its number on this tract. For example, the point on the gall bladder tract situated half-way between the neck and the tip of the shoulder at the highest point of the shoulder girdle has been named by the Chinese Jianjing but is more commonly referred to as Gall Bladder 21 (GB 21); the point situated between the head of the fibula and the upper end of the tibia called by the Chinese Zusanli is more usually known as Stomach 36 (St 36); and the point just above the web between the first and second toes known as Taichong is more often referred to as Liver 3 (Liv 3).

In the recently developed Western type of approach to acupuncture to be described in this book, acu-tracts and their alleged links with internal organs are not of themselves of any practical importance. However, because most of the trigger points employed in this Western form of acupuncture have been found to have a close spatial correlation with many of the traditional Chinese acu-points, some of the latter will be referred to in the text as a matter of interest.

In traditional Chinese acupuncture it is from an examination of the pulse that disease is mainly diagnosed. The *Nei Ching* contains a clear account of how, from a detailed study of the pulse at the wrist, it is possible to establish the nature of a disease, its location in the body and where best to insert needles to combat it.

The reason why the Chinese have placed such importance on examining the pulse is because they have always considered that it is at that site that the Yin chhi in the blood vessels and the Yang chhi in the tracts converge, and the pulse in some of their writings is referred to as *The Great Meeting Place*.

In the *Nan Ching* — The Manual of Explanations of Eighty-one Difficult Points in the Nei Ching — a work which first appeared some time around the 1st century AD it says:

The Yin chhi runs within the blood vessels, while the Yang chhi travels outside them (in the tracts). The Yin chhi circulates endlessly, never coming to a stop (save at death). After fifty revolutions the two chhi meet again and this is called a 'great meeting'. The Yin and Yang chhi go along with each other in close relation, travelling in circular paths which have no end. So one can see how the Yin and Yang mutually follow one another.

The Chinese method of examining the pulse consists of placing three fingers along the length of the radial artery at both wrists and by first applying superficial pressure to these points and then deep pressure 12 separate observations can be made. From this it is said to be possible to ascertain the state of chhi in the 12 main tracts, and when disease is present, to tell which organ is affected and into which tract needles have to be inserted.

Chinese sphygmology is therefore basically complicated and has been made even more complex over the centuries by the laying down of rules as to when the examination might most profitably

be carried out, including the taking into account of certain astrological considerations in determining the best day for it. Next, the right time of day has to be selected for according to the *Nei Ching* the examination must be done very early in the morning 'when the breath of Yin has not yet begun to stir and when the breath of Yang has not yet begun to diffuse, when food and drink have not yet been taken, when the twelve main vessels are not yet abundant, . . . when vigour and energy are not yet exerted'.

It is clear that the technique of pulse-diagnosis must always have been extremely difficult to master and yet it would seem that those who devised the procedure must have achieved some measure of agreement as to the significance of the various nuances that they considered they could detect at the wrist. Nevertheless their diagnostic interpretation of these was of necessity expressed in nosological terms quite irreconcilable with those based on our present-day knowledge of pathology, and therefore it is surprising to find that certain Western-trained doctors even to this day still try to base their practice of acupuncture on this archaic approach to diagnosis, and are quite unwilling to accept that such an anachronistic procedure should long ago have been relegated to the realms of history.

As the practice of acupuncture has of necessity always depended on the insertion of needles into the body it is of considerable interest to discover how primitive Asiatic man found objects of sufficient tensile strength and sharpness for this purpose.

Thorns of various plants, slivers of bamboo, and needles fashioned from bone have always been available. Bone needles have in fact been found in recent years in tombs from the neolithic age, and by the 6th century, which is about the date of the oldest existing reference to acupuncture, it would have been technically possible to make needles from bronze, copper, tin, silver and even gold. And certainly gold needles have recently been discovered in the tomb of the Han Prince, Liu-Shêng (113 BC). It is therefore somewhat surprising to find that seemingly needles in the early days of acupuncture were commonly made of stone, for in *Huang Ti Nei Ching* (2nd century BC), Chhi-Po says:

In the present age it is necessary to bring forward powerful drugs to combat internal illnesses, and to use acupuncture with sharp stone needles and moxa to control the external ones.

Also, in manuscripts written on silk before this and found in the tomb of the son of the Lord of Tai, there are two separate specific references to the use of stone needles.

It seems difficult to conceive how needles made of stone could have been sharpened sufficiently to penetrate the tissues of the body, but, included amongst the various mineral substances available in those far off days which it has been suggested might have been employed, are flint, mica, asbestos, and jade. However, there is no confirmatory evidence that any of these were utilized and the exact nature of the type of stone originally used still remains a matter for conjecture. The only certainty is that as iron and steel did not become available to the Chinese until the 5th century BC and as the practice of acupuncture was started long before this, it necessarily follows that materials other than iron must have initially been employed.

It is impossible in this brief review to mention all the various stages in the development of this technique over the centuries. Reference will however be made to the *Chen Chiu Chia I Ching* as this is the oldest existing book entirely devoted to acupuncture and moxibustion. It was written soon after the Chinese Empire became re-unified in AD 265 by one Huangfu Mi who apparently became interested in medicine partly because his mother was paralysed and partly because he himself suffered from rheumatism! In this book Huangfu Mi for the first time groups the various acu-points under the names of the various tracts to which they belong and, after numbering them, gives a detailed description of their positions and how to locate them. Further, he names specific acu-points recommended in the treatment of various illnesses and gives much advice as to how he considers acupuncture should best be practised. This is therefore an outstanding book in the history of acupuncture and one which was to exert a great influence of the practice of this technique throughout the East.

Mention must be made of the eminent physician Sun Ssu-mo (AD 581–673) as it was he who introduced the so-called module system for determining the exact position of acu-points on people's bodies irrespective of their various sizes by taking measurements using relative or modular inches. He defined a modular inch as being the distance between the upper ends of the distal and middle interphalangeal folds when a person flexes the middle finger; and recommended that measurements should be made by using strips of bamboo, paper, or straw, cut to the length of a person's individual modular inch.

Sun Ssu-mo was also the author of two outstanding books on acupuncture and moxibustion and was the first to draw attention to the importance of inserting needles into exquisitely tender points, particularly, he said, in treating low back pain. He called these ah-shih (oh-yes!) points, from the expletive often uttered by the patient when pressure is applied over them! This is of particular interest as he was clearly practising what is known now as trigger point acupuncture, and which having been rediscovered in recent years is described in Parts Two and Three of this book.

The Imperial Medical College, with a departmental professor of acupuncture, lecturers, and demonstrators, had been founded by AD 618, and by AD 629 a similar college of medicine had been established in each province.

From AD 1027 the teaching of acupuncture at these institutions was carried out with the help of life-size bronze figures of the human body. The walls of these figures had holes punched in them at the sites of all the known acu-points. The figures with their holes filled with water and covered by wax were then used for examining medical students in acupuncture. This was done by making the students insert needles into sites on these figures where they considered acu-points might exist, and if, on attempting this, no water poured out they failed their examination!

The Chinese have always had a deep conviction that the workings of the body are intimately linked with those of nature in general, and that various cyclical events external to the body have an important influence over matters of health and disease. Further, that for the successful eradication of disease by acupuncture it is necessary to perform the latter at a propitious time and one which can only be determined by taking into consideration the interrelationship of these various external factors. It is therefore not surprising to find that the *Nei Ching* clearly states that in order to discover the right time for both the application of acupuncture and moxibustion the physician must first establish the position of the sun, the moon, other planets, and the stars in addition to taking into account the season of the year and the prevailing weather conditions!

The following is a quotation from Chapter 26 of that book:

Therefore one should act in accordance with the weather and the seasons in order to have blood and breath thoroughly adjusted and harmonized — and consequently — when the weather is cold, one should not apply acupuncture. But when the days are warm there should not be any hesitation. . . .

In an earlier part of the same book there is a statement that when acupuncture is applied for an excess of Yang it has a draining effect, and when for a deficit of Yin it supplements vigour. Later on in the same chapter it states:

At the time of the new moon one should not drain, and when the moon is full one should not supplement. When the moon is empty to the rim one cannot heal diseases, hence one should consult the weather and the seasons and adjust the treatment to them.

This concept that cyclical events have an important controlling influence over matters of health and disease was still further developed with the introduction of the wu-yün liu-chhi system (the cyclical motions of the five elements and the six chhi) in AD 1099, and of the tzu-wu liu-chu system (noon and midnight differences in the flowing of the chhi) in about the middle of the 12th century.

These are complex systems the details of which will not be entered into. Suffice it to say that the first was based on the conviction that external cyclical, astronomical, meteorological, and climatic factors influence the workings of the body and that from a study of these the occurrence of disease and particularly epidemics of it may be predicted. And that the second was based on the idea that there are internal cyclical changes occurring inside the body and that these have to be taken into account when deciding upon ideal times for performing acupuncture and moxibustion. It is of great interest that such ideas concerning circadian rhythms in the body were put forward so long ago considering that it is only in very recent years that proof has been obtained of the existence of internal biological clocks.

From this brief review it may be seen that the Chinese did not discover the therapeutic effects of acupuncture as a result of some astute clinical observation nor alternatively were they inspired to use it by the logical development of some well-founded hypothesis. On the contrary, it would seem that it was very much by luck that they stumbled upon this valuable form of therapy because their original reasons for using it have subsequently been shown to be entirely fallacious. And further, to a very large extent they succeeded in obscuring the merits of this therapy by grafting upon it a somewhat esoteric set of rules for its application. The manner in which all this prevented acupuncture from becoming readily accepted in the Western world during the past 300 years will be discussed in detail in the next two chapters but before this it is necessary to say something about its changing fortunes in China itself.

From the time that acupuncture was first used in China it remained in the ascendance in that part of the world until reaching its zenith at about the end of the 16th century. From then onwards during the Ch'ing dynasty (1644–1911), when China was under Manchu rule, the practice of it went into a gradual decline. This initially was mainly because the Confucian religion practised by the Manchu people was associated with much prudishness so that the baring of the body, as clearly is so often necessary with treatment by acupuncture, was considered to be immoral. And also because the religion discouraged the inserting of needles into a person's body for fear that this might damage that which was considered to be sacred by virtue of it having been bestowed on that individual by loving parents. Another important reason was that from the 17th century onwards missionaries from Europe, with initially these mainly being Portugese Jesuits, in bringing the Christian religion to China, also brought with them the Western form of medical practice, and this over the next 300 years profoundly influenced the type of medicine practised in the Far East with the practice of acupuncture gradually being displaced.

Events moved so quickly that when Hsü Ling Thai, an eminent Chinese physician and medical historian, wrote about the history of Chinese medicine in 1757, he had to report that by that time acupuncture had become somewhat of a lost art with few experts left to teach it to medical students.

During the 19th century its status declined still further, with the Ch'ing emperors in 1822 ordering that it should no longer be taught at the Imperial Medical College. From then on an increasing number of colleges were opened by medical missionaries for the express purpose of teaching Chinese students Western medicine, until finally this ancient form of treatment reached its nadir in 1929 when the Chinese authorities officially outlawed the practice of it in that country.

It has to be remembered, however, that what has been said only really applied to a minority of the population because China has always been a land of the rich and poor, of the rulers and the oppressed, and whilst Western medicine increasingly displaced traditional Chinese medicine in the wealthy coastal cities the rural peasants that inhabited most of the country continued to depend on traditional forms of treatment including acupuncture, and increasingly, what health care system was available to them became more and more chaotic due to years of Japanese occupation, civil war, and lack of doctors trained in this type of medicine.

The Chinese communist victory in the so-called War of Liberation in 1949, however, changed all this with Mao Tse Tung being determined to improve the health service for the poor by ensuring that more doctors became trained in traditional Chinese medicine; and by ensuring that the practice of this form of medicine and Western medicine became closely integrated with both being taught in the medical colleges.

Following the Great Proletariat Cultural Revolution during the years 1966–69 there was even further emphasis placed on the importance of traditional Chinese medicine including acupuncture with the result that most hospitals offered both forms of treatment to their patients. It is therefore not surprising that when President Nixon and his entourage visited China in 1972, with acupuncture by then having been fully restored to its former prestigious position, its use in the treatment of disease and in particular as an anaesthetic was demonstrated to them with considerable pride. And it was because his personal physician was so impressed with what he saw that, on returning to America, he generated a wave of enthusiasm for it in the Western world that advances in knowledge concerning the neurophysiology of pain since that time have helped to sustain.

REFERENCES

Anon 1975 An outline of Chinese acupuncture. Foreign Language Press, Peking

Bonica J J 1974 Therapeutic acupuncture in the People's Republic of China. Journal of the American Medical Association 228 (12): 1544–1551

Lu Gwei-Djen, Needham J 1980 Celestial lancets. A history and rationale of acupuncture and moxa. Cambridge University Press, Cambridge

Macdonald A 1982 Acupuncture from ancient art to modern medicine. George Allen & Unwin, London

Mann F 1987 Acupuncture: The ancient Chinese art of healing (section 2). The meridians of acupuncture (section 3). In: Textbook of acupuncture. William Heinemann Medical Books, London

Needham J 1975 Science and civilization in China. Cambridge University Press, Cambridge

Porkert M 1974 The theoretical foundations of Chinese medicine. M.I.T. Press, Cambridge, Massachusetts

Veith I 1949 Huang Ti Nei Ching Su Wen The Yellow Emperor's classic of internal medicine. University of California Press, Berkeley

2. How news of acupuncture and moxibustion spread from China to the outside world

The Chinese had practised acupuncture and moxibustion for several centuries before news of it reached the outside world. The first people to hear about it were the Koreans and then not until about the beginning of the 6th century AD. It was not long after that, however, that both Chinese and Korean missionaries introduced it to Japan during the course of converting the people of that country to Buddhism.

The Western world, on the other hand, did not learn about these oriental practices until the 17th century when Jesuit missionaries, whilst attempting to convert the Chinese to Christianity, saw them being used in Canton, and when European doctors employed by the Dutch East Indian Company in and around Java saw them being used by the Japanese in that part of the world. Willem ten Rhijne (1647–1700), a physician born in the Dutch town of Deventer, and who received his medical education at Leyden University, must be given the credit for being the first person to give the Western world a relatively detailed, if unfortunately a somewhat misleading, account of the Chinese practice of acupuncture and moxibustion.

His opportunity to see orientals practising these techniques came when, soon after qualifying as a doctor, he joined the Dutch East India Company in 1673 and was sent to Java. During the latter part of his life there he was to become the director of the Leprosarium but as a young man he had no sooner arrived than he was ordered to go to the island of Deshima in Nagasaki Bay. It was during the 2 years he was stationed there that he first saw the techniques of Chinese acupuncture and moxibustion being practised by the Japanese, and managed to acquire four illustrations depicting acupuncture points lying along channels. He not

unnaturally assumed that the latter must be blood vessels, but found the matter confusing as the directions in which they appeared to run in no way conformed with those taken by any anatomical structures with which he was familiar. He was nevertheless very much impressed with the therapeutic effects of these two techniques and was therefore determined to learn more about them and in particular to get someone to explain the drawings to him. This however was not to prove easy because as he later said in his book on the subject,

The zealous Japanese are quite reluctant to share, especially with foreigners, the mysteries of their art which they conceal like most sacred treasures in their book cases.

It would seem, however, that the Japanese on the other hand had no such inhibitions when it came to them wanting to know all about Western medicine for, on the orders of the Governor of Nagasaki, a Chinese-speaking Japanese physician, Iwanaga Zoko, was sent to see ten Rhijne in order to question him closely about the way in which medicine was practised in Europe. Ten Rhijne however seemed to take all this in good part for when writing about it later he refers to the various questions put to him as nothing but 'bothersome trifles, to be sure', and moreover in return for the information he gave Zoko he managed to persuade the latter to attempt to explain to him the drawings in his possession. Unfortunately as ten Rhijne later pointed out in his book, in order for him to understand Zoko's explanations of the notes attached to the drawings it necessitated one interpreter having to translate the Chinese into Japanese and then another interpreter, whose command of the Dutch language was limited, having to translate the Japanese into Dutch. It therefore follows that the information ten Rhijne received was of necessity inaccurate and yet he himself then had to do his best to translate this into Latin, which was the universal language in the Western world at that time.

In spite of these difficulties there is no doubt that ten Rhijne convinced himself that he had sufficient understanding as to how the Japanese practised acupuncture for him to write an essay on it which he included with essays on other subjects in his book *Dissertatio de Arthritide; Mantissa Schematica; de Acupunctura . . .*, written some time after he had left Nagasaki on 27 October 1676 and returned to Java, and which was published simultaneously in London, The Hague, and in Leipzig in 1683.

In the introduction to this essay on acupuncture, in which he also included comments on moxibustion, he gave reasons why the Chinese and Japanese preferred these two particular forms of therapy to the therapeutic form of bleeding (phlebotomy; venesection) that was so widely practised in Europe in his time, by saying,

Burning and acupuncture are the two primary operations among the Chinese and Japanese who employ them to be free from every pain. If these two people (especially the Japanese) were deprived of the two techniques, their sick would be in a pitiful state without hope of cure or alleviation. Both nations detest phlebotomy because, in their judgement, venesection emits both healthy and diseased blood, and thereby shortens life. They have, accordingly, attempted to rid unhealthy blood of impurities by moxibustion; and to rid it of winds, the cause of all pain, with moxibustion and acupuncture.

It is interesting to learn from him that in Japan at that time therapy was mainly carried out by technicians working under the direction of medical practitioners, but as ten Rhijne said, 'For difficult illnesses the physicians themselves administer the needle.'

These technicians called by the Chinese Xinkieu, and by the Japanese Farritatte, must have had a fair degree of independence and clinical freedom for they had their own establishments with each of the latter having a distinctive sign outside it in the form of a wooden statue with acupuncture

and moxibustion points marked in different colours, an eye-catching device, similar to the multicoloured striped pole often seen outside a barber's shop in the Western world representing the splint for which the barber-surgeon in former times bound the arms of his patients during the process of blood-letting.

From ten Rhijne's account it would seem that the needles used by the Japanese in the 17th century were made of gold, or occasionally of silver, which is somewhat surprising considering that steel must have been readily available to them. The main indication for their use according to him was for the release of 'winds' for as he says,

The Japanese employ acupuncture especially for pain of the belly, stomach and head caused by winds . . . They perforate those parts in order to permit the confined wind to exit.

In an attempt to explain this further, he adds the following somewhat homely simile: 'in the same way, sausages, when they threaten to explode in a heated pan, are pierced to allow the expanding wind to go out'.

It would seem therefore that although the Chinese originally employed acupuncture for the purpose of clearing collections of 'wind' in acu-tracts (p. 7) in due course both they and the Japanese came to use it for the relief of abdominal pain brought about by the entrapment of a quite different type of 'wind' in the intestinal tract.

It is of particular interest in this respect that the only case history ten Rhijne includes in his book is of a Japanese soldier with some abdominal pain. The soldier believing this to be due to 'wind' produced as a result of drinking an excessive amount of water, is reported to have carried out his own treatment by inserting an acupuncture needle into his abdomen. Ten Rhijne was obviously present when he did this for he says,

. . . lying on his back, he drove the needle into the left side of his abdomen above the pylorus at four different locations . . . while he tapped the needle with a hammer (since his skin was rather tough) he held his breath. When the needle had been driven in about the width of a finger, he rotated its twisting-handle . . . Relieved of the pain and cured by this procedure, he regained his health.

Ten Rhijne whilst watching this demonstration of auto-acupuncture must have cast his mind back to his youth for by a strange coincidence the title of his dissertation for his doctorate in medicine was *De dolore intestinorum e flatu* ...! In his essay he also gives a long list of other disorders that the Japanese in those days were treating with acupuncture including such conditions as headaches, rheumatic pains, and arthritis that people all over the world are still using it for. The one notably bizarre and certainly very hazardous use for it at that time was in the field of obstetrics with the acupuncturist being advised to 'puncture the womb of a pregnant woman when the foetus moves excessively before the appropriate time for birth and causes the mother such severe pains that she frequently is in danger of death; puncture the foetus itself with a long and sharp needle, so as to terrify it and make it cease its abnormal movement fraught with danger for the mother'!

It is very unfortunate considering that ten Rhijne was sufficiently impressed with the practical value of acupuncture to feel that he wanted to pass on his knowledge of the subject to the Western world by writing an essay on it, that this should have proved to be a totally inaccurate account, due to his failure to understand that the Chinese believed in the existence of a system of channels (now referred to in the West as acu-tracts or meridians) completely separate from and yet closely associated with blood vessels. His knowledge of anatomy was extensive for at one stage in his life he taught the subject and therefore in all fairness there was no reason why it should have ever crossed his mind that the acu-tracts depicted in the illustrations he acquired could be anything but structures already well known to him from dissecting the human body. As a result he repeatedly refers to them as arteries, and to confuse the matter even more insists that the Chinese and Japanese use the terms artery, vein, and nerve interchangeably and so in some places he even refers to them as veins and in others as nerves.

His belief that these tracts were arteries is also readily understandable when it is remembered how much importance the Chinese placed on their long-held beliefs concerning the circulation of the blood in developing their practice of acupuncture. This is clearly expressed by ten Rhijne when he said,

Although Chinese physicians (who are the forerunners from whom Japanese physicians borrowed these systems of healing) are ignorant in anatomy, nonetheless they have perhaps devoted more effort over many centuries to learning and teaching with very great care the circulation of the blood, than have European physicians, individually or as a group. They base the foundation of their entire medicine upon the rules of the circulation, as if the rules were oracles of Apollo at Delphi.

He then goes on to point out how 'among the Chinese the masters employ hydraulic machines to demonstrate the circulation of the blood to their disciples who have earned the title of physician; in the absence of such machines the masters assist understanding with clear figures'. It is obvious that ten Rhijne was under the impression that the drawings he possessed were examples of such figures.

Another reason for his confusing acu-tracts with arteries was that he knew that the Chinese place considerable emphasis on the examination of the pulse in making a diagnosis before undertaking acupuncture or moxibustion. In referring to the latter for instance he says,

wherever pain has set in, burn; burn however in the location in which the arteries beat most strongly. For in that place the seat of the pain is lodged, where harmful winds inordinately move the blood. After prior examination of the pulse of the arteries, place the burning tow on the location marked with its own sign.

And in another place he says,

... wherever pain has lodged, burn. To which I add, when it is necessary puncture, puncture and burn where the arteries beat strongest. What the patient can detect by the sensation of pain the physician can detect by feeling the pulses in the affected part.

At the same time he is clearly aware that if the channels depicted in his illustrations and which he describes in the text of his book are arteries then they are a very inaccurate anatomical representation of the course known to be taken by such vessels. And it would seem that, fearing that for this reason alone authorities in the Western world might reject out of hand the whole system of acupuncture and moxibustion, he finds it necessary to apologize for the apparent ineptness of those who drew the illustrations by saying,

> In many instances, a person especially skilful at the art of anatomy will belittle the lines and the precise points of insertion, and will censure the awkward presentation of the short notes on the diagrams, when these should be more closely identified with walls of the blood vessels. But we must not on this account casually abandon our confidence in experiments undertaken by the very great number of superb and polished intellects of antiquity. Chinese physicians prefer to cast the blame for a mistake upon their own ignorance, rather than diminish in the slightest the authority of and trust in antiquity ...

Although the account of acupuncture in ten Rhijne's book was the first detailed one to appear in the Western world, a passing reference to the subject had already been made in a book written by Jacob de Bondt (1598–1631) who as surgeon-general to the Dutch East India Company in Java had also seen the technique being used in that part of the world. This book, *Historia Naturalis et Medica Indiae Orientalis*, published in 1658, is in the main an account of the natural history of animals and plants found in the East, but it contains a paragraph about acupuncture.

When ten Rhijne quotes this paragraph in his own book he cannot refrain from putting in parentheses his own critical comments thus causing de Bondt's description of acupuncture to read as follows:

> The results with acupuncture in Japan which I will relate even surpass miracles [without undermining belief in their authenticity]. For chronic pains of the head [and moreover for recent ones, especially those arising from winds], for obstruction of the liver and spleen, and also for pleurisy [and for other ailments, as is here made clear] they bore through [and they perforate] with a stylus [he should have said, with a needle] made of silver or bronze [more correctly, from gold] and not much thicker than ordinary lyre strings. The stylus [here the good author is quite in error] should be driven slowly and gently through the above mentioned vitals so as to emerge from another part.

One book that presumably ten Rhijne did not read, but which could have been a help to him in understanding something about acu-tracts, was written anonymously but almost certainly by a French Jesuit missionary working in Canton. This work was based on a translation of a 1st-century manual, the *Mo chüeh* (Sphygmological Instructions). This book printed at Grenoble in 1671 clearly refers to acu-tracts although admittedly there is very little detail about them or about the Chinese system of pulse-diagnosis in spite of its title *Les Secrets de la Médecine des Chinois, consistant en la parfaite Connoissance du Pouls, envoyez de la Chine par un Francois, Homme de grand mérite*.

It is more surprising that ten Rhijne did not learn about the belief of Chinese physicians in a system of channels or acu-tracts separate from the anatomically demonstrable circulatory system from the German Andreas Cleyer as they were together as medical officers in the service of the Dutch East India Company on Java. And Cleyer edited a book giving clear references to acu-tracts that was published in 1682, the year before ten Rhijne's book appeared.

Cleyer attributes several parts of this book *Specimen Médicinae Sinicae, sive Opuscula Medica ad mentem Sinesium* to an 'eruditus Europaeus' living in Canton. The possibility therefore exists that this was none other than the anonymous author of the book *Les Secrets de la Médecine des Chinois, consistant en la parfaite Connoissance du Pouls, envoyez de la Chine par un Francois, Homme de grand mérite* that appeared in 1671. Like the latter, Cleyer's book also includes translations from the *Mo chüeh* (Sphygmological Instructions) but is far more informative with a lengthy discussion of the various types of pulse found in health and disease; there are also no less than 30 drawings depicting the course of acu-tracts. In addition there are numerous references to acu-tracts, or viae (ways) as they are called in the text but unfortunately as might be expected the author is quite unable to explain how the Chinese believed that circulatory disturbances in these invisible tracts could be diagnosed from observations on the pulse.

Nevertheless the book certainly aroused the interest of Sir John Floyer (1649–1734) who included an abridged and paraphrased form of it in his famous two-volume work, *The Physician's Pulse-Watch or an Essay to Explain the Old Art of Feeling the Pulse, and to improve it by the help of a Pulse-Watch*, the first volume of which was published in 1707 and the second in 1710.

Floyer's pulse-watch was a portable instrument which he carried in a box, it having been made under his direction by a Mr Samuel Watson, a watchmaker in Long Acre, London. Its great virtue was that it ran for 60 seconds, and with it he studied the effects of a variety of different factors on the pulse rate including food, drink, tobacco, anxiety and fevers. He implored all young physicians to use the instrument 'to discern all those dangerous exorbitances which are caused by an irregular diet, violent passions, and a slothful life'.

His reference to Cleyer's observations on Chinese medicine comes in the first part of the second volume under the title of *An Essay to make a new Sphygmologia, by accommodating the Chinese and European observations about the Pulse into one System*. As may be gathered from the title this only discusses the Chinese method of pulse diagnosis and there is no mention of acupuncture in it. It would seem in fact that Floyer had no interest in the latter believing that the Chinese in the main treated most diseases pharmaceutically after having diagnosed them in the first place by means of observations on the pulse. Curiously enough he was not all that wrong because unbeknown to him, at the time his book was being written, acupuncture in China was going through one of its periodic phases of being out of fashion.

In spite of Floyer's enthusiasm for Chinese sphygmology his contemporaries failed to show any real interest in it, or for that matter in the practice of acupuncture itself. This perhaps is surprising considering that in the early part of the 17th century William Harvey dramatically changed long-held ideas in the Western world concerning the physiology of the circulatory system when in 1628 he published his famous book *Exercitatio Anatomica de Motu Cordis et Sanguinis in Animalibus*. In this he was at last able to refute the hitherto seemingly inviolable but erroneous teaching of Galen concerning the structure of the heart and the manner in which he had insisted that blood ebbs and flows in the vessels. Harvey proved by means of carefully conducted experiments what the Chinese had surmised centuries before that blood flows around the body in a continuous circle.

As might be expected, in view of the manner in which Galen's views had been revered for so many centuries, there was initially considerable opposition to Harvey's revolutionary discovery, but, based as it was on such sound evidence, its gradual acceptance over the course of years became inevitable.

Considering that the system of sphygmology devised by the Chinese and their practice of acupuncture were both firmly founded on the principle that blood circulates around the body one might therefore have thought that in the climate of opinion prevailing in the West towards the end of the 17th century that more interest might have been shown in them. Yet when the book *Clavis Medica ad Chinarum Doctrinam de Pulsibus*, which basically was yet another translation of the *Mo chüeh*, written by Michael Boym (1612–1659) a Polish Jesuit missionary in China, was published in 1686, it prompted Pierre Bayle in reviewing it that year in *Nouvelles de la République des Lettres* to say:

The Reverend Father expounds to us the Chinese system of medicine very clearly, and it is easy to see from what he says that the physicians of China are rather clever men. True, their theories and principles are not the clearest in the world, but if we had got hold of them under the reign of the philosophy of Aristotle, we should have admired them very much, and we should have found them at least as plausible and well based as our own. Unfortunately, they have reached us in Europe just at a time when the mechanick Principles invented, or revived, by our Modern Virtuosi have given us a great distaste for the 'faculties' of Galen, and for the calidum naturalis and the humidum radicale too, the great foundations of the Medicine of the Chinese no less than of that of the Peripateticks.

It should be noted that the Galenic-Aristotelian calidum naturalis or 'innate heat' was widely considered in the 17th century to correspond to the Chinese yang whilst the Galenic-Aristotelian humidum radicale or 'primigenial moisture' was considered to correspond to the Chinese yin.

It may therefore be seen from the sentiments expressed by Bayle that what really deterred most physicians in the Western world from taking any particular interest, either in the Chinese method of pulse-diagnosis, or in acupuncture itself, on first learning about them in the 17th century, at a time when they had only recently come to terms with Harvey's new and enlightened approach to anatomy and physiology after centuries of slavish adherence to Galenic dogma, was that the curiously esoteric and nebulous concepts including yin, yang, chhi and invisible acu-tracts upon which these Chinese practices seemed to be based, were all too reminiscent of some of the bizarre Graeco-Roman beliefs from which they had just been liberated.

Most European physicians also showed little or no enthusiasm for the Chinese practice of applying heat to the skin by burning moxa on it, when they first heard of this in the 17th century, in spite of the fact that at that time they were still firm believers in blistering their patients with strong irritants, and burning them with boiling oil and red hot irons! One person, however, who did advocate its use was Hermann Buschof, a Dutch Reformed Minister and a friend of ten Rhijne when they worked together in Java. He wrote a laudatory account of its use in gout and other arthritic conditions in a book published in 1674 entitled *Het Podagra*... Another protagonist was Sir William Temple the eminent 17th-century diplomat who wrote appreciatively about it in an essay 'The cure of gout by moxa' in his *Miscellanea* published in 1693, after having received this form of treatment for a painful attack of this affliction during an international conference at Nijmegen in 1677. Conversely that eminent physician Thomas Sydenham (1624–1689) when writing about gout some time earlier had referred disparagingly to the use of moxa in its treatment.

The most comprehensive account of moxibustion to reach the West however was that written by the German physician Englebert Kaempfer (1651–1716). Kaempfer, who was brought up in Germany at a time when it had recently been devastated by the ravages of the Thirty Years War (1618–1648), decided after qualifying as a doctor that rather than continue to live there he would prefer to seek work abroad. He therefore joined the United East India Company and became yet another of the surgeons to work at the Dutch trading station on the island of Deshima in Nagasaki Bay.

His observations on Japanese medical practice in that part of the world led him to write two essays, one 'Acupuncture, a Japanese cure for colic,' and the other 'Moxa, a Chinese and Japanese substance for cautery' that appeared together with a large number of essays on other subjects in his *Amoenitatum Exoticarum Politico-Physico-Medicarum Fasciculi V*... published in 1712.

The essay on acupuncture is of limited value because as may be seen from the title it confines itself to the use of this technique in one condition only, namely the relief of cramp-like pains occurring in association with a severe type of diarrhoea that was endemic in that part of the world at the time and known to the Japanese as senki. There is a detailed account of how needles should be inserted in this condition but all reference to acu-tracts is avoided, and it does not really add anything to that which had by that time already been written on the subject.

The essay on moxibustion, however, is far more wide ranging. His description of the sites at which he saw a moxa cautery applied, and the reasons for doing this make fascinating reading, as may be seen from the following quotation:

Considering the places cauterised, you would think the unexpected successes illusory. For example to facilitate birth, the tip of the small toe on the left foot; to prevent conception or to promote sterility, the navel; to relieve toothache, the adducting muscle of the thumb on the same side as the aching tooth.

The latter is a clear reference to the classical Chinese acupuncture and moxa point Ho-Ku, stimulation of which to this day is widely recognised as having a powerful analgesic effect.

From what has been said it will be clear that much information concerning acupuncture and moxibustion reached Europe during the 17th century but only limited use was made of these techniques either during that century or the following one because physicians in the Western world were completely mystified as to how these particular forms of therapy achieve their effects. One of the few men to think deeply about this matter was Gerhard van Swieten, the famous Dutch physician, who concluded that any beneficial effects that they may have must be for reasons entirely different from those that had been put forward by the Chinese, for as he said in 1755:

The acupuncture of the Japanese and the cautery of various parts of the body with (Chinese) moxa seems to stimulate the nerves and thereby to alleviate pains and cramps in quite different parts of the body in a most wonderful way. It would be an extraordinarily useful enterprise if someone would take the trouble to note and investigate the marvellous communion which the nerves have with one another, and at what points certain nerves lie which when stimulated can calm the pain at distant sites. The physicians of Asia, who knew no (modern) anatomy, have by long practical experience identified such points.

It was of course another 200 years before research into the neurophysiology of pain provided objective evidence in support of van Swieten's hypothesis.

It is now necessary to consider the attitudes of doctors, both in Europe and America, to acupuncture during the 19th century as this was a period when a few of the more courageous of them, in spite of not being able to accept the traditional theories upon which the Chinese based their practice of it, decided to explore empirically its clinical applications. And having convinced themselves of its merits in alleviating musculoskeletal pain, they attempted to popularize its use for this purpose. They were however to find their efforts thwarted by entrenched conservatism. Members of the medical profession at that time showed a strangely inconsistent attitude whereby they were more than willing to prescribe potentially toxic substances of uncertain efficacy whilst being quite unwilling to try out the relatively harmless procedure of inserting needles into people, presumably because they could not bring themselves to believe that anything so simple could have the effects claimed for it — an attitude of mind, regretfully, still adopted by some in the late 20th century!

REFERENCES

Bowers J Z 1966 Englebert Kaempfer; Physician, explorer, scholar and author. Journal of the History of Medicine and Allied Sciences 21: 237–259

Bowers J Z, Carrubba R W 1970 The doctoral thesis of Englebert Kaempfer on tropical diseases, oriental medicine and exotic natural phenomena. Journal of the History of Medicine and Allied Sciences 25: 270–310

Carrubba R W, Bowers J Z 1974 The Western world's first detailed treatise on acupuncture: Willem ten Rhijne's De Acupunctura. Journal of the History of Medicine and Allied Sciences 29: 391–397

Floyer Sir John 1707 The physician's pulse watch: or, an essay to explain the old art of feeling the pulse, and to improve it by the help of a pulse-watch. London

Harvey William 1628 Exercitatio anatomica de motu cordis et sanguinis in animalibus. London — an anatomical disquisition on the motion of the heart and blood in animals. Translated by Robert Willis, Barnes, Surrey, England 1847. In: Willius F A, Keys T E (eds) Classics of cardiology 1961 Vol 1. Dover Publications, New York

Lu Gwei-Djen, Needham J 1980 Celestial lancets. A history and rationale of acupuncture and moxa. Cambridge University Press, Cambridge

3. The practice of acupuncture in the Western world during the 19th century

There is good evidence to show that acupuncture came to be widely practised by the medical profession in Europe during the first half of the 19th century.

Its protagonists, however, turned their backs on the complexities of the traditional Chinese approach to the subject and, in a determined effort to shed it of all its mysticism, ignored the acutract system and refused to attempt to use the oriental system of pulse-diagnosis. They confined themselves for the most part to the treatment of painful conditions and the method adopted was simply a straightforward insertion of needles into painful areas, similar to the ah shih hsüeh type of acupuncture practised by Sun Ssu-mo in China in the 7th century (see Ch. 1). Both of these forms of acupuncture 'in loco dolenti', as Lu Gwei-Djen & Needham (1980) so aptly call it, were clearly the forerunners of the more sophisticated type of trigger point acupuncture recently developed in the Western world and described in detail later in this book.

The circumstances leading to this renewal of interest were not the same in every country. In Germany the somewhat unlikely source of inspiration was a letter published in 1806 by the playwright, August Von Kotzebue in his magazine *The Candid Observer (Funny and Serious)*. This letter ostensibly from his son travelling in Japan gave a somewhat satirical account of the way acupuncture was being practised there. This might have attracted no more than passing interest if it had not been for the fact that it caught the eye of some unknown physician who wrote a long rejoinder urging that the subject be treated with more seriousness. In spite of this it was some time before the clinical application of the technique

became widely adopted but in 1828 some important papers appeared including one by Bernstein, and another by Lohmayer reporting good results with this form of treatment in the alleviation of rheumatic pain.

In France, interest in acupuncture was reawakened in a far more direct manner. When Isaac Titsingh, a surgeon attached to the Dutch East India Company at Deshima, eventually returned to Europe, he brought with him among the memorabilia of his travels, an ebony case containing needles and moxa tinder; and also a teaching-aid in the form of a cardboard doll with acu-points and tracts painted on it that had been presented to him by a Japanese Imperial Physician. His friends in Europe showed considerable interest in these items, but what was to prove to be of even greater importance was his translation of an 18th-century Japanese treatise on acupuncture, for when this came to the attention of the Parisian physician Sarlandière he was so intrigued with it that he began to practise acupuncture himself and persuaded several other physicians in Paris to do likewise. Included among these were Berlioz, the father of the composer, who in 1816 wrote the first book on the subject in France; and Cloquet & Dantu who reported their results of treating patients with this technique in an article *Observations sur less Effets Thérapeutiques de l'Acupuncture* in Bayle's *Bibliothèque de Thérapeutique* published in 1828.

Sarlandière himself was the first to apply electric currents to implanted needles, and his book giving an account of this was published in 1825. This will no doubt surprise anyone who might have thought that electroacupuncture is a recent invention.

From their reports it is clear that these Parisian physicians were using acupuncture in the treatment of many different disorders but that their best results, as might be expected, were in the relief of musculoskeletal pain and migraine.

In Italy the first book to be published on the practice of acupuncture was that of Bozetti in 1820, but the one that was to become best known was that of Antonio Carraro published in 1825. Also of particular interest were two books, the first appearing in 1834 and the second in 1837, in which da Camin describes how following the example of Sarlandière he employed electroacupuncture and used Leyden jars as the source of electricity.

In England the medical practitioner who did most to interest his colleagues in the clinical application of acupuncture by writing two books on the subject was J. M. Churchill. The first, entitled *A Treatise on Acupuncturation, being a Description of a Surgical Operation originally peculiar to the Japanese and Chinese, and by them denominated Zin-King, now introduced into European Practice, with Directions for its Performance and Cases illustrating its Success*, was published in 1821; and the second consisting of a number of case histories was published in 1828. His treatise on acupuncturation, a modest volume of only 86 pages, was dedicated to the famous surgeon Astley Cooper as follows:

To Astley Cooper Esq. the steady friend and patron of humble merit the author respectfully inscribes this little treatise. Less from presumption of its deserving his approbation than as a mark of respect for splendid achievements and of gratitude towards a great master.

Churchill said it was his friend Mr Scott of Westminster, the first person as far as he knew to perform acupuncture in England, who initially drew his attention to the subject by demonstrating to him several successfully treated cases, and it was this which led him to study the technique himself.

From reading Churchill's books it is obvious that he restricted himself to treating cases of what he called 'rheumatalgia', and judging from the case histories this was invariably of short duration. This no doubt accounts for his uniformly excellent results and clearly because of this he

considered it only necessary to present a limited number of cases for as he said,

I would certainly add many others to the list but to minds open to conviction and truth no stronger impression would be made by multiplying examples, whilst the sceptical would not be persuaded though one rose from the dead!

He admits that he did not know how acupuncture works stating,

I have by no means made up my mind as to the nature of its action and rather than venture into speculations which may be received as doubtful by some and visionary by others I prefer to preserve a profound silence.

Such honesty has to be admired particularly as he clearly recognizes that his self-confessed ignorance concerning its action could seriously undermine his efforts to popularize the technique for he says '. . . if on the other hand, a rational theory, built on sound logical reasons, be the only evidence to which any value can be attached, then will my efforts have been unavailing and fruitless'. Such fears, however, proved groundless because his book undoubtedly aroused much interest with it, not only being translated into German in 1824 and into French in 1825, but it also inspired many of his English colleagues to take an interest in the subject. One such person was Mr Wansborough of Fulham, who writing in the *Lancet* in 1826 says,

As respects the modus operandi I have proceeded in every case according to the recommendation of Mr Churchill in his useful little work on acupuncturation to which I beg the readers of the Lancet to consult for further information on the subject.

In his paper he describes how by the use of acupuncture he alleviated the pain of various musculoskeletal disorders in eight patients. He says the latter were all so impressed with the result as to pronounce them as being magical!

He, like Churchill, was unwilling to commit himself as to how inserting needles into the body could have a therapeutic effect, but he clearly thought that the Chinese were wrong in believing that it was due to noxious air being released from the tissues for he says,

I shall not hazard a hypothesis of the modus operandi of acupuncturation but at the same time I am free to confess myself sceptical on the creed, that its effects are produced by the escape of air from the cellular membranes through the punctures made by needles.

He then proceeds to give three cogent reasons for his incredulity:

1. The very form of the needle is a barrier to the escape of air; 2. the cure is often performed before the needles are withdrawn; and 3. the cure is often performed by causing acute pain in the act of introducing them.

His first observation, being self-explanatory, needs no further comment; his second may sound farfetched to anyone who has not practised acupuncture but on occasions it is surprising how rapidly pain is relieved in response to needle stimulation; and his third is in line with the currently held view that for acupuncture to be successful in the relief of chronic pain the needling itself has to be such as to produce a brief intensely painful stimulus (see Ch. 8).

Another person whose interest in acupuncture was aroused by Churchill was John Elliotson, a physician who was originally on the staff at St Thomas's Hospital, London but who later became Professor of Medicine at University College Hospital. Elliotson writing in the *Medico-Chirurgical Transactions* in 1827 stated that the use of acupuncture both in his private practice and at St Thomas's Hospital over several years had led him to agree with Mr Churchill that it was mainly of value in the 'rheumatism of the fleshy parts' which he also in places referred to as 'rheumatalgia'.

In view of Elliotson's high standing as a teacher in a leading medical school it was unfortunate that his enthusiastic support for animal magnetism, a form of hypnosis introduced by Mesmer, caused him to suffer professional opprobrium, as this in turn served to undermine any influence he might otherwise have had in furthering the cause of acupuncture.

It is clear that in 19th-century Britain any interest which may have been shown in acupuncture both by the medical profession and the general public was intermittent, as may be seen from the following contribution to the subject by Dr T. Ogier Ward of Kensington, in the *British Medical Journal* on 28th August 1858:

. . . acupuncture is a remedy that seems to have its floods and ebbs in public estimation; for we see it much belauded in medical meetings every ten years or so, even to its recommendation in neuralgia of the heart, and then it again sinks into neglect or oblivion. And it is not unlikely that its disuse may be occasioned partly by fear of the pain, and partly by the difficulty the patient finds to believe so trifling an operation can produce such powerful effects. Its use is not as frequent as it deserves and now that we know the rationale of its operation I venture to bring forward a few cases in illustration of its remedial powers in order that others may be induced to give it a more extensive trial, and thus ascertain its true value in the treatment of neuralgia or rheumatic pains.

There then follows six case reports describing how muscle pain in various parts of the body including the shoulder, lower back and thigh was alleviated by inserting needles into the areas where the pain was most intensely felt. Acupuncture may not have been widely adopted by the British medical profession during the 19th century but there is evidence to show that at least one large provincial general hospital in this country favoured its use in the alleviation of musculoskeletal pain. T. Pridgin Teale, Surgeon to the General Infirmary at Leeds, writing in the *Lancet* in 1871, states,

In the present essay it is my wish to record some facts concerning a method of treatment of great antiquity which seems in a great measure to have dropped out of use, or at any rate to be at the present day but little employed or even known in many parts of the United Kingdom. It has however been for years a favourite traditional practice at the Leeds Infirmary.

He then goes on to say 'when it does succeed the relief it gives is almost instantaneous, generally permanent, and often in cases which for weeks or months have run the gauntlet of other treatments without benefit'.

He then proceeds to describe five cases including two with pain and restricted movement of the shoulder joint, one with pain around the coccyx following labour, one with persistent pain around the os calcis, and one with long-standing pain around the wrist following trauma. He expresses the opinion that cases suitable for acupuncture include trauma to muscle, stretching or tearing of muscle or tendon, and disuse pain. Certainly, even by today's standards, this is a reasonably comprehensive list of 'surgical' indications.

It is interesting to note that Teale from observing the area of redness which so frequently arises in the skin around the site where an acupuncture needle has been inserted was misled into thinking that acupuncture must work by producing some form of temporary congestion.

Another surgeon to write about the use of acupuncture in hospital practice at Leeds was Simeon Snell. Snell writing in the *Medical Times and Gazette* in 1880 at a time when he was ophthalmic surgeon to the Sheffield General Hospital says,

At the Leeds Infirmary the use of it is almost traditional. It was there that I both saw it employed, practised it myself and witnessed the remarkable benefits frequently resulting.

He then proceeds to describe five cases of pain with limitation of movement of the shoulder joint he had treated successfully at Leeds.

Presumably when he became an ophthalmic surgeon at Sheffield he had little opportunity to use the technique but one can be sure that he encouraged others to do so. And certainly he was more enlightened than Teale in his view as to how it works believing 'it may act as a stimulant to the nerve twigs'.

News concerning the manner in which acupuncture was being practised in Europe from the beginning of the 19th century quickly reached America. American physicians, however, at that time viewed this form of therapy with considerable suspicion and were reluctant to make use of it. An anonymous reviewer in admitting this, when reviewing Churchill's *Treatise on Acupuncturation* in the *Medical Repository* in 1822, was forced to say,

but we have probably been mistaken. Acupuncture is likely to become, employed with discrimination and directed with skill, a valuable resource.

In spite of these words of encouragement, and also that during the 1820s American medical journals published a number of European reports on the subject, the only physicians in the whole of that great continent who seemed to take any interest in it were a few in Philadelphia, with one of the most enthusiastic of these, as Cassedy (1974) has pointed out, being Franklin Bache.

Franklin Bache was the assistant physician at the Philadelphia State Penitentiary and in 1825 he decided to try the effects of acupuncture on prisoners suffering from various painful disorders, which as he said, when reporting his results a year later (Bache 1826), 'may be arranged into the four general heads of muscular rheumatism, chronic pains, neuralgia, and ophthalmia'. In his report in which he reviewed the results of the effects of acupuncture on 29 people, most of whom were convicts, he concluded that the treatment had much to offer in removing and mitigating pain, and that it was 'a proper remedy in almost all diseases, whose prominent symptom is pain'.

One cannot help but feel that if only more notice had been taken of this wise dictum that interest in acupuncture in 19th-century America might have become more widespread, but unfortunately certain other Philadelphian physicians decided to direct their energies to exploring its use in conditions of a far more dubious nature.

These included E. J. Coxe, D. T. Coxe, and Samuel Jackson, who having heard reports from Europe about it being possible to revive drowned kittens by inserting needles into their hearts, decided to investigate whether the same procedure had anything to offer in resuscitating drowned people! And finding, as might be expected, that it had not, they clearly became disillusioned with the therapeutic properties of acupuncture in general, for as Edward Coxe (1826) in reporting the results of their experiment remarked,

Whatever others may think of the possibility of resuscitating drowned persons by acupuncture, I can only say that I should think myself highly culpable, if, called to a case of asphyxia, I were to waste time, every moment of which is precious, in endeavouring to resuscitate by a means which I sincerely believe to be good for nothing.

This in my opinion is a very good example as to how acupuncture can so readily be brought into disrepute when it is not employed in a selective and discerning manner, and should serve as an object lesson to all those currently engaged in investigating the clinical applications of acupuncture. Despite this adverse report the cause of acupuncture in America received a boost when in 1833 the editors of the *Medical Magazine* reprinted a paper that John Elliotson, the physician at St Thomas's Hospital, London, had originally contributed to the *Cyclopaedia of Practical Medicine*. Also, in 1836 the editors of the prestigious and widely read *Boston Medical and Surgical Journal* reprinted an article that had appeared shortly before in the *Southern Medical and Surgical Journal*. In this paper, William M. Lee of South Carolina reported how he had used acupuncture for 6 years in the treatment of rheumatism and concluded that this method of treatment was 'entitled to far more attention than it has yet received in the United States'.

Such a view however does not seem to have been widely shared, for there continued to be a paucity of literature on acupuncture in America at that time with the only further outstanding contribution being that of Robley Dunglison, another Philadelphian physician. This took the form of an eight-page account of the subject in a compendium of his entitled *New Remedies*, and published in 1839. The same article was reproduced in subsequent editions of the book up to the last one which appeared in 1856, but in spite of this any interest that there may have been in this type of treatment was gradually fading leaving Samuel Gross in his book *A System of Surgery*, published in 1859 to state,

Its advantages have been much overrated and the practice . . . has fallen into disrepute.

This certainly may have been true so far as America was concerned but up in Canada none other than the famous physician Sir William Osler was using it in the late 19th and early 20th century, for in the eighth edition of his book *The Principles and Practice of Medicine* published in 1912 at the time when he was Regius Professor of Medicine at Oxford University he wrote,

For lumbago, acupuncture is, in acute cases, the most efficient treatment. Needles of from three to four inches in length (ordinary bonnet needles, sterilised, will do) are thrust into the lumbar muscles at the seat of pain, and withdrawn after five or ten minutes. In many instances the relief of pain is immediate, and I can corroborate the statements of Ringer, who taught me this practice, as to its extraordinary and prompt effect in many instances.

He had clearly been in the habit of using the technique for many years because Harvey Cushing (1925) in his book *The Life of Sir William Osler* refers to an unfortunate experience the great man had when he was a physician at the Montreal General Hospital.

It would seem that early in Osler's career at that hospital a certain Peter Redpath, a wealthy Montreal sugar refiner and member of the hospital's board, having suffered from intractable lumbago for some time, had high hopes that the newly appointed physician might be able to cure him.

Arrangements were therefore made for him to consult Osler in his office at the hospital and it is recounted that Redpath, having arrived exhausted from the effort of mounting the stairs, did not take kindly to being treated with acupuncture, for Cushing reports that:

at each jab the old gentleman is said to have rapped out a string of oaths, and in the end got up and hobbled out, no better of his pain, this to Osler's great distress, for he had expected to give him immediate relief which as he said 'meant a million for McGill'.

It should be noted that unlike the Chinese who have always attached much importance to manipulating needles such as twirling them between thumb and finger, once they have been inserted into the body, most 19th-century European exponents of acupuncture were content merely to insert their needles and then to leave them without touching them again for a short period of time. The actual time varied considerably and ranged from Mr Wansbrough of Fulham leaving them in situ for from 20 seconds to 4 minutes, and Mr Pridgin Teale leaving them on average for about 1 minute; up to Mr Churchill who advised leaving them for about 5–6 minutes, and Sir William Osler who recommended that they remain for 5–10 minutes.

This is of considerable practical interest for, during the present resurgence of interest in acupuncture in the latter part of the 20th century, many people including myself, for reasons to be explained in Chapter 8, favour the technique whereby needles, having been inserted, are left in position without any form of manipulation. However, it is also now realized that it is wrong to stipulate any particular period of time for which they should be left, as this varies widely from a few seconds to 10 minutes according to a patient's individual central nervous system's speed of reaction to peripheral nerve stimulation with dry needles.

It is also worth stressing once again that none of these physicians put needles into traditional Chinese acupuncture points, but so far as musculoskeletal disorders were concerned, which very sensibly is what in the main they used it for, simply inserted them into the painful areas. However, it is now realized that musculoskeletal pain does not necessarily originate at the site where it is felt, but is referred there via the central nervous

system from some focus of neural hyperactivity — now known as a trigger point — that is often situated some distance away, and that therefore rather than inserting a needle into the area where pain is felt, the latter is more likely to be relieved if the needle is inserted into the tissues overlying the trigger point for the purpose of stimulating A-delta nerve fibres in its vicinity.

This is the fundamental principle upon which the recently-developed Western approach to trigger point acupuncture is based, and the manner in which it was discovered will now be explained.

REFERENCES

Anon 1822 Review of James Churchill's treatise on acupuncturation. Medical Repository (New Series) 7: 441–449
Bache F 1826 Cases illustrative of the remedial effects of acupuncturation. North American Medical and Surgical Journal 1: 311–321
Berlioz L V J 1816 Mémoires sur les maladies chroniques, les évacuations sanguines et l'acupuncture, 2 vols. Croullebois, Paris
Bozetti S 1820 Memoria sull'agopuntura. Milan
Carraro A 1825 Saggio sull'agopuntura. Udine
Cassedy J H 1974 Early use of acupuncture in the United States. Bulletin of the New York Academy of Medicine 50 (8): 892–896
Churchill J M 1821 A treatise on acupuncturation being a description of a surgical operation originally peculiar to the Japanese and Chinese, and by them denominated zin-king, now introduced into European practice, with directions for its performance, and cases illustrating its success. Simpkins & Marshall, London (German trans 1824, French trans 1825)
Churchill J M 1828 Cases illustrative of the immediate effects of acupuncturation in rheumatism, lumbago, sciatica, anomalous muscular diseases and in dropsy of the cellular tissue, selected from various sources and intended as an appendix to the author's treatise on the subject. Callow & Wilson, London
Cloquet J, Dantu T M 1828 Observations sur les effets thérapeutiques de l'acupuncture. In: Bayle A L J (ed) Bibliotheque de Thérapeutique, vol 1, p 436
Coxe E J 1826 Observations on asphyxia from drowning. North American Medical and Surgical Journal 2: 292–293

Cushing H 1925 The life of Sir William Osler. Clarendon Press, Oxford
da Camin F S 1834 Sulla agopuntura, con alcuni cenni sulla puntura elettrica. Antonelli, Venice
da Camin F S 1837 Dell'agopuntura e della galvano-puntura. Osservazioni, Venice
Dunglison R 1839 Acupuncture. In: New remedies. Waldie, Philadelphia, p 23–30
Elliotson J 1827 The use of the sulphate of copper in chronic diarrhoea together with an essay on acupuncture. Medico-chirurgical transactions 13, part 2: 451–467
Elliotson J 1833 Acupuncture. Medical Magazine 1: 309–314
Gross S D 1859 A system of surgery, vol 1. Blanchard and Lea, Philadelphia, p 575–576
Lee W M 1836 Acupuncture as a remedy for rheumatism. Southern Medical and Surgical Journal 1: 129–133
Lu Gwei-Djen, Needham J 1980 Celestial lancets. Cambridge University Press, Cambridge, p 295
Osler Sir William 1912 The principles and practice of medicine, 8th edn. Appleton, New York, p 1131
Sarlandière le Chevalier J B 1825 Mémoires sur l'electropuncture . . . . . Private publication, Paris
Snell S 1880 Remarks on acupuncture. Medical Times and Gazette 1: 661–662
Teale T Pridgin 1871 Clinical essays no. III. On the relief of pain and muscular disability by acupuncture. Lancet 1: 567–568
Wansborough D 1826 Acupuncturation. Lancet 10: 846–848
Ward T Ogier 1858 On acupuncture. British Medical Journal (Aug 28): 728–729

PART TWO

Principles of trigger point acupuncture

4. Some basic observations leading to its development

INTRODUCTION

The traditional practice of Chinese acupuncture having become officially recognized once again in China during the 1950s, and it having since then been increasingly used by some doctors, and to an even greater extent by non-medically qualified practitioners in the West, there are at the present time many acupuncturists throughout the world who claim it to be of benefit in the treatment of a wide variety of different disorders. It is however only in the alleviation of pain, and in particular musculoskeletal pain, that there is any scientific basis for employing it. And, even when used within these strictly defined limits, the traditional Chinese approach to this form of therapy has serious drawbacks.

The principal disadvantage is that, for most practitioners of traditional Chinese acupuncture, needles have to be inserted somewhat arbitrarily in accordance with the numerous lists of points that are recommended for use in the treatment of various rather ill-defined clinical conditions in every standard textbook on the subject. Moreover, before a person is able to use these lists, recipes, or prescriptions, as they are sometimes called, it is first necessary to memorize the course taken by the various Chinese acu-tracts, and the exact anatomical position on them of the various acu-points. It can only be assumed that these traditional guides to point selection owe their origin to the time-honoured, but highly contentious, Chinese method of pulse-diagnosis, and for this reason alone they are unlikely to be acceptable to most doctors trained in 20th-century scientific Western medicine.

However, fortunately for those who wish to avoid this somewhat empirically determined and impersonal method of point selection and prefer to employ one based on a carefully conducted clinical examination of each individual patient, there is now a trigger point approach to acupuncture. This recently developed Western approach to acupuncture has as its main application the alleviation of pain that is referred to some part of the body from a focus or foci of neural hyperactivity in one or other of the structures which together form the musculoskeletal system. In order to explain the principles upon which it is based, it is first necessary to review the outstanding pioneer research into referred pain carried out by J.H. Kellgren at University College Hospital Medical School in the late 1930s.

THE REFERRAL OF MUSCULOSKELETAL PAIN — SOME EARLY OBSERVATIONS

It was Sir Thomas Lewis, the director of clinical research department at University College Hospital who, because of his particular interest in the subject of pain in general, prompted Kellgren to carry out clinical observations on the referral of musculoskeletal pain.

Lewis in his paper *Suggestions Relating to the Study of Somatic Pain* published in February 1938 states,

As an experimental method of producing muscle pain the injection of a minute quantity of a salt solution is the most satisfactory . . . In these observations I have noted that muscle pain is referred to a distance. Thus pain arising from the lower part of the triceps is often referred down the inner side of the forearm to the little

31

finger, from the trapezius it is usually referred to the occiput. I have been fortunate in interesting Dr Kellgren in this matter. In a long series of very careful researches carried out in my laboratory he has formulated some very striking principles underlying the reference of pain from muscle — principles which appear to have an important practical bearing.

Kellgren, in his paper *Observations on Referred Pain Arising from Muscle*, published later the same year, states that in taking on the task set him by Sir Thomas Lewis he was aware that the latter's experimental findings had already received support from the clinical observations made by several physicians, who, from 1925 onwards, had noted that certain painful conditions of the extremities are associated with tender areas in the muscles of the limb girdles and because of this had suggested the possibility that in such cases pain arising in muscle may be of the referred type.

In his experiments which he carried out on himself and healthy volunteers working in the same laboratory, he first anaesthetized the skin and then injected small amounts (0.1–0.3 cc) of hypertonic (6%) saline into various muscles; and then carefully observed the distribution of pain. For example, in studies involving the gluteus medius muscle the skin of the buttock was first anaesthetized with Novocain at three sites. Then intramuscular needles were inserted through these anaesthetized areas until they impinged upon the gluteal fascia. An injection of hypertonic saline into this fascia produced localized pain. The needles were then advanced into the muscle itself and a further injection into this produced a diffuse pain felt at some distance from the injection site in the lower part of the buttock, the back of the thigh, and on occasions as far down as the knee (Fig. 4.1). Injections into the fascia enveloping the tibialis anticus (anterior) muscle and into the muscle itself produced similar findings (Fig. 4.2).

Kellgren also points out in this paper that an injection of saline into muscle produces pain at some distance from the point stimulated and that, in certain cases, the maximal pain is not experienced in muscle itself but in other structures. From his experimental work he was able to show, for example, that when an injection is given into the occipital muscle, pain is felt diffusely as a

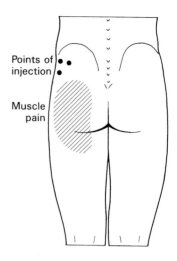

Fig. 4.1   The distribution of diffuse referred pain (hatched area) produced by injecting 6% saline into three points in the gluteus medius muscle. (Reproduced with permission of J. H. Kellgren from *Clinical Science*, vol. 3. pp 175–190 © 1938 The Biochemical Society, London.)

headache; when into the masseter muscle, it is felt in the mouth as toothache; when into the infraspinatus muscle, it is felt at the tip of the shoulder; when into the vastus intermedius, it is felt around the knee joint; when into the peroneus longus, it is felt at the ankle joint; and when into

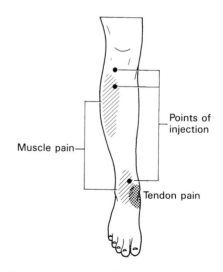

Fig. 4.2   The distribution of referred pain (hatched area) from injecting 6% saline into points in the tibialis anterior muscle. Also, the pattern of locally referred pain (stippled area) from injecting saline into the tendon of this muscle at the ankle. (Reproduced with permission of J. H. Kellgren from *Clinical Science*, vol. 3, pp 175–190 © 1938 The Biochemical Society, London.)

the multifidus muscle opposite the first and second lumbar vertebrae, it is felt in the scrotum.

His finding that referred pain from a focus of irritation in a muscle may be felt in such structures as joints, teeth, or the testicles is, of course, of considerable importance, and one which has constantly to be borne in mind in everyday clinical practice.

From these observations he decided that the distribution of referred pain, induced artificially in normal people, by injecting hypertonic saline into muscle broadly follows a spinal segmental pattern but that it does not correspond with the sensory segmental patterns of the skin.

Kellgren did not confine himself to laboratory experiments but applied knowledge gained from these to clinical medicine. And his paper, *A Preliminary Account of Referred Pains Arising from Muscle*, published in 1938, is of the greatest possible interest because, unbeknown to him, from his study of a number of cases of what he calls 'fibrositis' or 'myalgia' he laid down certain principles upon which the practice of modern Western acupuncture is now based. As his observations are therefore of such fundamental importance, part of his paper will be quoted in full:

During the last year I have made an extensive investigation of the character and distribution of muscular pain produced experimentally in normal subjects . . . Briefly I find that pain arising from muscle is always diffuse and is often referred, with a distribution which follows a spinal segmental pattern; and that this referred pain is associated with referred tenderness of the deep structures.

A number of cases of 'fibrositis' or 'myalgia' have been investigated from this point of view. The distribution of pain was noted as accurately as possible, and experience of the distribution of pain provoked from normal muscles guided me to the muscles from which spontaneous pain might have arisen. Such muscles almost always presented tender spots on palpation. Pressure on these spots sometimes reproduced the patient's pain; but a method more often successful was the injection of sterile saline into the tender muscle. The injection of Novocain may also reproduce the pain momentarily.

The search for the source of trouble by defining areas of tenderness is often confused by the patients calling attention to areas of referred tenderness. But referred tenderness is rarely conspicuous, and I have found it a useful guide to consider tenderness to be referred unless the patient winces under the palpation of a given spot. When these acutely tender spots were

not too extensive they were infiltrated with 1% Novocain . . . This infiltration often produced relief of the symptoms and signs, and sometimes abolished them completely.

It should be noted from this that Kellgren made a clear distinction between certain 'spots' in muscle so exquisitely tender that palpation of them makes the patient wince; and diffuse rather ill-defined areas of referred pain which on palpation are only slightly tender. Also, that he realized that such 'spots' as he called them, or trigger points as they are now termed, are the cause of this referred pain with it being possible to alleviate the latter by de-activating these acutely tender 'spots' or trigger points by infiltrating them with Novocain (Fig. 4.3).

Kellgren (1939) also investigated referred pain arising from experimentally-induced irritant foci in interspinous ligaments, tendons, joints and the periosteum. Two others who also made a valuable contribution to our understanding of skeletal pain were Verne Inman, an anatomist, and John Saunders, an orthopaedic surgeon working at the University of California Medical School. In their paper, *Referred Pain from Skeletal Structures*, published in 1944, they describe how they studied experimentally-induced pain in healthy volunteers by artificially stimulating periosteum, ligaments and tendons by mechanically traumatizing them either by scratching them with the point of a needle, or by drilling them with a special type of wire; and secondly by chemically stimulating them by injecting into them either normal isotonic Ringer's solution, or a weak solution of formic acid or hypertonic saline.

From these experiments they conclude,

Stimulation of the periosteum or the tendinous attachments of ligaments and tendons is accompanied by an extensive radiation of the pain, which, if sufficiently intense, radiates for considerable distances . . . so constant is the direction and locality to which the pain radiates that it has been found possible to chart and map out the extent of the areas to which the pain radiates, and an attempt has been made to relate them to areas of segmental innervation.

It should be noted that they refer to these areas of segmental innervation in the case of skeletal structures as sclerotomes in order to distinguish them from myotomes or dermatomes.

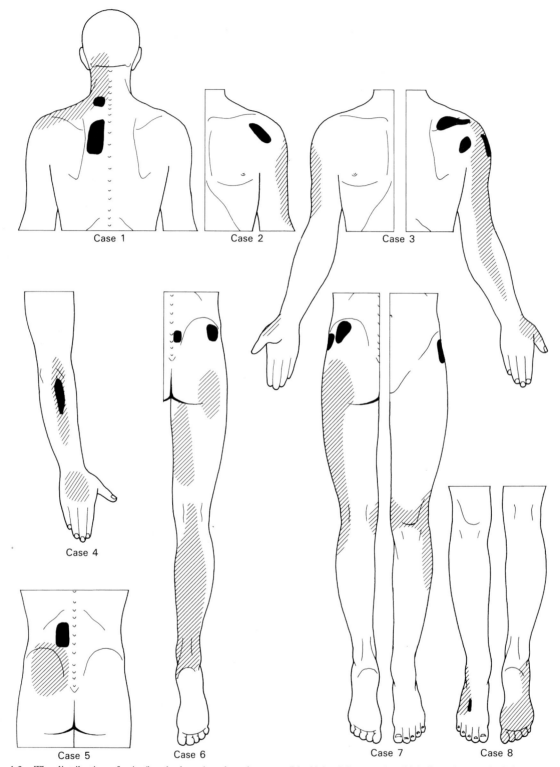

Fig. 4.3   The distribution of pain (hatched area) and tender spots (black) in eight cases in which the pain was abolished by injecting Novocain into the tender spots. (Reproduced with permission of J. H. Kellgren from the *British Medical Journal*, 1938.)

In this paper they also state that for several years they had been making detailed clinical observations on the radiation of pain from pathological disorders affecting bony and ligamentous structures. And they had found that in every case the type of pain was similar to that produced experimentally and that, like the latter, its radiation to distant areas had a distinctive pattern but one which could not be accounted for by reference to the distribution of peripheral nerves.

The anatomical distribution of referred musculoskeletal pain

It has to be admitted that there is much confusion concerning the anatomical distribution of referred pain in disorders of the musculoskeletal system. It will be remembered that Kellgren concluded that pain referred from skeletal muscle usually follows spinal segmental patterns but that this is not dermatomal, and that he also noted many exceptions when pain extended over several segments.

Travell & Bigelow (1946) also concluded from clinical observations on patients with referred pain from skeletal muscle that it does not follow a simple segmental pattern for, as they say, 'the reference from a single site may comprise fragments of several "segmental pain areas" without including any one entirely, or may take in a whole "segmental area", skip the adjacent one and reappear distally'.

Hockaday & Whitty (1967) in attempting to clarify the situation studied referred sensations produced by injecting 6% saline into interspinous ligaments in 28 normal subjects, and concluded that the

site of reference for a given site of stimulus was constant and replicable in the individual, but was not always confined to the segment of innervation in which the injection was given. Site of reference within a group of subjects varied widely and could not be interpreted as segmental or having a fixed anatomical substrate.

It is difficult however to be certain as to how much credence should be placed on conclusions drawn from any of the experiments carried out over the past 50 years in which hypertonic saline has been injected into various musculoskeletal structures in an attempt to map out the distribution of referred pain for as Wyke (1987) says, in discussing these during the course of considering various aspects of spinal ligamentous pain:

Although such saline solutions provide a very effective chemical irritant for connective tissue nociceptive receptors, it must be emphasised here that because of the diffuse distribution of this receptor system through the vertebral connective tissues, and because of the widespread intersegmental linkages between their afferent nerve fibres, attempts to use such a procedure as a means of delineating a supposed segmental nociceptive innervation of the spinal tissues are clearly fallacious, especially as it is impossible (even with the introduction of radio-opaque material into the injected solution) to be certain just how much of the diffuse nociceptive afferent system is being stimulated by any given volume of hypertonic saline.

The situation therefore is far from straightforward and Travell & Simons (1983) after years of extensively studying referred pain in patients with disorders of the musculoskeletal system have been forced somewhat negatively to conclude that referred pain of this type 'does not follow a simple segmental pattern. Neither does it follow familiar neurological patterns, nor the known patterns for referred pain of visceral origin'.

The relevance of these discoveries to the development of trigger point acupuncture

Kellgren's discovery that it is possible to alleviate referred musculoskeletal pain by injecting a local anaesthetic into what he called tender points has proved to be an important therapeutic advance. The relevance of this to the recent development of trigger point acupuncture might however at first sight seem to be somewhat obscure until it is explained that there are now sound neurophysiological grounds for believing that it is more rational as well as being simpler, safer and just as effective to alleviate this type of pain by stimulating with dry needles nerve endings in the superficial tissues directly overlying these intramuscularly situated tender points, or what, for reasons to be explained in the next chapter, are now called trigger points.

REFERENCES

Hockaday J M, Whitty C W M 1967 Patterns of referred pain in the normal subject. Brain 90: 481–496

Inman V T, Saunders J B de C M 1944 Referred pain from skeletal structures. Journal of Nervous and Mental Diseases 99: 660–667

Kellgren J H 1938 Observations on referred pain arising from muscle. Clinical Science 3: 175–190

Kellgren J H 1938 A preliminary account of referred pains arising from muscle. British Medical Journal 1: 325–327

Kellgren J H 1939 On the distribution of pain arising from deep somatic structures with charts of segmental pain areas. Clinical Science 4: 35–46

Lewis Sir Thomas 1938 Suggestions relating to the study of somatic pain. British Medical Journal 1: 321–325

Travell J, Bigelow N H 1946 Referred somatic pain does not follow a simple 'segmental' pattern. Federation Proceedings 5: 106

Travell J, Simons D G 1983 Myofascial pain and dysfunction. The trigger point manual. Williams and Wilkins, Baltimore

Wyke B 1987 The neurology of low back pain. In: Jayson M I V (ed) The lumbar spine and back pain, 3rd edn. Churchill Livingstone, Edinburgh, p 78

5. The myofascial pain syndrome and fibromyalgia

INTRODUCTION

Before turning to the neurophysiological principles upon which trigger point acupuncture is based, it is necessary to say something about the disorder for which it is mainly used, for unfortunately over the years there has been considerable controversy as to its nature and therefore over what to call it. It will have been noted that even Kellgren could not make up his mind about this, for he talks about having investigated a number of cases of 'fibrositis' or 'myalgia' (Ch. 4).

At the present time it is known as the myofascial pain syndrome (MPS). It is a disorder in which pain of a persistent and aching type is referred to a localized area of the body from trigger points in one or more muscles in that region. The erythrocyte sedimentation rate (ESR) is normal and there are no specific histological, biochemical or serological abnormalities.

In recent years it has become apparent that MPS has to be distinguished from what is currently known as the fibromyalgia syndrome (FS). Their clinical features are in many respects similar, but with the latter the pain is more widespread and it does not respond so readily to acupuncture. Their differential diagnosis will therefore have to be considered in some detail, but first the nosological confusion that preceded the introduction of these two terms will be discussed.

Nosological obfuscation

Before it was realized that MPS and FS are separate disorders they were known collectively over the past 200 years by a variety of different names. The original one was rheumatism, a term first introduced by Guillaume de Baillou in the latter part of the 16th century. Unfortunately, as Ruhmann (1940) has pointed out in his introduction to an English translation of De Baillou's book *Liber de Rheumatismo*, de Baillou used the term rheumatism not only when describing clinical manifestations of muscular rheumatism, but also when writing about what has since become known as acute rheumatic fever.

Thomas Sydenham then added to this terminological confusion when in his *Observationes Medicae* published in 1676 he included a chapter entitled 'Rheumatism' that dealt only with the characteristic migratory type of arthropathy seen in acute rheumatic fever. This confusion was further compounded when, in 1810, Wells called the carditis that develops in this febrile disorder rheumatism of the heart (Baldry 1971). Fortunately, Jean Bouillau helped to clarify the situation when in 1840 he made a clear distinction between the arthropathy and carditis of acute rheumatic fever and muscular rheumatism (Reynolds 1983).

By that time two British physicians, Balfour (1815) and Scudamore (1827) had put forward the idea that the pain of muscular rheumatism occurs as the result of inflammation developing in the fibrous connective tissue in muscle. This concept differed from the one held by 19th-century German and Scandinavian physicians who believed that the pain develops as the result of an inflammatory process in the muscle itself. Nevertheless it was one that was to persist throughout England and France for the rest of that century and in 1904 caused Sir William Gowers to recommend that the disorder hitherto known as muscular rheumatism should be called fibrositis.

Gowers did this during the course of a lecture on lumbago at what was then called the National Hospital for the Paralysed and Epileptic (National Hospital for Nervous Diseases, London). The arguments he put forward in support of his proposition were in retrospect distinctly specious, but nevertheless they led him to conclude: 'We are thus compelled to regard lumbago in particular, and muscular rheumatism in general, as a form of inflammation of the fibrous tissues of the muscles . . . (and thus) . . . we may conveniently follow the analogy of "cellulitis" and term it "fibrositis".'

Ralph Stockman, the then Professor of Medicine at Glasgow University, seemed to provide him with the pathological confirmation he required when, on examining microscopically some nodules removed from the muscles of patients affected by this disorder, he reported the presence of 'inflammatory hyperplasia . . . confined to white fibrous tissue' (Stockman 1904).

Although Stockman's findings have never subsequently been confirmed, their publication at that particular time helped to ensure that Gowers' term fibrositis became widely adopted. Any diagnostic specificity Gowers may have hoped to confer upon this term, however, was soon removed when in 1915 Llewellyn, a physician at the Royal Mineral Water Hospital in Bath, and Jones, a surgeon in that city, published a book entitled *Fibrositis*. In this they included under the term fibrositis a variety of disorders including gout and rheumatoid arthritis. Since that time the term has been used in such an imprecise manner as to make it virtually meaningless.

A search for a more suitable term for what was originally called muscular rheumatism has therefore continued, and some of the synonyms employed during this century include nodular fibromyositis (Telling 1911), myofascitis (Albee 1927), myofibrositis (Murray 1929), neurofibrositis (Clayton & Livingstone 1930), idiopathic myalgia (Gutstein-Good 1940), rheumatic myalgias (Good 1941) and even myodysneuria (Gutstein 1955).

Simons (1975, 1976) and Reynolds (1983), in their wide-ranging historical reviews of the subject, have shown that in addition to this longstanding terminological confusion there has also been much disagreement over the years concerning the diagnostic significance of the nodules, palpable bands and tender points found in this disorder.

Nodules and palpable bands

The Edinburgh physician William Balfour (1816), as a result of massaging muscles to relieve the pain of muscular rheumatism, was one of the first to report the presence of nodules in this disorder. However, it was not until the middle of the 19th century, when the Dutch physician Johan Mezger placed massage on a sound scientific basis (Haberling 1932), and this 'hands-on' technique then became widely adopted for the treatment of muscular rheumatism, that nodules and the elongated cord-like structures now known as palpable bands which are found in this disorder became generally recognized.

It was Mezger's Swedish and German students who were particularly influential in disseminating knowledge about these structures. In 1876, the Swedish physician Uno Helleday wrote extensively about nodules occurring in what he called chronic myitis (Helleday 1876). Following this, the German physician Strauss (1898) distinguished between nodules — which he described as being small, tender, apple-sized structures — and palpable bands — which he described as being painful, pencil-sized to little finger-sized elongated structures. The identification of these structures requires more than a cursory examination and, as Müller (1912) pointed out, the main reasons why so many doctors fail to identify them is because it requires a skilled technique, one which he considered difficult to learn but which he thought that could be made easier by the application of a lubricant to the skin.

He also thought that the reason why his contemporaries tended to deny the existence of nodules and palpable bands was because they did not bother to look for them conscientiously, unlike masseurs, who, according to him, had no difficulty in detecting them from palpating muscles systematically and then treating them appropriately. A similar state of affairs prevails today, with physiotherapists being far more practised in the art of palpating muscles than many doctors are.

Nodules

By the beginning of this century doctors in Britain were being taught to regard the presence of nodules as essential for the diagnosis of what was then called fibrositis. However, it soon became apparent that not only are nodules not always present in the disorder, but also that they are not infrequently present in people with no present or past history of it. It is because of their somewhat enigmatic and elusive nature and because of their distinctly nebulous morphology (Ch. 7) that over the course of this century their diagnostic significance has increasingly come to be questioned. Despite this, there is no doubt that when nodules are specifically sought they are frequently found in the lumbar region in patients with chronic low-back pain, and also to a less frequent extent in the neck and shoulder girdle of those affected by persistent musculoskeletal pain at that site. Moreover, the insertion of dry needles into these nodules helps to relieve this pain (Ch. 8).

Palpable bands

Unlike nodules which only develop in muscles in the lumbar and cervical regions, palpable bands are liable to develop in any muscle of the body. Like nodules, however, they are only discovered if conscientiously and skilfully looked for. When these elongated bands are carefully palpated they are found to contain one or more focal points of exquisite tenderness, now known as trigger points, but which Kellgren and others before him called tender points.

Tender points

Balfour (1824) not only found tender nodules in patients with muscular rheumatism but also observed that, separate from these, there are focal points of tenderness in the muscles. However, the first person to write at length about these was the French physician François Valleix.

Valleix, in his *Treatise on Neuralgia* published in 1841 described a disorder characterized by pain of a shooting nature and the finding of painful points (*points douloureux*) on palpation of the tissues. He realized that the pain emanated from these points for he states:

If, in the intervals of the shooting pains, one asks (a patient with neuralgia) what is the seat of the pain, he replies by designating limited points . . . . It is with the aid of pressure . . . that one discovers the extent of the painful points . . . .

Some of the pain syndromes he described would clearly be included in a present-day classification of neuralgias but others, such as what he termed femoropopliteal neuralgia, would not. Furthermore, 7 years later he somewhat confused the situation by calling muscular rheumatism a form of neuralgia (Valleix 1848). With reference to this he states:

I conclude that pain, capital symptom of neuralgia expresses itself . . . in different ways. If it remains concentrated in the nerves one finds characteristic, isolated, painful points; this is *neuralgia in the proper sense*. If the pain spreads into the muscles . . . this is *muscular rheumatism* . . . an obvious muscular rheumatism can transform itself into a true neuralgia . . . .

Despite his belief that neuralgia can turn itself into muscular rheumatism and vice versa, he must be given credit for recognizing that the pain in muscular rheumatism emanates primarily from focal points of neural hyperactivity, and also that it travels some distance from its source. He was wrong, however, in believing that this is because it is 'propagated along neighbouring nerves'.

Since then many other European physicians have erroneously subscribed to Valleix's idea that rheumatic pain spreads along the course of peripheral nerves, but they have differed in their views as to how this might occur. Stockman's (1904) explanation was that 'a branch of a nerve may be pressed upon by a nodule, or may even pass through it, hence the pain often radiates over a wide area perhaps far from a nodule'. Others believed that it occurred as a result of pressure on a nerve when a muscle goes into spasm. A third hypothesis, and one which was widely held well into the 20th century, was that it is due to rheumatic inflammation of connective tissue in or around nerves, and it was for this reason that the terms neurofibrositis and perineuritis were introduced (Gowers 1904, Llewellyn & Jones 1915, Clayton & Livingstone 1930).

Those who put forward such ideas seem to have been oblivious of the fact that the British physician

Thomas Inman, as long ago as 1858, had shrewdly noted that the radiation of pain in muscular rheumatism 'is independent entirely of the course of nerves'. They also seem to have ignored the observations made by the German physician Cornelius, who at the beginning of this century noted that 'this radiation often enough absolutely does not keep to the individual nerve trunks' and is bound 'to no anatomical law' (Cornelius 1903).

Cornelius not only confirmed Inman's observation that the radiation of pain is not along the course of peripheral nerves and therefore cannot be due to compression of these structures, but went further than this by showing that pressure on tender points in muscles evokes this type of pain and that the latter must therefore emanate from these points. He clearly realized that the reason why these points are tender is because they are sites where nerve endings are in a state of hyperactivity and for this reason he called them nerve points (*nervenpunkte*). He also stated that he thought this neural hyperactivity occurred as a result of external factors such as changes of temperature, alterations in weather conditions, physical exertion and emotional upsets, or alternatively because of 'heightened excitability' of the nervous system occurring as the result of such influences as heredity, intemperance and illness in general.

He was therefore beginning to formulate ideas concerning the pathogenesis of muscular rheumatism which were very much in line with the modern view that the pain develops as a result of nerve endings at tender points (or what today are more often called trigger points) becoming sensitized for one or other of a variety of different reasons. In the light of all this, it may be seen that Valleix may not have been so far off the mark as at first sight might be thought when he called muscular rheumatism a type of neuralgia. There is also no doubt that Sir William Osler (1909), with his customary perspicacity, must have had Valleix and Cornelius in mind when, in writing about what he called muscular rheumatism or myalgia in his famous textbook of medicine, he said:

It is by no means certain that the muscular tissues are the seat of the disease. Many writers claim, perhaps correctly, that it is a neuralgia of the sensory nerves of the muscles.

Early 20th-century physicians, however, had difficulty in explaining why pain occurring as the result of the sensitization of nerve endings at tender points should be felt some distance away from them. Cornelius (1903) stated it was due to 'reflex mechanisms' but did not enlarge much on the nature of these. Nobody else seems to have been able to take the matter much further until 1952, when Neufeld attributed the heterotopic nature of rheumatic pain to cortical misinterpretation of sensation. It was, however, the 3rd decade of the 20th century which was particularly notable for studies concerning the clinical aspects of rheumatic heterotopic pain.

Hunter (1933) described cases in which there was referral of pain from tender points in the muscles of the abdominal wall. Edeiken & Wolferth (1936) described how, in some patients with coronary thrombosis who had developed pain in the shoulder during the course of strict bed rest, pressure on tender points in muscles over the left scapula caused the spontaneously occurring shoulder pain to be reproduced. Then, in 1938 there were no less than three important contributions to the subject.

One of these was Kellgren's experimental and clinical observations concerning the referral of pain from tender points, which were of such considerable importance, both from a diagnostic and therapeutic point of view, that they have already been considered at some length in Chapter 4. A second was that of the Czechoslovakian physician Reichart, who was one of the first to describe and illustrate diagramatically specific patterns of radiating pains from tender points in muscles. The third came from a Polish physician, Gutstein, following his arrival in England as a political refugee.

Gutstein, unlike Kellgren, who in 1938 published his clinical observations in the British Medical Journal, published his findings that year in the less widely read British Journal of Physical Medicine, and that is possibly one of the reasons why it did not receive the attention it deserved. Nevertheless, in an attempt to get the medical profession to take notice of what he had to say about musculoskeletal pain, he wrote a number of papers on the subject over the next 10 years. Confusingly, however, during the course of this he changed his name three times and even more confusingly kept giving the musculoskeletal pain disorder he was discussing a different name. Thus in 1938 and again in 1940, under the name of M. Gutstein, he wrote about what he called muscular or common rheumatism. In 1940 under the name of Gutstein-Good he called the disorder idiopathic myalgia. Then, a year later, by which time he had changed his name yet again to Good, he wrote about rheumatic myalgias! In 1950 he called it fibrositis, and in 1951 non-articular rheumatism. To add to the confusion, there was at about the same time an R. R. Gutstein (1955) calling this disorder myodysneuria!

Despite all this, Good made the valuable observation that pressure applied to tender points, or what he called myalgic spots in a muscle or tendon, gives rise to both local and referred pain, and he must be given the credit for being the first person to stress that the patterns of pain referral from tender points in individual muscles are the same in everyone; these patterns he illustrated in well-executed drawings. In a similar manner to Kellgren he alleviated this type of pain by injecting a local anaesthetic into these tender points.

Sadly, the medical profession in Britain largely ignored Kellgren's and Good's valuable observations. One reason for this was that by the 1950s many of its leading rheumatologists had come to the conclusion that fibrositis, or non-articular rheumatism as it was by that time more commonly called, is not an organic disorder and that a more appropriate name for it is psychogenic rheumatism. They were led to believe this because of doubts concerning the significance of its physical signs, the absence of any characteristic histological appearances and the lack of any specific laboratory tests for it. Typical of this view was the one expressed by Ellman & Shaw (1950) who, during the course of discussing patients with this disorder stated:

From the striking disparity between the gross nature of their symptoms and the poverty of the physical findings . . . it seems clear that the nature of this often very prolonged incapacity is psychiatric in the majority of cases . . . the patient aches in his limbs because in fact he aches in his mind.

Another reason was that by the 1950s specialists in the field of physical medicine were of the opinion that there is no such disorder as muscular rheumatism and that the pain, said to be associated with it, occurs as the result of disorders in the vertebral column with, in particular, degenerative discs impinging upon nerve roots (Cyriax 1948, de Blecourt 1954, Christie 1958).

Fortunately, there were physicians in other parts of the world who were sufficiently perspicacious to recognize the merits of Kellgren's observations. One of these was Michael Kelly in Australia. Kelly not only adopted Kellgren's methods of diagnosing and relieving referred pain from tender points in muscles but recorded his clinical observations in a series of valuable papers published over a period of 21 years from 1941 onwards. References to the majority of these are to be found in his last paper (Kelly 1962).

The physician, however, who from the 1940s onwards has done the most to further the subject is Janet Travell. She first began to take an interest in it after reading how Edeiken & Wolferth (1936) had been able to reproduce spontaneously occurring shoulder pain by applying pressure to tender points in muscles around the scapula, and then reading about observations made both by Kellgren and by the American orthopaedic surgeon Steindler (1940).

It was Steindler who, during the course of reporting how he was able to relieve 'sciatica' by injecting Novocain into tender points in muscles in the lumbar and gluteal regions, first called these points 'trigger points'. It was, however, Travell who brought this term into general use when, in the early 1950s, she introduced the adjective myofascial and began to refer to myofascial trigger points and to describe the pain coming from these as myofascial pain. She adopted the term myofascial as a result of observing, whilst doing an infraspinatus muscle biopsy, that the pain pattern evoked by stretching or pinching the fascia enveloping the muscle is similar to that when the same is done to the muscle itself. Following this, she realized that each muscle in the body has its own specific pattern of myofascial trigger point pain referral and she introduced the term myofascial pain syndromes — a term which has since been generally accepted.

By 1951, Travell & Rinzler had had sufficient experience in recognizing these patterns of pain referral to enable them to give a detailed description of a large number of them at that year's meeting of the American Medical Association. In the following year they published an account of them in a classic contribution to the subject, 'The Myofascial Genesis of Pain', which is particularly notable for the clarity of its illustrations (Travell & Rinzler 1952). Thirty-one years later, Travell and her colleague David Simons had gained such considerable experience in the diagnosis and management of the myofascial pain syndromes that they were able to produce the first authoritative textbook on the subject (Travell & Simons 1983).

FIBROMYALGIA

In 1965 Smythe, a rheumatologist, and Moldofsky, a psychiatrist in Toronto, Canada, began to take a fresh look at so-called fibrositis and investigated electroencephalographically sleep disturbances in patients suffering from this disorder (Moldofsky et al 1975, Smythe 1986, Moldofsky 1986). They found that the rapid 8–10 c/sec alpha rhythm normally found in rapid eye movement (REM) sleep intrudes into the usual slow 1–2 c/sec delta rhythm of non-REM stage IV deep sleep. It is for this reason that 60–90% of patients with fibromyalgia complain of a non-restorative sleep that causes them to wake feeling tired and with generalized muscle stiffness (Goldenberg 1987).

It was this renewed interest in fibrositis that eventually led to the recognition of a syndrome characterized by persistent generalized muscle pain, non-restorative sleep, early morning stiffness, marked fatigue, and multiple tender points scattered over the body at certain specific sites.

When Smythe & Moldofsky (1977) first drew attention to this syndrome they somewhat confusingly referred to it as the 'fibrositis' syndrome, but, for the same reason that made this term unacceptable earlier in this century, it was soon abandoned and in 1981 it was re-named the fibromyalgia syndrome (Yunus et al 1981). Since then it has been the subject of several comprehensive reviews (Simons 1986, Bennett 1986 a & b, Smythe 1986, Bennett 1987, Goldenberg 1987,

McCain & Scudds 1988, Simons 1988, Wolfe 1988, Yunus 1989, Simons 1990, Bennett 1990).

The optimum criteria for the diagnosis of this syndrome have gradually evolved over the years as a result of controlled studies. The latest, very extensive study carried out by the American College of Rheumatology's Multicenter Fibromyalgia Criteria Committee (Wolfe et al 1989) showed that the best criteria are simply widespread pain and the finding of 11 or more tender points on digital palpation at 18 possible sites.

The three main differences between the myofascial pain syndrome (MPS) and the fibromyalgia syndrome (FS) are as follows. With MPS the pain is characteristically localized to one area of the body, although at times several separate sites are affected simultaneously; it is equally common in males and females; and it is principally traumatic in origin. In contrast to this, with FS, the pain is generalized; 90% of those affected are females; and the cause is unknown.

The relationship between tender points and trigger points in FS

The American rheumatologists who in recent years have made a special study of FS, state that one of its characteristic features is the presence of tender points. In contrast to this, the American specialists in physical medicine (physiatrists), such as Travell and Simons who write authoritatively about MPS, emphasize that one of its characteristic features is the presence of trigger points. From this it might be thought that tender points and trigger points are distinctive features of these two disorders but this is not necessarily so, for, as Simons (1988) has said, 'rheumatologists rarely examine tender points for taut bands, local twitch responses, or for referral of pain to distant sites on palpation'. The truth would seem to be that whilst some tender points do not have all the characteristic features of trigger points, what the two types of points have in common is that they are both actual or potential sources of pain. As Margoles (1989) has stated from the study of a large number of patients with FS, it is the rule rather than the exception with this syndrome to find both tender points and trigger points. This conclusion is in keeping with the view recently expressed by Bennett (1990) that many patients with FS have active trigger points and that many of the so-called tender points are in reality latent trigger points.

The question therefore that has to be asked is whether MPS and FS represent two extremes of a single disorder (Thompson 1990). Bennett (1990) believes they are distinctive syndromes, but there is no doubt that they are closely inter-related, for it is not uncommon for a patient with MPS to progress with time to a clinical picture identical to that of FS (Bennett 1986a & b). Moreover, in attempting to distinguish clinically between MPS and FS it has to be remembered that MPS is not always localized to one area but may at times develop in several separate areas simultaneously. In such cases it closely resembles FS. The clinical characteristics of these two syndromes are summarized in Table 5.1.

Table 5.1 Clinical characteristics of MPS and FS

	MPS	*FS*
Sex	Equally common in males and females	Predominantly females — over 4/5ths of patients are women (Yunus 1989)
Pathogenesis	Trauma	Unknown. ? Some systemic biochemical disorder. In a minority of cases a traumatically induced MPS may lead to the development of FS (Bennett 1986a, b)
Distribution of pain	Usually localized, but may affect several parts of the body when multiple syndromes are present simultaneously	Generalized
Sleep disturbance	Pain causing arousal from sleep is common	Tiredness on waking as a result of non-restorative sleep is a characteristic feature
Morning stiffness	No	Yes in 75% of cases
Fatigue	No	Yes in 75% of cases
Cold weather sensitivity	Yes	Yes
Sympathetic overactivity	Myofascial trigger points are often responsible for this, causing the distal part of a limb to become cold	Raynaud's phenomenon has been reported in 53% of cases in one series (Vaerøy et al 1988) 30% in another (Dinerman et al 1986)
Psychological disturbances	Anxiety and/or depression may develop as a result of persistent pain	Yes — in a minority, but not as frequent as originally thought, with psychological testing not showing neurotiscism, hypochondriasis or depression to be common (Clark et al 1985). However, emotional upsets and stress seem capable of bringing it on (Moldofsky 1986)
Other associated disorders	Tension headaches Parathesiae	The following are commonly associated (Yunus 1989): irritable bowel syndrome tension headaches parathesiae subjective swelling of joints primary dysmenorrhoea
Administration of: NSAIDS	No effect	No effect (Dinerman et al 1986)
Corticosteroids by mouth	No effect	No effect (Clark et al 1985)
by local injection	Only indicated when there is marked local inflammatory reaction (see Ch. 7)	Not indicated
Tricyclic antidepressants in sub-antidepressant dosage	Not indicated	Very helpful in improving quality of sleep, in reducing morning stiffness and in alleviating pain (Goldenberg et al 1986)
Cardiovascular fitness training	Not indicated	Said to confer some benefit (McCain & Scudds 1988)
Prognosis	Very good if trigger points are identified and deactivated	Poor. Disease tends to take protracted course in spite of treatment

From Table 5.1 it may be seen that MPS and FS, whilst having many features in common, are separate entities with different prognoses and with each requiring its own particular type of management.

Acupuncture for the relief of fibromyalgia pain

The reason why it is important to distinguish between FS and MPS is that their management is different. It would clearly not be appropriate in a book on acupuncture to enter into a detailed discussion concerning the management of FS. This has recently been comprehensively reviewed by Russell (1990) and McCain (1990). My remarks will therefore be confined to considering what place, if any, acupuncture has in its management.

The pain in FS — which would seem to be due to some as yet unidentified noxious substance in the circulation giving rise to neural hyperactivity at tender points and trigger points — takes a protracted course and it is only possible by means of acupuncture to suppress this neural hyperactivity for short periods. This means, therefore, that this form of treatment has to be repeated every 2–3 weeks for months or even years. Such treatment therefore is far from satisfactory, but nevertheless some patients insist that it improves the quality of their lives.

Acupuncture for the relief of the myofascial pain syndromes

The main indication for trigger point acupuncture is in the treatment of the trauma-induced myofascial pain syndromes described in Part III of this book. However, in order to understand how trigger point pain develops in these syndromes and how, by means of acupuncture, it is often possible to obtain long-term relief from this type of pain, it is first necessary to consider the various pain-arousing and pain-suppressing mechanisms that are present in the peripheral and central nervous system.

REFERENCES

Albee F H 1927 Myofascitis. A pathological explanation of many apparently dissimilar conditions. American Journal of Surgery 3: 523–533
Baldry P E 1971 The battle against heart disease. University Press, Cambridge
Balfour 1815 Observations on the pathology and cure of rheumatism. Edinburgh Medical and Surgical Journal 11: 168–187
Balfour 1816 Observations with cases illustrative of new simple and expeditious mode of curing rheumatism and sprains . . . . Adam Black, Edinburgh
Balfour 1824 Illustrations of the efficacy of compression and percussion in the cure of rheumatism and sprains. The London Medical and Physical Journal 51: 446–462, 52: 104–115, 200–208, 284–291
Bennett R M 1986a Current issues concerning management of the fibrositis/fibromyalgia syndrome. The American Journal of Medicine 81 (suppl 3A): 15–18
Bennett R M 1986b Fibrositis: Evolution of an enigma. The Journal of Rheumatology 13(4): 676–678
Bennett R M 1987 Fibromyalgia. Journal of the American Medical Association. 257(20): 2802–2803
Bennett R M 1990 Myofascial pain syndromes and the fibromyalgia syndrome. A comparative analysis. In: Fricton R, Awad E (eds) Advances in pain research and therapy. Raven Press, New York, vol 17, p 43–65

Christie B G 1958 Discussion on non-articular rheumatism. Proceedings of the Royal Society of Medicine 51: 251–255
Clark S, Campbell S M, Forehand M E et al 1985 Clinical characteristics of fibrositis II. A blinded controlled study using standard psychological tests. Arthritis & Rheumatism 28: 132–137
Clayton E G, Livingstone J L 1930 Fibrositis. Lancet 1: 1420–1423
Cornelius A 1903 Narben und Nerven. Deutsche Militärärztliche Zeitschrift 32: 657–673
Cyriax J 1948 Fibrositis. British Medical Journal 2: 251–255
de Blecourt J J 1954 Screening of the population for rheumatic diseases. Annals of Rheumatic Diseases 13: 338–340
Dinerman H, Goldenberg D L, Felson D T 1986 A prospective evaluation of 118 patients with the Fibromyalgia Syndrome: Prevalence of Raynaud's phenomenon . . . . . . The Journal of Rheumatology 13(2): 368–373
Edeiken J, Wolferth C C 1936 Persistent pain in the shoulder region following myocardial infarction. American Journal of Medical Science 191: 201–210
Ellman P, Shaw D 1950 The chronic 'rheumatic' and his pains. Psychosomatic aspects of chronic non-articular rheumatism. Annals of Rheumatic Diseases 9: 341–357

Goldenberg D L, Felson D T, Dinerman H A 1986 A randomized controlled trial of amitriptyline and naproxen in the treatment of patients with fibromyalgia. Arthritis and Rheumatism 29: 1371–1377

Goldenberg D L 1987 Fibromyalgia syndrome. An emerging but controversial condition. Journal of the American Medical Association 257 (20): 2782–2787

Good M G 1941 Rheumatic myalgias. Practitioner 146: 167–174

Good M G 1950 The role of skeletal muscle in the pathogenesis of diseases. Acta Medica Scandinavica 138: 285–292

Good M G 1951 Objective diagnosis and curability of non-articular rheumatism. British Journal of Physical Medicine and Industrial Hygiene 14: 1–7

Gowers W R 1904 Lumbago: Its lessons and analogues. British Medical Journal 1: 117–121

Gutstein M 1938 Diagnosis and treatment of muscular rheumatism. British Journal of Physical Medicine 1: 302–321

Gutstein M 1940 Common rheumatism and physiotherapy. British Journal of Physical Medicine 3: 46–50

Gutstein R R 1955 A review of myodysneuria (fibrositis). American Practitioner 6: 570–577

Gutstein-Good M 1940 Idiopathic myalgia simulating visceral and other diseases. Lancet 2: 326–328

Haberling W 1932 Johan Georg Mezger of Amsterdam. The founder of scientific massage (translated by Emilie Recht). Medical Life 39: 190–207

Helleday U 1876 Nordiskt medicinskt arkiv 6 and 8 Nr 8. P A Norstedtosöner, Stockholm

Hunter C 1933 Myalgia of the abdominal wall. Canadian Medical Association Journal 28: 157–161

Inman T 1858 Remarks on myalgia or muscular pain. British Medical Journal 407–408 & 866–868

Kelly M 1962 Local injections for rheumatism. Medical Journal of Australia 1: 45–50

Llewellyn L J, Jones A B 1915 Fibrositis. Rebman, New York

McCain G A 1990 Management of the fibromyalgia syndrome. In: Fricton J R, Awad E (eds) Advances in pain research and therapy. Raven Press, New York, vol 17, p 289–303

McCain G A, Scudds R H 1988 The concept of primary fibromyalgia (fibrositis) clinical value, relation and significance to other chronic musculoskeletal pain syndromes. Pain 33: 273–287

Margoles M S 1989 The concept of fibromyalgia. Pain 36: 391

Moldofsky H 1986 Sleep and musculoskeletal pain. The American Journal of Medicine 81 (suppl 3A): 85–89

Moldofsky H, Scarisbrick P, England R, Smythe H 1975 Musculoskeletal symptoms and non-rem sleep disturbance in patients with fibrositis syndrome and healthy subjects. Psychosomatic Medicine 371: 341–351

Müller A 1912 Untersuchungsbefund am rheumatisch erkranten muskel. Zeitschift Klinische Medizin 74: 34–73

Murray G R 1929 Myofibrositis as a simulator of other maladies. Lancet 1: 113–116

Neufeld I 1952 Pathogenetic concepts of 'fibrositis' — fibropathic syndromes. Archives of Physical Medicine 33: 363–369

Osler W 1909 The principles and practice of medicine, 7th edn. S. Appleton & Co, New York, p 396

Reichart A 1938 Reflexschmerzen auf grund von myogelosen. Deutsch Medizinische Wochenshrift 64: 823–824

Reynolds M D 1983 The development of the concept of fibrositis. The Journal of the History of Medical and Allied Sciences 38: 5–35

Ruhmann W 1940 The earliest book on rheumatism. The British Journal of Rheumatism II (3): 140–162 (This paper includes an original translation of de Baillou's *Liber de Rheumatismo* which, originally written in medieval Latin, was first published by a descendant M J Thevart in 1736, i.e. 120 years after the author's death.)

Russell I J 1990 Treatment of patients with fibromyalgia syndrome. In: Fricton J R, Awad E (eds) Advances in pain research and therapy. Raven Press, New York, vol 17, p 305–314

Scudamore C 1827 A treatise on the nature and cure of rheumatism. Longman, London, p 11

Simons D G 1975 Muscle pain syndromes — Part I. American Journal of Physical Medicine 54: 289–311

Simons D G 1976 Muscle pain syndromes — Part II. American Journal of Physical Medicine 55: 15–42

Simons D G 1986 Fibrositis/fibromyalgia: A form of myofascial trigger points? The American Journal of Medicine 81 (suppl 3A): 93–98

Simons D G 1988 Myofascial pain syndromes: Where are we? Where are we going? Archives of Physical Medicine and Rehabilitation 69: 207–211

Simons D G 1990 Muscular pain syndromes. In: Fricton J R, Awad E (eds) Advances in pain research and therapy. Raven Press, New York, vol 17, p 1–41

Smythe H 1986 Tender points: Evolution of concepts of the fibrositis/fibromyalgia syndrome. The American Journal of Medicine 81 (suppl 3A): 2–6

Smythe H A, Moldofsky H 1977 Two contributions to understanding of the 'fibrositis' syndrome. Bulletin of Rheumatic Diseases 28: 928–931

Steindler A 1940 The interpretation of sciatic radiation and the syndrome of low-back pain. Journal of Bone and Joint Surgery 22: 28–34

Stockman R 1904 The causes, pathology and treatment of chronic rheumatism. Edinburgh Medical Journal 15: 107–116, 223–225

Strauss H 1898 Über die sogenannte 'rheumatische muskelschwiele'. Klinische Wochenshrift 35: 89–91, 121–123

Sydenham Thomas 1676 Observationes Medicae. The works of Thomas Sydenham translated by R G Latham in 1848. Sydenham Society, London.

Telling W H 1911 Nodular fibromyositis, an everyday affliction, and its identity with so-called muscular rheumatism. Lancet 1: 154–158

Thompson J M 1990 Tension myalgia as a diagnosis at the Mayo Clinic and its relationship to fibrositis, fibromyalgia and myofascial pain syndrome. Mayo Clinic Proceedings 65: 1237–1248

Travell J, Rinzler S H 1952 The myofascial genesis of pain. Postgraduate Medicine 11: 425–434

Travell J, Simons D G 1983 Myofascial pain and dysfunction. The trigger point manual. Williams and Wilkins, Baltimore

Vaerøy H, Helle R, Førre O, Kåsse, Terenius L 1988
Elevated CSF levels of substance P and high incidence of
Raynaud's phenomenon in patients with fibromyalgia. New
features for diagnosis. Pain 32: 21–26

Valleix F 1841 Traité des Neuralgies; ou, affections
douloureuses des nerfs. Ballière, Paris.

Valleix F 1848 Études sur le rhumatisme musculaire, et en
particulier sur son diagnostic et sur son traitement. Bulletin
général de thérapeutique médicale et chirurgicale
35: 296–307

Wolfe F 1988 Fibrositis, Fibromyalgia and Musculoskeletal
Disease. The current status of the fibrositis syndrome.

Archives of Physical Medicine and Rehabilitation
69: 527–531

Wolfe F, Smythe H A, Yunus M B et al 1989 Multicenter
Fibromyalgia Criteria Committee. Arthritis & Rheumatism
32(4) (suppl): 547

Yunus M, Masi A T, Calabro J J, Miller K A, Feigenbaum
S L 1981 Primary fibromyalgia (fibrositis) clinical study of
50 patients with matched controls. Seminars in Arthritis
and Rheumatism 11, 151–171

Yunus M B 1989 Fibromyalgia syndrome: new research on
an old malady. British Medical Journal 298: 474–475

6. Neurophysiology of pain

INTRODUCTION

The purpose of this brief, and therefore somewhat superficial, account of the neurophysiology of pain is simply to provide a certain amount of insight into its complexities. It should therefore serve as a basis for discussing, in subsequent chapters, the various physiological mechanisms which are involved in the development of myofascial trigger point pain and in its alleviation by means of stimulating peripheral nerve endings with dry needles.

As space does not permit the neurophysiology of pain to be considered at length, anyone interested to learn more about this fascinating subject is recommended to read an extremely lucid account of it in Melzack & Wall's book *The Challenge of Pain* (1988a) or an even more detailed presentation of its various aspects by a number of authorities in their *Textbook of Pain* (Wall & Melzack 1989).

Modern concepts concerning the transmission of noxious impulses from the periphery to the cortex and how the sensation of pain may be modulated by various physiochemical mechanisms in the central nervous system have been profoundly influenced by the gate-control theory first put forward by Melzack & Wall (1965). Although this theory, as might be expected, has had to be revised over the years in the light of further knowledge, it nevertheless remains a remarkably useful hypothesis and as Liebskind & Paul (1977) have said, when discussing reasons for the current interest in pain research,

Probably the most important was the appearance in 1965 of the gate control theory of pain by Melzack & Wall. This theory, like none before it, has proved

enormously heuristic. It continues to inspire basic research and clinical applications.

It will therefore be necessary to consider this particular theory at some length but, in order fully to understand its ingenuity and implications, it is first necessary to say something about the nature of pain, and the parts of the central nervous system in which pain-modulating mechanisms are to be found.

The nature of pain

Pain is not a simple, straightforward sensory experience, in the manner as, for example, is seeing or hearing, since it has both emotional and physical components. The definition of pain put forward by the International Association for the Study of Pain (1980) is that it is 'an unpleasant sensory and emotional experience associated with actual or potential tissue damage, or described in terms of such damage' (Merskey 1979).

As Hannington-Kiff (1974) points out, pain has three main components: physical, emotional and rational. The physical component is determined by the responsiveness of an individual's nociceptive system to a given stimulus; the rational component is derived from an objective interpretation of pain in the cerebral cortex; the emotional component is determined by the responsiveness of an individual's limbic system to any particular noxious stimulus.

It therefore follows that for a given noxious stimulus the intensity with which pain is felt varies from person to person, and with regard to this a distinction has to be made between an individual's pain threshold and pain tolerance.

The pain threshold is the least stimulus intensity at which a subject perceives pain and, contrary to popular belief, this is much the same in everyone (Thompson 1984a). As Wyke (1979) has pointed out, it is an all too common misconception:

that measuring pain thresholds tells one something about the mechanisms that influence the intensity of a patient's experience of pain. On the contrary, of course, what one should assess in this regard is not a patient's pain threshold but his pain tolerance, because what brings patients to doctors to seek relief is not the occurrence of some minor pain of which they are just aware when their pain threshold is reached (we have this every day of our lives) but is when the limit of their individual pain tolerance is reached.

This, of course, is of considerable practical importance when attempting to assess pain and the effect of any particular form of treatment on it, for it is not changes in pain threshold that have to be measured but rather changes in pain tolerance.

Pain tolerance clearly depends on a person's emotional response to a noxious stimulus. It is very interesting with respect to this to note that the 17th-century Dutch philosopher Benedict Spinoza (1632–1677) referred to pain as 'a localized form of sorrow'.

It therefore follows that throughout a person's life the intensity with which pain is felt depends on his or her psychological make-up, cultural background, parental influence and ethnic origin (Zborwski 1952, Bond 1979). The manner in which perception of, and reaction to, noxious stimuli is influenced by past experiences has been demonstrated in ingenious experiments carried out on various animals, including dogs (Melzack & Scott 1957, Melzack 1969) and monkeys (Lichstein & Sackett 1971).

A person's reaction to pain at any specific time is also dependent on the current mood — with anxiety or depression intensifying it — and on prevailing circumstances. A severe wound sustained in the heat of battle, for example, may hardly be noticed, whereas a similar injury incurred in a less stressful environment may be the cause of severe pain (Beecher 1959). Conversely, the intensity with which pain is felt is diminished by distraction of attention. It is for this reason that some people find background music helpful whilst undergoing some painful experience such as at the dentist (Gardner & Licklider, 1959). This is also why chronic pain sufferers find that their pain is far less intrusive if the mind is occupied by carrying out some absorbing task (Wynn Parry 1980).

Types of pain

Pain is occasionally purely psychogenic but more often it is an organic physio-emotional experience occurring either as a result of the primary activation of visceral or somatic nociceptors (nocigenic or nociceptive pain) or as a result of damage to the peripheral or central nervous system (neurogenic or neuropathic pain).

NOCIGENIC (NOCICEPTIVE) PAIN

Our understanding of the psychological and physical components of nocigenic pain has been greatly advanced by recent detailed studies showing that the behavioural and physiological response to it is dependent on a number of facilitatory and inhibitory modulating mechanisms in various parts of the central nervous system. The structures that are of particular importance in this complex process are certainly sensory receptors, their associated afferent nerve fibres, the dorsal horns, ascending and descending tracts in the neuraxis, the reticular formation in the midbrain and medulla, the thalamus, the limbic system and the cerebral cortex. Each of these will be considered in turn.

Sensory receptors

Nociceptors

Although the experience of nocigenic pain ultimately depends on interpretative processes in the neurons of the cerebral cortex, it occurs primarily as a result of a noxious stimulus activating myelinated and unmyelinated nociceptors.

Myelinated nociceptors

These nociceptors are connected to the spinal cord's dorsal horns via medium diameter (1–5μm) myelinated A-delta nerve fibres with a conduction velocity of 5–15 m/s (11–33.5 mph).

These A-delta nociceptors are activated by any noxious mechanical stimulus such as that delivered by a sharp pointed instrument or needle and for this reason are also known as high-threshold mechanonociceptors. Approximately 20–50% of them, in addition, respond to suddenly applied heat in the noxious range of from 45° upwards and, because of this, are known as mechanothermal nociceptors.

A-delta myelinated nociceptors are found mainly in and just under the skin and, as will be discussed in Chapters 8 and 10, it is these receptors which are stimulated when needles are inserted into acupuncture points.

The receptive field of a high-threshold mechanonociceptor in the skin (Fig. 6.1) consists of a number of sensitive spots about 1 mm in diameter grouped together in a cluster covering on average a total area of 5 mm² (Georgopoulos 1974).

There are also a certain number of A-delta nerve fibres in muscle, in which situation, they are also called Group III fibres. It would seem, however, that most of these are concentrated in the fascia rather than the muscle itself because, as Edwards (1990) has pointed out, the latter is relatively insensitive to needle prick or knife cut. This is why percutaneous needle biopsy of muscle only gives a sensation of deep pressure and why it is only when the instrument gets caught in the fascia that there is any acute discomfort (Edwards et al 1983).

Stimulation of A-delta nociceptors gives rise to an immediate, sharp, relatively brief pricking sensation — the so-called first or fast pain (Fig. 6.3). This sensation serves to provide a warning of impending tissue damage and is accompanied by reflex withdrawal movements designed to avoid or minimize such damage.

Unmyelinated nociceptors

These receptors, known as C-polymodal nociceptors, are connected to the spinal cord's dorsal horns via small diameter (0.25–1.5μm) unmyelinated C afferent nerve fibres. The conduction velocity rate of these is only 0.5–2 m/s (1–4.5 mph). These receptors are termed polymodal because under experimental conditions it is possible to activate them by applying either a mechanical, thermal or chemical stimulus (Fig. 6.2). However, it is somewhat of a misnomer as, clinically, such activation is invariably

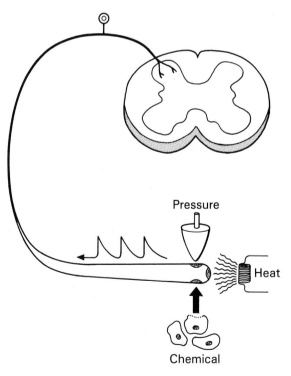

Fig. 6.2 Sensitivity range of the C-polymodal nociceptor. Its terminals are sensitive to direct heat or mechanical distortion, and to chemicals released from damaged cells. Reproduced with permission from Howard Field's *Pain*. McGraw-Hill 1987

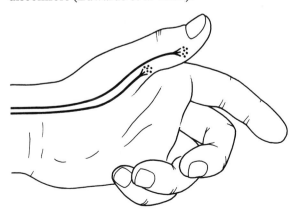

Fig. 6.1 The multipunctate receptive field of an A-delta nociceptor. Reproduced with permission from Howard Field's *Pain*. McGraw-Hill 1987

only produced by chemicals released as a result of tissue damage.

The receptive field of C-polymodal nociceptors is usually a single area rather than a cluster of spots as in the case of A-delta nociceptors. These nociceptors are present everywhere in the body except the nervous system. The C nerve fibres connected to those present in muscle are also called Group IV fibres.

Among the various places in muscle where Group IV fibres are to be found are their motor points. A muscle's motor point is by definition the point where its motor nerve enters. However, in the fasciculus containing the motor nerve are also various sensory afferents. These include spindle fibres (Group I); A-beta fibres (Group

II); A-delta nociceptive fibres (Group III) and C nociceptive fibres (Group IV).

In addition, throughout a muscle's connective tissue, in the walls of its blood vessels and in tendons, there are a large number of C (Group IV) sensory afferent free nerve endings, and some A-delta (Group III) ones. It has been estimated that nociceptive afferents constitute 75% of the sensory innervation of skeletal muscle (Stacey 1969).

It is the stimulation of C-polymodal nociceptors in any deeply situated tissue such as muscle that leads to the development of pain which, because its onset is delayed beyond the first few seconds, is known as 'second' or 'slow' pain (Fig. 6.3). This type of pain takes the form

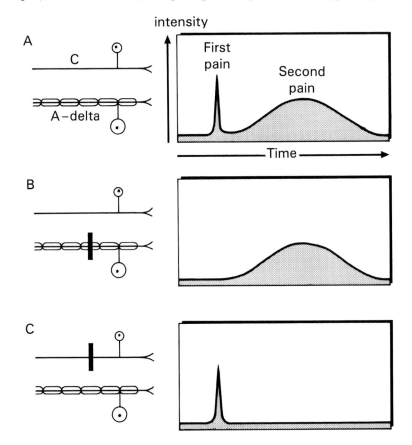

Fig. 6.3   A. First pain — produced by stimulation of A-delta afferent nerve fibres. Second pain — produced by stimulation of C afferent nerve fibres.
B. First pain suppressed by the selective application of pressure to the A-delta afferent fibres.
C. Second pain suppressed by selectively blocking, with low concentrations of local anaesthetic, the C afferent fibres
Reproduced with permission from Howard Field's *Pain*. McGraw-Hill 1987

of a widespread, ill-defined, deep-seated dull aching associated with much tenderness and the development of muscle spasm, rigidity and tonic contraction.

The pain which emanates from trigger points in the myofascial pain syndromes described in Part Three of this book is of this 'second' or 'slow' type. Therefore, despite the fact that sensory nerve fibres at a trigger point site are not all of one type, it necessarily follows that with respect to its pain-producing property a trigger point is essentially a plexus of sensitized C-polymodal nociceptors.

TRAUMA-INDUCED SENSITIZATION OF NOCICEPTIVE SENSORY AFFERENTS

The main aetiological factor responsible for the production of the various primary myofascial pain syndromes is trauma. When a muscle is subjected to trauma, there is an inflammatory reaction as the result of tissue damage. As a part of this process, a number of chemical substances appear in the inflammatory exudate that are capable of sensitizing Group III and Group IV nociceptive sensory afferents and making them electrically active (Mense 1977).

One of the most potent of these algesic substances is bradykinin, a 9-amino acids peptide produced in damaged tissue by enzymatic cleavage from large plasma proteins (Fields 1987a).

Others that appear in the inflammatory exudate come from the mast cells present in the connective tissue in and around peripheral nerves (Olsson 1968). Trauma causes mast cells to undergo degranulation (Nennesmo & Reinholt 1986), and when this happens histamine is liberated into the tissue together with two groups of substances derived from the fatty acid arachidonic acid present in the mast cell membrane. These arachidonic metabolites are the leukotrienes and the prostaglandins. The former are produced by the action of the enzyme lipoxygenase on arachidonic acid, and the latter by the action of cyclooxygenase on it. With respect to this, it is of interest to recall that aspirin and other non-steroidal anti-inflammatory drugs owe their analgesic effect to being cyclooxygenase inhibitors.

Mast cells, on degranulation, also release a platelet-activating factor which in turn causes platelets to release serotonin, a substance known to potentiate the action of bradykinin on Group IV muscle afferent fibres (Mense 1981).

Once C-sensory afferents have become chemically sensitized, they release the 11-amino acid polypeptide substance P. Substance P is a vasodilator and causes tissues to become oedematous. In addition, it also facilitates the release of histamine from mast cells and serotonin from platelets.

It is because vasodilation, oedema and pain are the principal signs of inflammation and are also produced by activity in unmyelinated primary afferents that Fields (1987b) has been led to make the following interesting observation:

In a sense, then, nociceptor activity is not merely a passive signal indicating that tissue damage has occurred, but may play an active role in body defences by participating in the inflammatory process. In fact, destruction of the small-diameter primary afferents of a limb can markedly slow experimental inflammatory arthritis. Although the clinical significance of this neurogenic component of inflammation has yet to be determined, there is no doubt that it exists.

Low-threshold mechanoreceptors

These mechanoreceptors, situated in the skin, muscles, tendons and joints are not responsive to noxious stimuli but, on the contrary, are activated by innocuous ones. Those in the skin for example are stimulated when the latter is stretched or lightly touched and also when its hairs are bent. Proprioceptors in muscle are present in the form of specially designed spindles; and in the tendinous parts of muscles they are called tendon organs. These receptors provide information concerning a muscle's passive tension and active contraction. Those in a joint provide information concerning its position and speed of movement.

These low-threshold mechanoreceptors are connected to the spinal cord's dorsal horns via large diameter A-beta myelinated nerve fibres. These A-beta nerve fibres have a diameter of 5–15µm and the relatively fast conduction velocity of 30–100 m/s.

The dorsal horn

Laminae

It was the Swedish anatomist, Bror Rexed (1952), who established that the cells of the spinal cord are arranged in layers or laminae. There are six laminae in the dorsal (Lamina I–VI); three in the ventral horn (Lamina VII–IX) and an additional column of cells clustered around the central canal known as Lamina X (Fig. 6.4).

At the outer part of the dorsal horn there is a clear zone visible to the naked eye and it was because of this appearance that the Italian anatomist Luigi Rolando (1773–1831) in 1824 named it the substantia gelatinosa. Some neurophysiologists (Wall 1990) state that the substantia gelatinosa includes both Lamina I and II whilst others (Bowsher 1990, Fields 1987c) call Lamina II the substantia gelatinosa and Lamina I the marginal zone.

The thin unmyelinated C nociceptive afferents terminate mainly in Laminae I and II where their axon terminals secrete Substance P (SP) or vasoactive intestinal polypeptide (VIP) according to whether they arise from somatic structures or visceral ones respectively (Thompson 1988).

The medium-sized myelinated A-delta nociceptive afferents terminate chiefly in Laminae I, II and V.

In contrast to this, most of the large diameter myelinated A-beta low-threshold mechanoreceptive afferent fibres, on entering the spinal cord, pass directly up the dorsal column to end in the medulla oblongata's gracile and cuneate nuclei. Axons from these nuclei then form the medial leminiscus and this, after decussating in the medulla, terminates principally in the ventrobasal thalamus. However, what is of particular importance as far as the pain modulating effect of A-beta afferent activity is concerned is that the medial leminiscus is connected, via the anterior pretectal nucleus, to the periaqueductal grey area in the midbrain at the upper end of the opioid peptide mediated serotinergic descending inhibitory system (see p. 64).

Therefore, as a result of these connections, A-beta afferent activity is enabled to block the C afferent input to the spinal cord by promoting activity in this descending system (Bowsher 1991). In addition, Todd & Mackenzie (1989) have shown that large diameter A-beta nerve fibres, on entering the spinal cord, give off branches which make contact with gamma-aminobutyric acid mediated interneurons (GABA-ergic interneurons) in Lamina II. These also exert an inhibitory effect on the C afferent input to the cord.

It therefore follows that high-frequency, low intensity transcutaneous nerve stimulation (TENS) which exerts its pain modulating effect by recruiting A-beta nerve fibres (Ch. 9), achieves this effect partly by these fibres, when stimulated, evoking activity in the opioid peptide mediated descending inhibitory system and partly by them evoking activity in dorsal horn GABA-ergic interneurons (Fig. 6.6).

Dorsal horn transmission cells

The neurons in the dorsal horn responsible for transmitting sensory afferent information to the brain are of three main types — low-threshold mechanoreceptor cells, nociceptive-specific cells, and wide dynamic range cells.

Low-threshold mechanoreceptor cells, found chiefly in Laminae III and IV, transmit to the brain information received via large diameter low-threshold A-beta afferents that have become activated by some innocuous stimulus such as light touch to the skin.

Nociceptive-specific cells, principally present in Lamina I but also to a lesser extent in Lamina IV and V (Christensen & Perl 1970), as their name implies, are only excited by nociceptive primary afferents. Somewhat paradoxically, a study by Mayer et al (1975) suggests that interpretation of pain is related more closely to activity in wide dynamic range cells than it is to that in nociceptive-specific ones.

Wide dynamic range cells, which are present in all laminae but are mainly concentrated in Lamina V and to a lesser extent in Lamina I, transmit to higher centres information received via A-beta, A-delta and C afferents. The message they pass on to the higher centres therefore varies according to whether the peripherally applied stimulus is innocuous or noxious. It thus follows that the sensation ultimately experienced may be one of touch, or the brief localized pricking type of so-called first pain, or the persistent widespread aching type of so-called second pain.

The wide-dynamic range cells which receive small diameter afferents from the heart and abdominal organs also receive low-threshold afferents from the skin (Cervero 1983). Melzack & Wall (1988b) suggest that this may be the reason why pain from a pathological lesion in some internal structure may appear to be coming from the surface of the body and why in such circumstances the skin is liable to be tender.

It needs to be understood that none of these transmission cells possess physiological specificity, as they are capable of changing from one to another depending on the excitability of the spinal cord. For example, animal experiments have shown that, under light barbiturate anaesthesia, nociceptive-specific cells become wide dynamic range ones (Collins & Ren 1987) and that under deeper anaesthesia the latter become nociceptive-specific (Dickhaus et al 1985).

Dorsal horn excitatory and inhibitory interneurons

As will be discussed in greater detail when considering the gate-control system, before C afferent nociceptive information received by these dorsal horn transmission cells is projected centripetally, it undergoes modification as a result of activity in excitatory and inhibitory interneurons situated in Lamina II.

ASCENDING PATHWAYS

The long-held belief that nociceptive information is transmitted centripetally via a single contralateral spinothalamic tract had to be revised in the 1950s when it was shown that the transmission is through a number of pathways each of which has its own conduction velocity and termination in the brain (Kerr et al 1955).

It is now recognized that these pathways have developed over the course of time as part of an evolutionary process (Melzack & Wall 1988c) and that their relative importance varies from one species to another (Willis 1989).

Two major ascending systems have been identified, one phylogenetically much older than

the other. The principal pathway in the newer of the two systems is the neospinothalamic pathway and the main one in the earlier developed system is the paleo-spino-reticulo-diencephalic pathway (Bowsher 1987).

The neospinothalamic pathway (Fig. 6.4)

The neospinothalamic pathway arises from the dorsal horn's Laminae I and V, where the majority of the small myelinated A-delta nociceptive fibres terminate. It ascends in the contralateral anterolateral tract to reach the ventrobasal nucleus in the lateral part of the thalamus, and from there it projects to the somatosensory cortex in the postcentral gyrus. This topographically organized lateral pathway subserves the sensory-discriminative process responsible for the localization and identification of a noxious stimulus (Melzack & Casey 1968) and for determining when such a stimulus reaches the pain threshold.

The paleo-spino-reticulo-diencephalic pathway (Fig. 6.4)

This pathway, which Melzack & Casey (1968) call the paramedian pathway, arises from the dorsal horn's Laminae VII and VIII and to a lesser extent from Lamina V. As this pathway carries information ultimately interpreted as 'second' or 'slow' pain which is conveyed to the dorsal horn by C afferent fibres, and as these terminate in neurons in Laminae I and II, it follows that electrical impulses from these neurons have to pass through several internuncial relays before reaching Laminae V, VII and VIII. From the dorsal horn, it ascends in the contralateral anterolateral tract alongside the neospinothalamic pathway until it reaches the base of the brain where it separates from this by passing medially into the brainstem's reticular tissue. From there, C afferent nociceptive information is projected to the cerebral cortex via the medially situated intralaminar nuclei of the thalamus.

Brainstem's reticular formation

The reticular formation which ramifies throughout the medulla and midbrain is so-called because

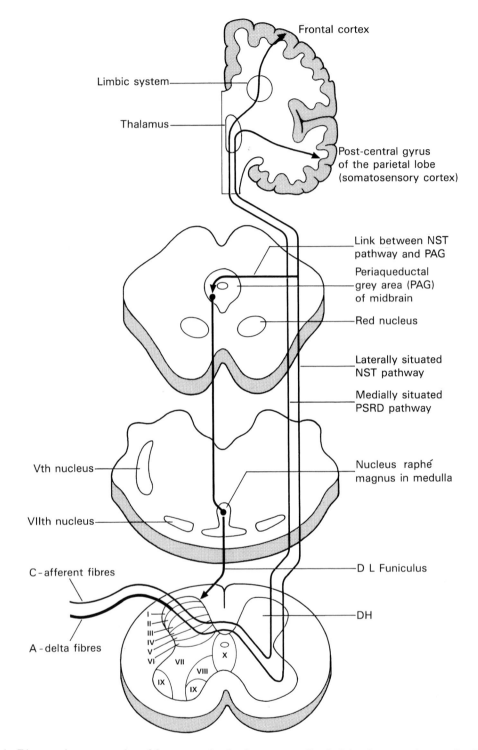

Fig. 6.4 Diagramatic representation of the course taken by the two ascending 'pain' pathways — the neospinothalamic (NST) pathway carrying A-delta 'pin prick' information, and the paleo-spino-reticulo-diencephalic pathway carrying C 'tissue damage' information. It also shows the descending inhibitory pathway — the dorsolateral funiculus (DLF) which links the periaqueductal grey area (PAG) and the nucleus raphé magnus (NRM) with the dorsal horn (DH).

its dense mass of neurons with overlapping and intertwining dendrites give it a net-like appearance.

As Casey (1980) has pointed out, it is because neurons in the reticular formation have bifurcating axons which project downwards to the spinal cord and upwards to the thalamus and hypothalamus that this structure is so extremely well adapted to playing a major integrating role in pain experience and behaviour.

Its links with the motor neurons of muscle spindles enable it to bring about alterations in muscle tone. With respect to this, it is because people who are psychologically tense have an overactive reticular system that they tend to hold certain groups of their muscles persistently taut (Nathan 1982). When this happens, pain is liable to develop in these muscles as a result of trigger points in them becoming activated (see Ch. 7). As Mense (1990) has succinctly put it, 'skeletal muscle is a tool for expressing emotional state in higher mammals and, thus, psychogenic changes of muscle tone may become a source of pain'.

The reticular formation contains several nuclei which make important contributions to the experience of pain and the behavioural activities associated with this. One of these is the nucleus reticularis gigantocellularis situated in the medulla. This nucleus, which receives a large input from the paramedian pathway and which has an upwards projection to the intralaminar part of the thalamus, contains neurons whose discharge in response to a noxious stimulus, as Casey has shown in a series of experiments on cats, sets off aversive escape behaviour (Casey 1971 a & b; Casey et al 1974). In addition, serotonin-containing cells in this nucleus and the adjacent nucleus raphe magnus, together with neurons in the periaqueductal grey area of the midbrain from which they receive an excitatory input, form the upper part of the opioid peptide mediated descending inhibitory system that is of such considerable importance in the control of pain.

Most of the fibres in the paramedian pathway terminate at the reticular formation but some continue upwards to the medially situated intralaminar nuclei of the thalamus. There are also separate ascending projections from the reticular formation that reach both these thalamic

nuclei and the hypothalamus. It is because of this link between the reticular formation and the hypothalamus that so-called second or slow C afferent tissue damage type pain has autonomic concomitants.

From the intralaminar nuclei of the thalamus there are projections to a number of structures clustered around the thalamus which collectively form the limbic system, as well as projections to other parts of the brain including, in particular, the frontal lobe.

The limbic system

The limbic system consists of a group of structures clustered around the thalamus. These include the hypothalamus; the hippocampus (Greek, *sea horse*); the amygdala (Latin, *almond*); and the cingulum bundle connecting the hippocampus with the frontal cortex.

There is evidence that the limbic structures control the motivational or behavioural responses to pain together with the emotional response to it or what may be called its affective dimension. With respect to the latter, it is the extent to which the limbic system becomes activated in response to any given noxious stimulus that determines how much any particular individual suffers from it — in other words, the degree to which it hurts that person. It is therefore activity in the limbic system which governs a person's pain tolerance.

The frontal cortex

As mentioned when discussing the nature of pain, this physico-emotional experience is considerably influenced by cognitive activities such as memories of past experiences, mood and prevailing circumstances. By virtue of the frontal cortex having a two-way communication system not only with all sensory cortical areas but also with the limbic and reticular structures, it controls both of these cognitive activities as well as the paramedian system's motivational-affective ones. (Melzack & Casey 1968).

In the past, extensive resections of the frontal lobes were performed as a last resort for intractable pain. Patients who underwent this, because the sensory component of pain subserved by the somatosensory cortex was still present, remained aware of the pain and often said it was as intense as before, but they were no longer worried about it and no longer needed medication for it. The effect of a lobotomy, therefore, was to reduce the motivational-affective and aversive dimensions of the pain experience. As Freeman & Watts (1950) remarked, 'Prefrontal lobotomy changes the attitude of the individual towards his pain, but does not alter the perception of pain.'

The discovery of a descending inhibitory system.

In 1954 Hagbarth & Kerr found that stimulation of either the reticular formation, the cerebellum, or the cerebral cortex, has a controlling influence on the flow of nociceptive impulses up the anterolateral tract, and concluded that this must be because each of these structures is capable of exerting a descending inhibitory effect on dorsal horn transmission cells. Then, in 1958, Melzack, Stotler & Livingston quite unexpectedly discovered, during the course of experiments on cats, that damage to a small area of reticular tissue, known as the central tegmental tract and situated near the midbrain's periaqueductal grey area, markedly enhances pain perception in these animals. It was presumed that this must be because tissue damage at this site interferes with a naturally occurring inhibitory system.

ADVANCES IN KNOWLEDGE DURING THE 1950s AND 1960s

There were several important advances concerning the neurophysiology of pain during the 1950s and 1960s. The Swedish anatomist, Bror Rexed (1952), established that the cells of the spinal cord are arranged in layers or laminae; Hagbarth & Kerr (1954) found evidence of a descending inhibitory system; Kerr et al (1955) established that there are a number of ascending pathways related to pain. In addition, Noordenbos (1959) furthered the theory first put forward by Head in 1920 that a rapidly conducting afferent fibre system inhibits transmission in a more slowly conducting one by establishing that the fast system is made up of large diameter myelinated fibres and

the slow one by small diameter unmyelinated ones. In referring to the interaction between these two systems, he pithily commented; 'stated in the most simple terms, this interaction could be described as fast blocks slow'.

This comment, as Wall (1990) has recently admitted, profoundly influenced Melzack's and his thinking when eventually they came to formulate their gate-control theory. Also influential was the fact that Wall (1960), by a series of ingenious recordings from single dorsal horn cells, was able to confirm Noordenbos's observations concerning this interaction, and was able to show that it is strongly influenced by descending inhibitory systems first identified by Melzack, Stotler & Livingston in 1958.

The gate-control theory

It was thus in the light of knowledge acquired by a number of different workers during the 1950s that Melzack & Wall in 1965 developed their now-famous theory that in each dorsal horn of the spinal cord there is a 'gate-like mechanism which inhibits or facilitates the flow of afferent impulses into the spinal cord'. The theory, as originally propounded, stated that the opening or closing of the 'gate' is dependent on the relative activity in the large diameter (A-beta) and small diameter fibres (A-delta and C), with activity in the large diameter fibres tending to close the 'gate', and activity in the small diameter fibres tending to open it. Also, an essential part of the theory ever since the time it was first put forward is that the position of the 'gate' is in addition influenced by the brain's descending inhibitory system.

Substantia gelatinosa

From the start, Melzack & Wall envisaged the gate as being situated in the substantia gelatinosa where, as they said, inhibitory interneurons are to be found in Lamina II. They also premised that the interaction between the large and small diameter fibres influences activity both in these interneurons and in the dorsal horn transmission cells (T cells). It was thought and subsequently confirmed that the large diameter myelinated afferents excite the inhibitory interneurons, and that the effect of this is to presynaptically reduce the input to the T cells and thereby to inhibit pain. They further postulated that activity in small diameter unmyelinated fibres, by inhibiting activity in the inhibitory interneurons, facilitates the flow of noxious impulses to the T cells and by so doing enhances pain.

By the time that Melzack & Wall introduced their theory, there was already good evidence to support their belief that it is the substantia gelatinosa (i.e. Laminae I & II) which acts as the 'gate'. Szentagothai (1964) and Wall (1964) had shown that it receives axons directly and indirectly from large and small diameter fibres, that it has connections with cells in deeper laminae and, that its cells connect with one another and are connected to similar cells at distant sites — on the ipsilateral side by means of Lissauer's tract and on the opposite side by means of fibres that cross the cord.

Although it remains reasonable to assume that it is the substantia gelatinosa which acts as the spinal gating mechanism, Melzack & Wall (1982a) have found it necessary to emphasize that there is still no absolute proof of this. They also posed the question rhetorically, 'If the substantia gelatinosa is a gate control, why is it so complex?', and answered this by saying that it would be wrong to consider that this structure is only concerned with the modulation of nociceptive impulses, but rather that it has to monitor all forms of incoming information and that it is likely to have 'to control and emphasize different aspects of the arriving messages with the emphasis changing from moment to moment'.

There can be no doubt, therefore, that the substantia gelatinosa has the properties of a complex computer and, the greater the detail in which its structure and function are studied, the more intricate the mechanisms contained in it are found to be. There is now experimental evidence to show that the cells which make up this structure, together with those in the underlying laminae, are somatotopically organized (Melzack & Wall 1982b) in the same way as cells in the dorsal column-medial lemniscus system (Millar & Basbaum 1975) and cells in midbrain structures (Soper & Melzack 1982).

It is also now known that the afferent nociceptive input into the substantia gelatinosa is influenced by several descending inhibitory systems linking cortical and brain stem structures with the dorsal horn via the dorsolateral funiculus.

It is obvious from the number of peptides found in the substantia gelatinosa in recent years that its function must be extremely complicated. It is now known that nerve terminals at this site contain at least five peptides, these being vasoactive intestinal peptide, somatostatin, angiotensin, cholecystokinin and substance P (Jessell 1982). Endogenous opioids are to be found in the dorsal horn of the spinal cord in the same areas as small diameter primary pain afferents containing substance P neurons and opiate receptors (Clement-Jones 1983). Now that it is known that morphine inhibits the release of substance P — a primary afferent nociceptor transmitter — it has been proposed that, in addition to the opioid mediated descending inhibitory system, opioid containing interneurons presynaptically control the afferent nociceptive input (Jessell & Iversen 1977). Such a hypothesis would certainly provide a neurochemical basis for the 'gate' theory of pain control.

There are thus strong arguments in support of Melzack & Wall's original idea that the substantia gelatinosa acts as a complex 'gating' mechanism which modulates input signals to the spinal cord by means of decreasing their effect on other highly specialized transmission cells (T cells), the function of which is to pass on these messages to various centres in the brain. For a more detailed account of the evidence in support of the substantia gelatinosa's role as a controlling 'gate', reference should be made to Wall's (1980a, 1980b, 1989) comprehensive reviews of the subject.

Revision of the gate-control theory

Advances in knowledge since 1965 have inevitably led to the theory being revised. For example, Melzack & Wall soon came to the conclusion that there are excitatory as well as inhibitory interneurons in the substantia gelatinosa and that inhibition not only occurs presynaptically, as originally thought, but also takes place postsynaptically.

Furthermore, when the gate-control theory was first put forward, it was considered that the flow of centripetal impulses into the dorsal horn and from it up to the brain is influenced partly by descending inhibitory mechanisms and partly by the relative activity in small diameter and large diameter afferent nerve fibres and that it is always the net result of these various facilitatory and inhibitory effects which control the activation of T cells.

When Wall, however, re-examined the theory in 1978, he pointed out that the situation was not as straightforward as might have appeared at first, and that large diameter fibre activity is, in certain circumstances, capable of firing T cells, so that the inputs from large and small fibres may at times summate with each other. He also admitted that their original ideas concerning the inhibitory effects of large diameter fibres was much influenced by Noordenbos (1959) who, having shown that in post-herpetic neuralgia there is a loss of large myelinated fibres, generalized from this observation by proposing that pain in general is due to a loss of inhibition normally provided by large fibres. As Wall (1978) then goes on to say, 'We now know that loss of large fibres is not necessarily followed by pain. In Friedreich's ataxia there is just such a preferential large-fibre defect without pain' ... (and) 'the polyneuropathy of renal failure in adults is not associated with complaints of pain although there is preferential destruction of large fibres.' He then cites many other examples to show that 'any attempt to correlate the remaining fibre diameter spectrum with the symptomatology of neuropathies is no longer possible'.

This notwithstanding, it would seem that when the central nervous system is intact and unaffected by disease, the balance between the large and small diameter fibres in determining the output of T cells remains an acceptable hypothesis. The theory has also been subjected to criticism by others for neglecting the known facts about stimulus specificity of nerve fibres which have emerged since Von Frey first developed his theory about this in the closing years of the last century (Nathan 1976).

For all these various reasons and others including advances in knowledge concerning the rela-

tive functions of A-delta and C nerve fibres (to be discussed later), Melzack & Wall have had to subject their theory to certain modifications (Wall 1978, Melzack & Wall 1982c, 1988d). Nevertheless, it remains remarkably useful and has been considerably enriched by subsequent biochemical discoveries. Much, however, remains to be explained. For example, the descending control system has turned out to be not one system but a number of systems involving a complexity of chemical substances yet to be unravelled. And when enkephalin-containing terminals and opiate receptor-bearing axons were discovered, it was assumed that they must make contact but, surprisingly, this apparently is not so (Hunt et al 1980).

Despite all this, 20 years after Melzack & Wall first put forward their gate-control theory, Verrill (1990) reviewed its influence on current ideas concerning pain modulation and was led to conclude that:

despite continuing controversy over details, the fundamental concept underlying the gate theory has survived in a modified and stronger state accommodating and harmonizing with rather than supplanting specificity and pattern theories. It has stimulated multidisciplinary activity, opened minds and benefited patients.

The relevance of the gate-control system to the 1st and 2nd phases of nociceptive pain

As stated earlier, when some deep-seated structure such as muscle is damaged, the resultant inflammatory reaction leads to the release of chemical substances which sensitize A-delta and C afferents. The outcome of this is that two types of pain develop one after the other. Initially there is a sharp, well-defined sensation — the first pain — brought on as a result of activity in the A-delta afferent nerve fibres. The pain during this first phase is only of brief duration and is followed by a less well-defined and more prolonged second pain which develops as a result of activity in C afferent nerve fibres. Melzack & Wall (1988d) have now pointed out that the gate-control pain modulating mechanisms only operate during the 1st phase and that the prolongation of the pain during the 2nd phase is due to C afferent fibres, where they terminate intraspinally, liberating a variety of peptides including substance P, cholecystokinin, neurokinins, vasoactive intestinal peptide and others, giving rise to immediate neuronal excitation in the dorsal horn followed by a slow-onset, prolonged facilitation.

It should be noted with respect to this that the peptide content of C fibres is not the same in every type of tissue. The peptide make-up of C fibres in muscle, for example, is very different from that of C fibres in the skin. That is why C afferents from damaged muscle produce prolonged facilitation where those from skin do not.

ADVANCE IN KNOWLEDGE DURING THE 1970s AND 1980s.

Opiate receptors

During the 1970s, biochemists and pharmacologists were becoming increasingly convinced that the reason why morphine is such a powerful analgesic is because there must be highly specialized chemical receptors in the central nervous system to which this substance can readily attach itself. In 1973, Solomon Snyder of the Johns Hopkins School of Medicine, Baltimore, and Candice Pert of the U.S. National Institute of Mental Health discovered during the course of basic research on drug addiction that there are clusters of cells in certain parts of the brain, including the brain stem nuclei, the thalamus and hypothalamus, which serve as opiate receptors (Pert & Snyder 1973). A number of cells in the dorsal horn were then also found to have the same function (Atweh & Kuhar 1977). The finding of opiate receptors in the midbrain perhaps was not so surprising as it had already been shown that an injection of only a small amount of morphine into the area has a considerable analgesic effect. However, of particular interest was the discovery that there are also cells with the same function in the substantia gelatinosa of the dorsal horn and that a local injection of a small amount of morphine into this structure (laminae I and II) has a markedly inhibitory effect on the response of lamina V transmission cells to afferent nociceptive stimuli (Duggan et al 1976); this lent considerable

support to the idea that the substantia gelatinosa has an important pain-modulating function. It is now known that there are at least three distinct types of opioid receptors termed mu, kappa and delta (Paterson et al 1983).

The distribution of opiate receptors in the CNS is of considerable interest. There are numerous ones in the paramedian system's intralaminar (medial) thalamic nuclei, reticular formation and limbic structures. In contrast, however, there are only a few in the neospinothalamic system's ventrobasal thalamus and post-central gyrus. This explains why a microinjection of morphine into structures in the paramedian system has a powerful analgesic effect but not when injected into the ventrobasal thalamus. It also explains why morphine suppresses so-called second or 'slow' tissue damage type of pain but not the so-called first or 'rapid' type of pain produced, for example, by a pinprick.

In the dorsal horn there are large numbers of opiate receptors situated postsynaptically on neuronal membranes. There are also some situated presynaptically on the intraspinal part of C afferent nerve fibres, but at present the biological significance of these remains unknown (Fields & Basbaum 1989).

It is beause of a particularly high concentration of opiate receptors in the substantia gelatinosa that a micro-injection of morphine into this structure has a marked pain-suppressing effect. It is also why lumbar intrathecal injections of opiates produce profound analgesia in animals (Yaksh & Rudy 1976) and man (Wang et al 1979).

In addition, there is a high concentration of opiate receptors in the corpus striatum, where their function is unknown. They are also extremely numerous in the brain stem's respiratory centre, thus explaining why morphine is such a powerful respiratory depressant.

Opioid peptides

Once these opiate receptors had been located, it was argued that nature was hardly likely to have provided animals, including man, with them for the sole purpose of having somewhere for opium and its derivatives to latch on to should they happen to be introduced into the body. It was far more likely that they are there because morphine-like substances (opioid substances) are produced endogenously.

A search for physiologically occurring morphine-like substances was therefore instituted. Many scientists took part in this, including Snyder and his colleagues at Baltimore; Terenius & Wahlstrom in Uppsala; and Hughes et al in Aberdeen.

The big breakthrough occurred in 1975 when Hughes et al in the Unit for Research on Addictive Drugs at Aberdeen University in collaboration with a research team at Reckitt & Colman isolated a substance from the brains of pigs which appeared to act like morphine and which latched on to opiate receptors in the brain. They named it enkephalin ('in the head'). It was a major discovery, and Lewin (1976) showed considerable prescience by commenting in the *New Scientist*:

With the structure of enkephalin now at hand ... we are now poised for an exciting breakthrough in the complete understanding of opiate analgesia, addiction and tolerance. Probably the most intriguing aspect of all this is the inescapable implication of the existence of an unexpected chemical transmitter system in the brain, a system which may have something to do with dampening pain, but almost certainly has more general effects also.

Enkephalin having been isolated, Linda Fothergil at Aberdeen and Barry Morgan at Reckitt & Colman attempted to analyse its structure and soon established that it was a peptide, but came up against certain technical difficulties in establishing the exact sequence of its amino acids. Therefore they enlisted the help of a spectroscopist, Howard Morris at the Imperial College, London. Morris was able to show that in fact there are two enkephalin polypeptides — leucine (leu) and methionine (met) enkephalin — but for a time the chemical source from which

these substances are made in the body remained a mystery.

By a strange chance, about the time that Morris was considering this, he attended a lecture at Imperial College given by Derek Smythe of the National Institute for Medical Research on beta-lipotrophin, a 91 amino acid peptide which, had been isolated from the pituitary glands of sheep 10 years previously (Li et al 1965). Smythe showed a series of slides illustrating its chemical structure and as Morris sat there looking at these, he suddenly saw to his amazement the amino acid sequence of met enkephalin hidden away in the 61–65 position of the betalipotrophin structure. It subsequently became apparent however that met and leu enkephalin are derived by enzyme cleavage not from this substance but from the precursor proenkephalin A. Since the discovery of the enkephalins, opioid bioactivity has been found in various beta-lipotrophin fragments with the most potent of these being one in the 61–91 position known as beta-endorphin (Fig. 6.5).

It is now known that beta-endorphin, together with beta-lipotrophin and ACTH (corticotrophin) are all derived by enzyme cleavage from a large precursor pro-opiomelancortin but that of these three polypeptides only beta-endorphin has known analgesic activity, and also that ACTH acts as a physiological antagonist of this (Smock & Fields 1980).

Recently two other opioid peptides with N-terminals identical to that of leuenkephalin have been isolated. These are dynorphin, a 17 amino acid peptide (Goldstein et al 1979), and the decapeptide alpha-neoendorphin (Weber et al 1981), both of which are cleaved from yet another precursor pro-enkephalin B (prodynorphin).

These various substances are sometimes referred to collectively as the endorphins (endo-

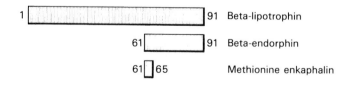

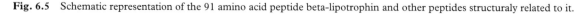

Fig. 6.5   Schematic representation of the 91 amino acid peptide beta-lipotrophin and other peptides structuraly related to it.

genous morphine-like substances) but as may be seen there are three distinct families of these peptides — the enkephalins, the dynorphins, and the endorphins — and therefore it is better simply to call them opioid peptides (Thompson 1984b).

Distribution of endogenous opioid peptides

Studies using radioimmunoassays and immuno-histochemical techniques have demonstrated high levels of enkaphalins and dynorphins in the limbic structures, the periaqueductal grey, the nucleus raphe magnus and the substantia gelatinosa of the dorsal horn. From these sites, opioid peptides spill over into the cerebrospinal fluid. In addition, opioid peptides are released from the anterior pituitary and adrenal medulla into the plasma.

By means of radioimmunoassays and gel filtration techniques, it has been possible to demonstrate the presence of beta-endorphin and metenkephalin in human plasma (Clement-Jones 1983). Beta-endorphin is found there in asso-ciation with beta-lipotrophin and ACTH with all three showing the same pattern of circadian secretion from the anterior pituitary (Shanks et al 1981). Plasma metenkephalin levels, however, show no relationship to those of the other peptides just mentioned during circadian studies and corticosteroid suppression tests. It is not derived from the pituitary, as levels are detectable in subjects with pan-hypopituitarism (Clement-Jones & Besser 1983) but released from the adrenal gland into the circulation (Clement-Jones et al 1980). It is also derived from the gut, sympathetic ganglia and peripheral autonomic neurons (Smith et al 1981).

When opioid peptides were first discovered, it was assumed that any structure containing them must have a pain-modulating function. It is clear however that this is not so because there is, for example, a very high concentration of them in the basal ganglia where their function has yet to be explained (Bowsher 1987). They are also present in vagal nuclei in the medulla where they presumably contribute to various reflexes such as those associated with the control of coughing.

DESCENDING SYSTEMS

During the 1970s, exciting discoveries were made concerning the biochemistry of the descending inhibitory system, although it was observations made in the 1950s, firstly by Hagbarth & Kerr (1954) and then by Melzack et al (1958) — with their unexpected discovery in experiments on cats that damage to the central tegmental tract in the midbrain markedly enhances pain in these animals — which set the stage for these discoveries.

It was because of their observations that David Reynolds, a young psychologist at the University of Windsor, Ontario, decided to investigate whether, by electrically stimulating this central tegmental-lateral periaqueductal grey area, it might be possible to increase the effects of any inhibitory system that might be present there to such an extent as to bring about pain sup-pression. In 1969 he was able to report that such stimulation did in fact produce such a profound degree of analgesia that it was possible to carry out surgical operations on conscious rats without any other from of anaesthesia, and later he reported being able to control pain by this method during operations on higher species of animals.

Unfortunately, although Reynolds' observ-ations were of the utmost importance, regrettably they were viewed with considerable scepticism and largely ignored. It was not until Mayer, Liebeskind and their colleagues (Mayer et al 1971), with no knowledge of Reynolds' contri-butions to the subject, independently carried out similar experiments on rats, that any notice was taken of the remarkable phenomenon, now generally referred to as stimulation-produced analgesia.

Stimulation-produced analgesia

It has been found possible to produce analgesia by electrically stimulating one or other of several sites, but the most consistently effective manner of doing this is to place electrodes either on the periaqueductal grey area in the midbrain or on the nucleus raphé magnus in the medulla (Liebskind & Paul 1977).

Although stimulation-produced analgesia was first demonstrated in experimental animals, it was quickly shown to have considerable therapeutic value in relieving humans of persistent severe pain. In fact, man has been shown to obtain more lasting analgesia using this method than do many types of animals (Adams 1976, Hosobuchi et al 1977).

Electrical stimulation of the brain stem for the purpose of suppressing pain had not been in use for long before it was discovered that its analgesic effect could be abolished by the morphine-antagonist naloxone (Akil et al 1976) and that the injection of a small amount of morphine directly into the periaqueductal grey area produces analgesia (Herz et al 1970, Mayer & Price 1976, Mayer & Watkins 1981). It was therefore concluded that the morphine must act by activating neurons in the descending inhibitory system situated in the brain stem, and it raised the possibility that stimulation-produced analgesia might also occur as a result of the release of endogenous opioids. Melzack & Melinkoff's observation (1974), that the analgesic effect of electrically stimulating the brain stem is enhanced by carrying this out for several minutes before a painful stimulus is administered, provided support for this idea.

Dorsolateral funiculus

The supposition that this descending inhibitory system exerts its effect on neurons in the dorsal horn was confirmed when it was shown that neither opiate-induced nor stimulation-produced analgesia occurs when the dorsolateral funiculus which serves as the link between the nucleus raphe magnus and these neurons is cut (Basbaum et al 1977).

It is now known that 5-hydroxytryptamine (5HT; serotonin) is the main transmitting agent in this pathway (Basbaum & Fields 1978), and that para-chlorophenylalanine, a serotonin inhibitor, suppresses analgesia brought about either by electrical stimulation of the periaqueductal grey area or the nucleus raphé magnus, or by the microinjection of morphine into either of these structures (Anderson & Proudfit 1981). It should

incidentally also be noted that the pain-suppressing effect of certain tricyclic antidepressants is probably also because of their ability to enhance transmission down this descending pathway by blocking the re-uptake of 5HT (Thompson 1984a).

It will be remembered from what was said earlier that Melzack & Wall (1965) in their original gate-control theory of pain put forward the supposition that the 'gate' in the dorsal horn has, as one of its main controls, a descending inhibitory system. This hypothesis received strong support once the phenomenon of stimulation-produced analgesia was discovered.

Opioid peptide mediated descending inhibitory system

It is now realized that there are several descending inhibitory systems but the one about which most is known is the one mediated by opioid peptides. In this system, the midbrain's periaqueductal grey, which has inputs from the thalamus, the hypothalamus, the amygdala and the frontal cortex, projects to the medullary-situated nucleus raphé magnus and nucleus reticularis gigantocellularis. Serotinergic axons from these latter structures descend in the dorsolateral funiculus to end in synaptic contact with enkephalinergic interneurons situated on the border of Lamina I and Lamina II of the dorsal horn. These interneurons, when activated in this manner, exert an inhibitory effect on the dorsal horn tranmission cells responsible for projecting centripetally, via the paramedian pathway, nociceptive information received from C-polymodal afferents (Fig. 6.6).

Clinically, this descending inhibitory system may be brought into action as a result of activity in the frontal cortex. Mainly, however, this happens either as a result of A-delta nerve stimulation setting up activity in the neo-spinothalamic ascending pathway, which at the midbrain level gives off a collateral to the periaqueductal grey area, or as a result of A-beta nerve stimulation setting up activity in the dorsal column-medial leminisus ascending pathway which also projects to the periaqueductal grey area. (see Fig. 6.6).

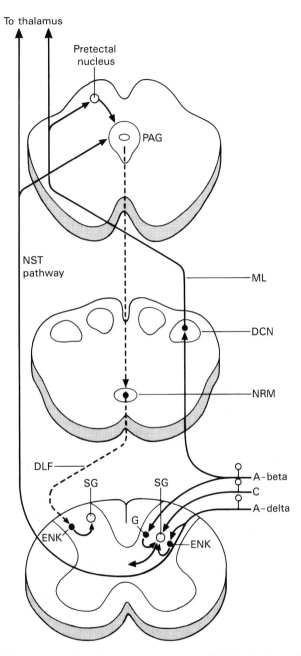

Fig. 6.6 Tissue damage nociceptive information reaches the substantia gelatinosa (SG) vis C afferent fibres. The onward transmission of this information is inhibited by enkephalinergic interneurons (ENK) which are activated via A-delta 'pin prick' fibres as they enter the cord and via serotinergic inhibitory fibres that descend in the dorsolateral funiculus (DLF) from the nucleus raphé magnus (NRM) in the medulla and periaqueductal grey area (PAG) in the midbrain (the descending inhibitory system). The descending inhibitory system is brought into action either via collaterals which link the neospinothalamic 'A-delta pin prick' ascending pathway (NST) with the PAG: or via collaterals which form a link between the PAG and the medial leminiscus (ML), which arises from dorsal column nuclei (DCN) connected to A-beta fibres in the dorsal column. The onward transmission of tissue damage nociceptive information in C afferent fibres is also inhibited by inhibitory GABA-ergic interneurons (G) which are activated by the A-beta fibres that enter the substantia gelatinosa.

(Based on Dr David Bowsher's diagram in the Journal of the British Medical Acupuncture Society (1991). Reproduced with permission).

Opioid peptide mediated analgesia system (OMAS)

The enkephalinergic inhibitory interneurons situated on the border of Laminae I and II of the dorsal horn not only block C afferent transmission as a result of A-delta afferent activity causing the descending inhibitory system to come into action in the manner just described. These interneurons also do this because A-delta nerve fibres make direct intraspinal contact with them in the dorsal horn (Fig. 6.6). In addition, enkephalinergic interneurons present on the terminals of C afferent fibres exert a presynaptic inhibitory effect (Bowsher 1990). It therefore follows that the acupuncture technique of stimulating A-delta nerve fibres with dry needles relieves C-afferent-transmitted tissue damage-type pain as a result of this kind of stimulus evoking activity in opioid peptide mediated pain modulating mechanisms situated at both supraspinal and spinal levels.

These two endogenous pain control mechanisms collectively constitute what Fields and Basbaum (1989) refer to as the opioid mediated analgesia system (OMAS).

The physiological activation of the opioid mediated analgesia system (OMAS)

When opiate receptors and their opioid peptides were found to be present in the central nervous system it was assumed, because the administration of naturally occurring opium and its derivatives has for long been known to have an analgesic effect, that the body's own opioid peptides must be capable of modulating pain. Support for this idea came from finding that a microinjection of morphine either into certain midline nuclei in the brain stem or into the substantia gelatinosa produces analgesia (Herz et al 1970), and from the fact that the administration of high doses of beta-endorphin into the cerebrospinal fluid (Oyama et al 1980) and the intravenous injection of an enkephalin analogue (Calimlim et al 1982) has an analgesic effect.

Although it is now accepted that opioid peptides exert their analgesic effect both at supraspinal and spinal levels the question that

has to be addressed is under what circumstances this OMAS is activated.

It was thought that, because naloxone is an opiate receptor antagonist with a particular affinity for μ receptors, that observations on the effects of this substance on pain produced by various means might throw some light on the matter. Unfortunately, the results of experiments designed to study the effects of naloxone on pain in man have proved to be bewilderingly conflicting. As Woolf & Wall (1983) point out, 'each positive result is matched by negative ones', and they go on to say:

the hodge-podge of conflicting results cannot be explained by the use of inadequate doses since many of the negative studies used higher doses than the positive ones. It is obvious that there must be an uncontrolled naloxone-reversible variable unrelated to pain in these studies, which may well be the degree of the subjects' stress.

Now this would seem to be the nub of the matter — that both noxious inputs and stress activate the OMAS. Whilst there is no doubt that a noxious input brought about by stimulating A-delta afferent nerve fibres, with, for example, acupuncture needles, may activate the system, so also may this be achieved either by environmental or surgical stress (Gracely et al 1983).

Many experiments have been conducted by Lewis et al (1980, 1981, 1982) on stress-produced analgesia in rats. The rats were stressed by having electric currents applied to their feet. Lewis and his colleagues found that what determines whether or not the analgesia produced by this type of shock is naloxone reversible, and therefore opioid peptide mediated or not, depends on its duration. Thus the analgesia produced by foot shock applied for 30 minutes is naloxone reversible, whereas that produced by foot shock applied for 3 minutes is not.

It is important to note that it was only when stress, such as that produced in these experiments on rats with an electric shock, is applied for a relatively long period that the OMAS is activated, because Levine et al (1979) have similarly shown, with respect to noxious stimuli, that this analgesia producing system also only operates when such a stimulus is of long duration. They demonstrated this by showing that naloxone has little or no effect on relatively brief, experimentally produced pain but markedly increases the intensity of any protracted pain such as that which may be experienced following a dental operation.

In summary, therefore, it has now been established that the OMAS is physiologically activated either by a prolonged, intense, noxious stimulus or some form of prolonged stress. A briefly applied noxious or stressful stimulus is also capable of producing analgesia. However, the question that has been asked is whether they do so by activating some less well-understood, non-opioid mediated system, because as will be discussed in Chapter 10, the possibility that different analgesia-producing systems are activated according to whether the noxious stimulus is strong or weak is of considerable relevance when it comes to considering whether or not the pain suppressing mechanisms involved with either prolonged or brief stimulation with acupuncture needles are different.

Finally, it has to be said that the exact manner in which endogenous opioid peptides achieve their analgesic effect is not known. It is particularly confusing that electrical stimulation, which presumably has an excitatory action, and an opiate microinjection, which presumably has an inhibitory action, both produce analgesia when applied to certain midline brain stem nuclei. Fields & Basbaum (1989) suggest that this is because 'the opioid peptides may act by inhibiting inhibitory interneurons, thus disinhibiting the output neurons in these analgesia-producing regions'.

Non-opioid peptide mediated descending systems

For many years now the morphine antagonist naloxone has been used to investigate brain stem stimulation-analgesia, the action of opiates introduced into the central nervous system and the role of endogenous opioid peptides in suppressing pain.

As long ago as 1965, Lasagna showed that naloxone seemed to increase pain when administered to experimental subjects already experiencing some level of clinical pain. A more recent double-blind clinical study of postoperative dental pain (Levine et al 1978) has demonstrated that compared with a placebo, naloxone considerably increased the intensity of pain.

However, it was not long before contradictory reports started to appear, with Lindblom & Tegner (1979) even questioning whether the endogenous opioids are active in suppressing chronic pain as the administration of naloxone in their patients did not make the pain worse. Also, Dennis et al (1980) found that the adminstration of naloxone does not impair the analgesia produced by midbrain stimulation in rats suffering pain produced by injecting formalin subcutaneously.

Furthermore, as will be discussed again in Chapter 10, despite the fact that there have been many reports of acupuncture-induced analgesia being suppressed by naloxone, Chapman et al (1980) was unable to confirm this in a trial designed to study the effects of acupuncture on experimentally induced dental pain.

It is now accepted that one of the reasons for these conflicting reports must be that there are several descending control systems and that, whereas one of these is opioid peptide mediated, others must be mediated by various other transmitters. Most of these have yet to be discovered and their transmitters identified. However, it is now known that one such system has its origin in the dorsolateral pons where noradrenalin-containing cells project into the spinal cord (Melzack & Wall 1988e).

Another reason put forward for the contradictory evidence concerning these various descending inhibitory pain-modulating mechanisms is the likelihood that in some of the experiments more than one of these systems is active at any given time (Watkins & Mayer 1982).

THE DISTINCTION BETWEEN NOCIGENIC AND NEUROGENIC PAIN

Because the tissue-damage type of pain described earlier in this chapter occurs as a result of trauma-induced chemical sensitization of C-polymodal nociceptors, it may be described as nocigenic in order to distinguish it from the neurogenic or neuropathic type of pain which develops as a result of structural damage to the peripheral or central nervous system.

Neurogenic pain is very much less responsive than nocigenic pain to the acupuncture technique of evoking activity in endogenous opioid peptide mediated pain modulating mechanisms by means of stimulating A-delta nerve fibres with dry needles, which is hardly surprising considering that this type of pain is extremely resistant to the effects of opioid drugs (Portenoy et al 1990).

Therefore, before considering the use of acupuncture (or for that matter any other form of therapy) for the alleviation of chronic pain, it is essential to establish whether it is nocigenic or neurogenic in type.

With certain types of pain, such as, for example, post-herpetic neuralgia, trigeminal neuralgia and central pain from spinal cord or brain stem damage, there is usually no difficulty in recognizing its neurogenic origin. However, when pain develops during the course of some neurological disorder such as a stroke, multiple sclerosis, or subacute combined degeneration, whilst it may be neurogenic, it should not automatically be assumed to be so, for not infrequently myofascial trigger point nocigenic pain develops in such disorders as the result of strain imposed upon weakened muscles. Similarly, with post-herpetic neuralgia, it has to be remembered that this neurogenic type of pain is difficult to alleviate and may cause a patient to tense muscles in the vicinity of the affected area; this may lead to the development of acupuncture-responsive nocigenic trigger point pain.

Cancer is another commonly occurring disorder where pain may be either nocigenic or neurogenic and it is necessary to take this into consideration when deciding how best to alleviate it (Banning et al 1991), including whether or not to attempt to do this with acupuncture (Filshie 1990).

Because it is so essential to distinguish between these two types of pain in the assessment and management of persistent neck and low-back pain, this subject will be discussed again at some length in Chapters 14 and 17 respectively.

In order to differentiate between nocigenic and neurogenic pain it is essential to pay close attention to the patient's description of the pain and to carry out a carefully conducted clinical examination.

Nocigenic pain of myofascial origin takes the form of a widespread, dull, aching sensation with tenderness of the tissues in the affected area. Systematic examination reveals the presence of well-demarcated, exquisitely-tender trigger points some distance from this.

In contrast to this, neurogenic pain occurring as a result of peripheral nerve injury or dysfunction is commonly described as being of a burning nature and is often associated with shooting electrical sensations which, though not necessarily painful, are extremely distressing (dysaesthesia). In addition, there is characteristically a latent interval between the time that the neural damage occurs and the onset of the pain. The intensity of the pain usually increases gradually to reach its maximum some weeks or months after onset. During this time, the skin becomes markedly hypersensitive so that it only requires a slight breeze or the rubbing of clothes to being on an episode of pain (allodynia).

With neurogenic pain occurring as a result of nerve injury or dysfunction, there is inevitably some activation of nociceptors but the reason why this type of pain differs from that which is entirely nocigenic must be that the structural damage, as pointed out by Fields (1987d), causes 'disruption of the sensory apparatus so that a normal pattern of neural activity is no longer transmitted to the perceptual centers'. Melzack & Wall (1988f), with reference to this, state:

the presence of peripheral nerve damage is signalled rapidly by nerve impulses and slowly by chemical transport. The long-term end result is that central cells whose input has been cut in the periphery increase their excitability and expand their receptive fields... The duty of sensory cells is to receive information. When cut off from the source of their information, the cells react by increasing their excitability to such an extent that they begin to fire both spontaneously and to distant inappropriate inputs.

From experiments with the C nerve inactivator capsaicin, it has been shown that it is due to damage to C fibres that the prolonged central effects develop (Melzack & Wall 1988g). It is this central cell hyperexcitability which is responsible for various sensory abnormalities detectable on clinical examination.

When the skin over an area of the body affected by neurogenic pain and over a non-painful area (preferably the contralateral mirror-image region) are in turn gently brushed with strands of cotton wool the sensation produced over the affected area is abnormally intense (hyperaesthesia). It may also be unpleasant (dysaesthesia) or even painful (alloydynia). The noxious sensation produced by sticking a pin into the skin overlying an area affected by this type of pain is also far more intense than when such a stimulus is applied to skin in a non-painful area (hyperalgesia).

In addition, with neurogenic pain the phenomena of summation, spatial spread, and after discharge are often present. When the skin over an area affected by neurogenic pain is repeatedly pricked with a pin for 30 seconds or more the perceived intensity grows with successive stimuli (summation); this unpleasant sensation may also spread beyond the area stimulated (spatial spread); also, it may persist after the stimulation has been discontinued (after discharge).

Reflex sympathetic dystrophy syndrome

Nerve injury is occasionally associated with the development of a particularly intense burning type of pain known as causalgia. Causalgia is associated with efferent hyperactivity in the sympathetic nervous system and is one of the manifestations of what is now called the reflex sympathetic dystrophy syndrome (RSD syndrome) (De Takats 1937). Nerve injury is only one of the causes of this; others include myocardial infarction, cerebrovascular accidents, surgical trauma and, as Livingston pointed out in his classical monograph on the subject published in 1943, also fractures and such relatively minor soft tissue injuries as lacerations and sprains.

One of the most distressing features of the RSD syndrome is marked allodynia. It is thought that this may partly be brought about by sympathetic efferent activation of low-threshold mechanoreceptors. Other features include hyperaesthesia, hyperalgesia, dysaesthesia, and hyperpathia, as well as a non-pitting oedema of the soft tissues, and a smooth, cyanosed, sweaty, extremely cold skin showing evidence of pilomotor hyperactivity (goose flesh).

Relief from the pain may be obtained by repeated injections of a local anaesthetic into a nearby sympathetic ganglion, or by repeated peripheral sympathetic blockade produced by intravenous injections of guanethidine into an affected limb after its arterial blood supply has been cut off by the application of a tourniquet (Hannington-Kiff 1989).

As a myofascial trigger point pain syndrome may also have sympathetic concomitants such as coldness of an extremity, hyperhidrosis and pilomotor hyperactivity, it is clearly important to distinguish between this and the RSD syndrome, particularly as both of them can be brought on by the same type of relatively minor soft tissue trauma, and their treatment is entirely different. At the same time, it has to be remembered that both syndromes may occur together and that in every case of the RSD syndrome it is important to carry out a systemic search for myofascial trigger points. This has clearly been demonstrated by Filner (1989) who, in a series of 36 patients referred to him over a 16-month period with the typical thermographic appearance of the RSD syndrome, found that there was not only evidence of sympathetic overactivity but also of myofascial trigger point hyperactivity. In order to give the patients long-lasting relief from their pain, it was necessary not only to carry out a sympathetic blockade but also to deactivate the trigger points.

REFERRAL OF PAIN

As previously discussed, it was during the 1930s that John Kellgren was able to demonstrate that pain emanating from what would now be called a myofascial trigger point is referred to a site some distance from it. Not only, as might be expected, is the trigger point exquisitely tender, but there is also, surprisingly, some tenderness of the healthy tissues in the area of the body where the pain is felt. Since then many suggestions have been put forward to explain this referral of the pain and the tenderness at the site affected by it. These include two hypotheses — convergence-facilitation and convergence-projection — and the possible effects of two observed phenomena, namely the peripheral branching of nociceptive afferents and sympathetic overactivity. Each of these will now be discussed.

Convergence-facilitation

The convergence-facilitation hypothesis (Ruch 1965) embraces the idea that whilst the somatic afferent spinal input from nociceptors in the skin is not normally sufficient to activate dorsal horn transmission cells, it does so when it is facilitated by sensory impulses arising from some more deeply situated structure.

It is not only with myofascial trigger point pain that there is pain of a referred type and tenderness of the tissues in the zone of pain referral. It will be recalled that a similar phenomenon occurs with ischaemic heart disease. During an episode of angina, not only is pain referred down the left arm but the area affected becomes tender despite the fact that the tissues at that site are healthy. Melzack & Wall (1988h), in discussing this, state:

the tenderness of the arm suggests that nerve impulses from the heart and from the region where the pain is referred must converge and summate and thereby increase the pain.

This convergence-facilitation theory may well explain how referred pain may become augmented and why, because of this, the tissues at the affected site become tender, but it does not seem to explain as satisfactorily as the convergence-projection theory why the pain in the first place should be felt some distance from its primary source.

Convergence-projection

The convergence-projection theory (Ruch 1965) takes into account the fact that when nociceptive sensory afferent fibres innervating a visceral organ and those innervating somatic structures enter the spine at the same segmental level, they converge on the same dorsal horn transmission cells. The consequence of this is that the brain, having no way of telling from which of these two sites a noxious stimulus has arisen, and because the transmission cells are more frequently activated by somatic stimuli than they are by visceral ones, tends to mislocate pain of visceral origin and to project it erroneously to somatic structures.

It may readily be seen how this mechanism works in the case of pain of cardiac origin, for part of the afferent input from the heart, together with the sensory input from somatic structures on the left side of the chest and ulnar aspect of the left arm, is to the dorsal horn at the level of the first thoracic segment. It would seem to be that for this reason the brain mislocates myocardial ischaemic pain and projects it to the praecordium and inner side of the left arm.

A similar mechanism may well operate with respect to myofascial trigger point pain.

Peripheral branching of nociceptive sensory afferents

Another possible way in which the brain may mislocate pain is as a result of the peripheral branching of nociceptive sensory afferents. Recent animal studies have shown that, because of this, a small number of dorsal root ganglion cells have two branches supplying structures as far apart as the shoulder and diaphragm (Laurberg & Sorensen 1985) and the arm and pericardium (Alles & Dom 1985).

At present, there is no information as to whether similar branched afferents are present elsewhere in the body and therefore whether this anatomical variant contributes to the referral of pain in general.

Sympathetic hyperactivity

The area affected by pain from an activated myofascial trigger point sometimes has a decreased skin temperature occurring as a result of induced sympathetic hyperactivity (Travell & Simons 1983). As the latter, by its ability to bring about the release of sensory afferent sensitizing substances, is capable of causing pain to develop in a zone of pain referral, this may be yet another mechanism responsible for myofascial trigger point pain referral.

Convergence at the supraspinal level

As Fields (1987e) has pointed out, the fact that nociceptive afferents converge both peripherally and at the spinal level makes it not unreasonable to suggest that they may also converge in the higher centres of the brain, particularly as it is a major function of the cerebral cortex to formulate and project images.

Despite the various hypotheses and anatomical observations just described, there is still much work to be done before there can be any certainty as to exactly how pain referral from myofascial trigger points, or for that matter from any other source, takes place. After discussing this matter at some length, Simons (1990) concludes by saying:

We see that there is much evidence for many mechanisms that refer pain, tenderness and autonomic phenomena . . . the fact that at this time we are unable to identify which mechanism(s) contribute to the clinical pain phenomena with which we are concerned does not mean that their recognition is unimportant. It does suggest that this is one of the important gaps in our knowledge that must be filled before we can hope to truly understand muscle pain syndromes.

THE EMOTIONAL ASPECTS OF PAIN

Finally, it is necessary to examine the emotional aspects of pain and to discuss what influence these may have on the assessment and treatment of chronic pain. Pain is a complex physico-emotional experience with its emotional component largely determining how much suffering it causes. It is, therefore, not surprising that in describing pain, no matter whether it is nocigenic, neurogenic (neurophathic) or psychogenic, patients are liable to include not only adjectives like aching, tingling or burning to describe its sensory qualities, but also adjectives like depressing, horrible or excruciating to convey the suffering caused by it.

Melzack & Torgerson (1971), in recognizing that there are three main categories of pain experience — sensory, affective and evaluative — drew up the McGill Pain Questionnaire and this, together with a more recently introduced shortened version (Melzack 1987) has been shown to be of considerable value in the assessment of pain. It is, however, because all types of pain experience have an emotional component that it must never be assumed that pain is due to some primary psychological disturbance simply because a patient uses a predominance of affective terms to describe it.

Pain may very occasionally be a hallucinatory sensation experienced by schizophrenics. It may also be a manifestation of conversion hysteria or hypochondriasis. It therefore has to be admitted that there is such an entity as psychogenic pain (Feinmann 1990) but there are good grounds for believing that this is relatively rare and that affective disorders such as anxiety or depression are mostly the result of chronic pain rather than the cause of it.

The relationship of emotional factors to chronic pain can be assessed by giving patients with it specially designed standardized questionnaires such as the Minnesota Multiphasic Personality Inventory (MMPI). Sternbach et al (1973) used this inventory to compare the relative significance of psychological symptoms occurring in patients with acute (i.e. less than 6 months' duration) and chronic low-back pain. They found that although those with the shorter history of pain had elevated scores on the scales for depression, anxiety, hysteria and hypochondriasis, the scores were significantly higher in those with chronic pain. The MMPI was also used by Sternbach & Timmermans (1975) in their study of 113 patients with low-back pain of at least 6 months' duration. An assessment was made before and after either surgery followed by rehabilitation or rehabilitation only. From this assessment it was found that there was a significant decrease in the hysteria, depression, anxiety and hypochondriasis scales following successful alleviation of the pain.

Observations such as these confirm that chronic pain is usually the cause rather than the result of neurotic symptoms and Melzack & Wall (1988i) in discussing this conclude:

It is evident from studies such as these that it is unreasonable to ascribe chronic pain to neurotic symptoms. The patients with the thick hospital charts are all too often prey to the physicians' innuendos that they are neurotic and that their neuroses are the cause of the pain. Whilst psychological processes contribute to pain, they are only part of the activity in a complex nervous system. All too often, the diagnosis of neurosis as the cause of pain hides our ignorance of many aspects of pain mechanisms.

The error of failing to recognize pain as being organic in origin and considering it to be entirely psychological most commonly occurs in my experience when myofascial trigger point activity causes pain to persist long after all clinical evidence of tissue damage has disappeared in the post-traumatic persistent myofascial trigger point pain syndrome (Ch. 7). This error, of course, is particularly likely to be made when the pain has led to the development of appreciable anxiety or depression or both. The reason why this mistake is so frequently made is clearly because doctors in general, when investigating pain, fail to search for myofascial trigger points.

It is as a result of this that many injustices are committed concerning the cause of persistent pain in accident compensation cases. Accidents undoubtedly give rise to much psychological distress (Muse 1985, 1986) but this does not mean that post-accident pain which does not respond readily to some of the more conventional methods of treating organic pain is necessarily psychological in origin and in some way associated with an unconscious or even at times a conscious desire for compensation.

Such an assumption is all too prevalent and in the past has led experienced physicians such as Henry Miller (1961, 1966) to believe that once compensation is awarded, persistent post-accident pain invariably starts to improve. That this is not so has recently been demonstrated by Mendleson (1982, 1984) who, from a study of accident compensation cases in Australia, concludes that 'patients are not cured by the verdict'. and that, in general, the pain remains as intense after the financial settlement as before. This is confirmed by Melzack et al (1985) who, in commenting both on Mendelson's findings and their own psychological studies of accident compensation cases, states:

... the phrase 'compensation neurosis' is an unwarranted, biased diagnosis. Not only are the disability and pain not cured by the verdict but

compensation patients do not exaggerate their pain or show evidence of neurosis or other psychopathological symptoms greater than those seen in pain patients without compensation.

From serving on medical appeal tribunals which deal with people seeking compensation for post-accident disablement, it has become evident to me that of those who seek financial assistance because of persistent pain only relatively few are malingerers. This observation is in keeping with that of Leavitt & Sweet (1986) in their study of the frequency of malingering amongst patients with low-back pain.

What, however, has become apparent to me is that a disturbingly large number of these claimants are allowed to suffer from potentially treatable nocigenic pain for unnecessarily long periods of time simply because the dictum laid down by Livingston as long ago as 1943 is so frequently ignored. He said that in every case of persistent pain following trauma it is essential to search for trigger points. It was because Crue & Pinskey (1984) did not do this that they failed to find a nociceptive peripheral input in a group of patients with chronic back pain; introduced the totally inept diagnostic term 'chronic intractable benign pain'; and made the unwarranted assumption that such pain is a central phenomenon — a polite way of saying 'it is all in the mind!' As Rosonoff et al (1989) have now shown, in 96–100% of patients with chronic low-back or neck pain of the type studied by Crue & Pinskey, the pain emanates from trigger points.

Finally, it is necessary to reiterate that whilst anxiety is rarely the cause of pain, persistent pain is commonly associated with the development of anxiety. When this happens, the anxiety causes muscles to be held in a state of tension and with musculoskeletal pain this results in an increase in trigger point activity with a consequent exacerbation of the pain (Craig 1989). In all such cases it is not sufficient simply to deactivate the trigger points but it is also necessary to reduce the anxiety. The most satisfactory way of achieving this is by the use of hypnotherapy (Orne & Dinges 1989) and by teaching the patient how to practise autohypnosis on a regular daily basis.

REFERENCES

Adams J E 1976 Naloxone reversal of analgesia produced by brain stimulation in the human. Pain 2: 161–166

Akil H, Mayer D J, Liebeskind J C 1976 Antagonism of stimulation produced analgesia by naloxone, a narcotic antagonist. Science 191: 961–962

Alles A, Dom R M 1985 Peripheral sensory nerve fibres that dichotomize to supply the brachium and the pericardium in the rat: A possible morphological explanation for referred cardiac pain? Brain Research 342: 382–385

Anderson E G, Proudfit H K 1981 The functional role of the bulbospinal serotonergic system. In: Jacobs B L, Gelperin A (eds) Serotonin neurotransmission and behaviour. M.I.T. Press, Cambridge, Massachusetts, p 307–338

Atweh S F, Kuhar M J 1977 Autodiographic localization of opiate receptors in rat brain 1. Spinal cord and lower medulla. Brain Research 22: 471–493

Banning A, Sjøgren P, Henreksen H 1991 Pain causes in 200 patients referred to a multidisciplinary cancer pain clinic. Pain 45: 45–48

Basbaum A I, Fields H L 1978 Endogenous pain control mechanisms: review and hypothesis. Annals of Neurology 4: 451–462

Basbaum A I, Marley J J E, O'Keefe J, Clanton C H 1977 Reversal of morphine and stimulus-produced analgesia by subtotal spinal cord lesions. Pain 3: 43–56

Beecher H K 1959 Measurements of subjective responses. Oxford University Press, Oxford

Bond M R 1979 Pain. Its nature, analysis and treatment. Churchill Livingstone, Edinburgh

Bowsher D 1987 Mechanisms of pain in man. ICI Pharmaceuticals Division

Bowsher D 1990 Physiology and pathophysiology of pain. Journal of the British Medical Acupuncture Society 7: 17–20

Bowsher D 1991 The physiology of stimulation-produced analgesia. Journal of the British Medical Acupuncture Society IX(2): 58–62

Calimlim J F, Wardell W M, Sriwatanakue K et al 1982 Analgesic effect of parenteral metkephamid acetate in treatment of postoperative pain. Lancet 1: 1374–1375

Casey K L 1971a Somatosensory responses of bulboreticular units in awake cat: relation to escape-producing stimuli. Science 173: 77–80

Casey K L 1971b Responses of bulboreticular units to somatic stimuli eliciting escape behavior in the cat. International Journal of Neuroscience 2: 15–28

Casey K L 1980 Reticular formation and pain: towards a unifying concept. In: Bonical J J (ed) Pain. Raven Press, New York p 93–105

Casey K L, Keene J J, Morrow T 1974 Bulboreticular and medial thalamic unit activity in relation to aversive behavior and pain. In: Bonica J J (ed) Pain, Advances in neurology. Raven Press, New York, vol 4 p 197–205

Cervero F 1983 Somatic and visceral inputs to the thoracic spinal cord of the cat. Journal of Physiology 337: 51–67

Chapman C R, Colpitts Y M, Benedetti C, Kitaeff R, Gehrig J D 1980 Evoked potential assessment of acupuncture analgesia: attempted reversal with naloxone. Pain 9: 183–197

Christensen B N, Perl E R 1970 Spinal neurons specifically excited by noxious or thermal stimuli: marginal zone of the dorsal horn. Journal of Neurophysiology 33: 293–307

Clement-Jones V 1983 Role of the endorphins in neurology. Practitioner 227: 487–495

Clement-Jones V, Besser G M 1983 Clinical perspectives in opioid peptides. British Medical Bulletin 39(1): 95–100

Clement-Jones V, Lowry P J, Rees L H et al 1980 Met-enkaphalin circulates in human plasma. Nature 283: 295–297

Collins J G, Ren K 1987 WDR response profiles of spinal dorsal horn neurons may be unmasked by barbiturate anesthesia. Pain: 28: 369–378

Craig K D 1989 Emotional aspects of pain. In: Wall P D, Melzack R (eds) Textbook of pain, 2nd edn. Churchill Livingstone, Edinburgh, p 220–230

Crue B L, Pinskey J J 1984 An approach to chronic pain of non-malignant origin. Postgraduate Medical Journal 60: 858–864

De Takats G 1937 Reflex dystrophy of the extremities. Archives of Surgery 34: 939–956

Dennis S G, Choinière M, Melzack R 1980 Stimulation-produced analgesia in rats: assessment by two pain tests and correlation with self-stimulation. Experimental Neurology 68: 295–309

Dickhaus H, Pauser G, Zimmerman M 1985 Tonic descending inhibition affects intensity coding of nociceptive responses in spinal dorsal horn neurones in the cat. Pain 23: 145–158

Duggan A W, Hall J G, Headley P M 1976 Morphine, enkephalin and the substantia gelatinosa. Nature 264: 456–458

Edwards R H T 1990 Pathophysiology of muscle pain. In: Lipton S, Tunks E, Zoppi M (eds) Advances in pain research and therapy. Raven Press, New York, vol 13 p 157–163

Edwards R H T, Round J M, Jones D A 1983 Needle biopsy of skeletal muscle. A review of 10 years' experience. Muscle Nerve 6(9) 676–683

Feinmann C 1990 Psychogenic regional pain. British Journal of Hospital Medicine 43: 123–127

Fields H L 1987a Pain. McGraw-Hill, New York p 31, b p 35, c p 44, d p 216 e p 82–94

Fields H L, Basbaum A I 1989 Endogenous pain control mechanisms In: Wall P D, Melzack R (eds) Textbook of pain, Churchill Livingstone, Edinburgh, p 206–220

Filner B E 1989 Role of myofascial pain syndrome treatment in the management of reflex sympathetic dystrophy syndrome. Communication to the 1st international symposium on myofascial pain and fibromyalgia. Minneapolis

Filshie 1990 Acupuncture for malignant pain. Journal of the British Medical Acupuncture Society 8: 38–39

Freeman W, Watts J W 1950 Psychosurgery in the treatment of mental disorders and intractable pain. C C Thomas, Springfield, Illinois, USA

Gardner W J, Licklider J C R 1959 Auditory analgesia in dental operations. Journal of the American Dental Association 59: 1144–1149

Georgopoulos A P 1974 Functional properties of primary afferent units probably related to pain mechanisms in primate glabrous skin. Journal of Neurophysiology 39: 71–83

Goldstein A, Tachibana S, Lowney L I, Hunkapiller M, Hood L 1979 Dynorphin (1–13) an extraordinarily potent opioid peptide. Proceedings of the National Academy of Sciences of the United States of America 76: 6666–6670

Graceley R H, Dubner R, Wolskee P J, Dector W R 1983 Placebo and naloxone can alter post-surgical pain by separate mechanisms. Nature 306: 264–265

Hagbarth K E, Kerr D I B 1954 Central influences on spinal afferent conduction. Journal of Neurophysiology 17: 295–307

Hannington-Kiff J F 1974 Pain relief. Heinemann Medical, London

Hannington-Kiff J G 1989 Pharmacological target blocks in painful dystrophic limbs. In: Wall P D, Melzack R (eds) Textbook of pain. Churchill Livingstone, Edinburgh, p 754–766

Herz A, Albus K, Metys J, Schubert P, Teschemacher H 1970 On the sites for the anti-nociceptive action of morphine and fentanyl. Neuropharmacology 9: 539–551

Hosobuchi Y, Adams J E, Linchitz R 1977 Pain relief by electrical stimulation of the central gray matter in humans and its reversal by naloxone. Science 177: 183–186

Hughes J, Smith T W, Kosterlitz H W, Fothergill L A, Morgan B A, Morris H R 1975 Identification of two related pentapeptides from the brain with potent opiate agonist activity. Nature 258: 577–579

Hunt S P, Kelly J S, Emson P C 1980 The electron microscope localization of methionine enkephalin within the superficial layers of the spinal cord. Neuroscience 5, 1871–1890

Jessell T W 1982 Neurotransmitters and CNS disease — Pain. Lancet 2: 1084–1087

Jessell T W, Iversen L L 1977 Opiate analgesics inhibit substance P release from rat spinal trigeminal nucleus. Nature 268: 549–551

Kerr D I B, Haughen F P, Melzack R 1955 Responses evoked in the brain stem by tooth stimulation. American Journal of Physiology 183: 253–258

Lasagna L 1965 Drug interaction in the field of analgesic drugs. Proceedings of the Royal Society of Medicine 58: 978–983

Laurberg S, Sorensen K E 1985 Cervical dorsal root ganglion cells with collaterals to both shoulder skin and the diaphragm. A fluorescent double labelling study on the rat. A model for referred pain? Brain Research 331: 160–163

Leavitt F, Sweet J J 1986 Characteristics and frequency of malingering among patients with low back pain. Pain 25: 357–364

Levine J D, Gordon N C, Jones R T, Fields H L 1978 The narcotic antagonist naloxone enhances clinical pain. Nature 272: 826–827

Levine J D, Gordon N C, Fields H L 1979 Naloxone dose dependently produces analgesia and hyperalgesia in postoperative pain. Nature 278: 740–741

Lewin R 1976 The brain's own opiate. New Scientist 69: 13

Lewis J W, Cannon J T, Liebeskind J E 1980 Opioid and non-opioid mechanisms of stress analgesia. Science 208: 623–625

Lewis J W, Sherman J E, Liebeskind J C 1981 Opioid and non-opioid stress analgesia: assessment of tolerance and cross tolerance with morphine. Journal of Neuroscience 1: 358–363

Lewis J W, Tordoff M G, Sherman J E, Liebeskind J C 1982 Adrenal medullary enkephalin-like peptides may mediate opioid stress analgesia. Science: 217: 557–559

Li C H, Barnafi L, Chrétien M, Chung D 1965 Isolation and amino-acid sequences of Beta-LPA from sheep pituitary glands. Nature 208: 1093–1094

Lichstein L, Sackett G P 1971 Reactions by differentially raised rhesus monkeys to noxious stimulation. Developmental Psychobiology 4: 339–352

Liebeskind J C, Paul L A 1977 Psychological and physiological mechanisms of pain. American Review of Psychology 28: 41–60

Lindblom U, Tegner R 1979 Are the endorphins active in clinical pain states? Narcotic antagonism in chronic pain patients. Pain 7: 65–68

Livingston W K 1943 Pain mechanisms. Macmillan, New York

Mayer D J, Price D D 1976 Central nervous system mechanisms of analgesia. Pain 2: 379–404

Mayer D J, Price D D 1975 Neurophysiological characterization of the anterolateral spinal cord neurons contributing to pain in man. Pain 1: 51–58

Mayer D J, Watkins L R 1981 The role of endorphins in endogenous pain control systems. In: Emrich H M (ed) Modern problems in pharmpsychiatry: The role of endorphins in neuropsychiatry. S Karger, Basel

Mayer D J, Wolfle T H, Akil H, Carder B, Liebeskind J C 1971 Analgesia from electrical stimulation in the brainstem of the rat. Science 174: 1351–1354

Melzack R 1969 The role of early experience in emotional arousal. Annals of New York Academy of Science 159: 721–730

Melzack R 1987 The short-term McGill Pain Questionnaire. Pain 30: 191–197

Melzack R, Casey K L 1968 Sensory, motivational, and central control determinants of pain: a new conceptual model. In: Kenshalo D (ed) The skin senses. C C Thomas, Springfield, Illinois, p 423–443

Melzack R, Katz J, Jeans M E 1985 The role of compensation in chronic pain. Analysis using a new method of scoring the McGill Pain Questionnaire. Pain 23: 101–112

Melzack R, Melinkoff D F 1974 Analgesia produced by brain stimulation: evidence of a prolonged onset period. Experimental Neurology 43: 369–374

Melzack R, Scott T H 1957 The effects of early experience on the response to pain. Journal of Comparative Physiology and Psychology 50: 155–161

Melzack R, Stotler W A, Livingston W K 1958 Effects of discrete brainstem lesions in cats on perception of noxious stimulation. Journal of Neurophysiology 21: 353–367

Melzack R, Torgenson W S 1971 On the language of pain. Anesthesiology 34, 50–59

Melzack R, Wall P D 1965 Pain mechanisms. A new theory. Science 150: 971–979

Melzack R, Wall P D 1982a The challenge of pain. Penguin, Harmondsworth, Middlesex, p 236, b p 237, c p 260

Melzack R, Wall P D 1988a The challenge of pain, Penguin, Harmondsworth, Middlesex, 2nd ed, b p 173, c p 125, d p 165–193, e p 141, f p 118, g p 181, h p 56, i p 32

Mendelson G 1982 Not 'cured by a verdict': effect of legal settlement on compensation claimants. Medical Journal of Australia 2: 132–134

Mendleson G 1984 Compensation, Pain Complaints and Psychological Disturbance. Pain 20: 169–177

Mense S 1977 Neurons outflow from skeletal muscle following chemical noxious stimulation. Journal of Physiology 267: 75–88

Mense S 1981 Sensitization of Group IV muscle receptors to bradykinin by 5-hydroxytryptamine and prostaglandin E $_2$ Brain Research 225: 95–105

Mense S 1990 Physiology of nociception in muscles. In: Fricton J R, Awad E (eds) Advances in pain research and therapy, Vol 17. Raven Press, New York

Merskey H 1979 Pain terms: a list with definitions and notes on usage. Recommended by the IASP sub-committee on taxonomy. Pain 6: 249–252

Millar J, Basbaum A I 1975 Topography of the projection of the body surface of the cat to cuneate and gracile nuclei. Experimental Neurology 49: 281–290

Miller H 1961 Accident neurosis. British Medical Journal 1: 919–925

Miller H 1966 Accident neurosis. Proceedings of the Medico-Legal Society, Victoria 10: 71–82

Muse M 1985 Stress-related, post-traumatic chronic pain syndrome: criteria for diagnosis and preliminary report on prevalence. Pain 23: 295–300

Muse M 1986 Stress-related post-traumatic chronic pain syndrome: behavioral treatment approach. Pain 25: 389–394

Nathan P W 1976 The gate-control theory of pain. A critical review. Brain 99: 123–158

Nathan P 1982 The nervous system, 2nd edn. Oxford University Press, Oxford, p 104–113

Nennesmo I, Reinholt F 1986 Mast cells in nerve end neuromas of mice. Neuroscience letters 69: 296–301

Noordenbos W 1959 Pain. Elsevier, Amsterdam.

Olsson Y 1968 Mast cells in the nervous system. In: Bourne G H, Danielli J F, Jeow K W (eds) International review of eytology. Academic Press, New York p 27–70

Orne M T, Dinges D F 1989 Hypnosis. In: Wall P D, Melzack R (eds) Textbook of pain, 2nd edn. Churchill Livingstone, Edinburgh, p 1021–1031

Oyama T, Jin T, Yamaya R 1980 Profound analgesic effects of beta-endorphin in man. Lancet 1: 122–124

Paterson S J, Robson L E, Kosterlitz H W 1983 Classification of opioid receptors. British Medical Bulletin 39: 31–36

Pert C D, Snyder S H 1973 Opiate receptor: demonstration in nervous tissue. Science 179: 1011–1014

Portenoy R K, Foley K M, Inturrisi C E 1990 The nature of opioid responsiveness and its implications for neuropathic pain: new hypotheses derived from studies of opioid infusions. Pain 43: 273–286

Rexed B 1952 The cytoarchitectonic organization of the spinal cord in the cat. Journal of Comparative Neurology 96: 415–495

Reynolds D V 1969 Surgery in the cat during electrical analgesia induced by focal brain stimulation. Science 164: 444–445

Rosonoff H L, Fishbain D A, Goldberg M, Santana R, Rosonoff R S 1989 Physical findings in patients with chronic intractable benign pain of the neck and/or back. Pain 37: 279–287

Ruch T C 1965 Pathophysiology of pain. In: Ruch T C, Patton H D (eds) Physiology and biophysics. Saunders, Philadelphia, p 345–363

Shanks M F, Clement-Jones V, Linsell C J et al 1981 A study of 24 hour profiles of plasma mentenkaphalin in man. Brain Research 212: 403–409

Simons D 1990 Muscular pain syndromes. In: Fricton J R, Awad E (eds) Advances in pain research, Raven Press, New York vol 17 p 1–41

Smith R, Grossman A, Gaillard R et al 1981 Studies on circulating metenkephalin and beta-endorphin: normal subjects and patients with renal and adrenal disease. Clinical Endocrinology 15: 291–300

Smock T, Fields H L 1980 ACTH (1–24) blocks opiate-induced analgesia in the rat. Brain Research 212: 202–206

Soper W Y, Melzack R 1982 Stimulation-produced analgesia. Evidence for somatotopic organization in the midbrain. Brain Research 251: 301–311

Stacey J J 1969 Free nerve endings in skeletal muscle of the cat. Journal of Anatomy (London) 105: 231–254

Sternbach R A, Timmermans G 1975 Personality changes associated with reduction of pain. Pain 1: 177–181

Sternbach R A, Wolf S R, Murphy R W, Akeson W H 1973 Traits of pain patients: The low-back 'loser'. Psychosomatics 14: 226–229

Szentagothai J 1964 Neuronal and synaptic arrangement in the substantia gelatinosa rolandi. Journal of Comparative Neurology 122: 219–239

Thompson J W 1984a Pain mechanisms and principles of management. In: Evans J, Grimley, Laird F I (eds) Advanced geriatric medicine 4. Pitman, London

Thompson J W 1984b Opioid peptides. British Medical Journal 288 (6413): 259–260

Thompson J W 1988 Acupuncture or TENS for pain relief? Scientific and clinical comparisons. New Zealand Journal of Acupuncture. August 21–33

Todd A J, McKenzie J 1989 GABA — immunoreactive neurons in the dorsal horn of the rat spinal cord. Neuroscience 32: 799–806

Travell J G, Simons D G 1983 Myofascial Pain and Dysfunction. The Trigger Point Manual. Williams & Wilkins, Baltimore

Verrill P 1990 Does the gate theory of pain supplant all others? British Journal of Hospital Medicine. 43: 325

Wall P D 1960 Cord cells responding to touch, damage and temperature of skin. Journal of Neurophysiology 23: 197–210

Wall P D 1964 Presynaptic control of impulses at the first central synapse in the cutaneous pathway. In: Physiology of spinal neurons. Progress in Brain Research 12. Elsevier, Amsterdam, p 92–118

Wall P D 1978 The gate-control theory of pain mechanisms. A re-examination and a re-statement. Brain 101: 1–18

Wall P D 1980a The role of substantia gelatinosa as a gate control. In: Bonica J J (ed) Pain. Raven Press, New York, p 205–231

Wall P D 1980b The substantia gelatinosa. A gate control mechanism set across a sensory pathway. Trends in Neurosciences (Sept): 221–224

Wall P D 1989 The dorsal horn. In: Wall P D, Melzack R (eds) Textbook of pain. Churchill Livingstone, Edinburgh

Wall P D 1990 Obituary — William Noordenbos (1910–1990) Pain 42: 265–266

Wall P D, Melzack R (eds) 1989 Textbook of pain, 2nd edn. Churchill Livingstone, Edinburgh

Wang J K, Nauss L A, Thomas J E 1979 Pain relief by intrathecally applied morphine in man. Anesthesiology 50: 149–151

Watkins L R, Mayer D J 1982 Organization of endogenous opiate and non-opiate pain control systems. Science 216: 1185–1192

Weber E, Roth K A, Barchas J 1981 Colocalisation of alpha-neo-endorphin and dynorphin immunoreactivity in hypothalamic neurons. Biochemical and Biophysical Research Communications 103: 951–958

Willis W D 1989 The origin and destination of pathways involved in pain transmission In: Wall P, Melzack (eds)

Textbook of pain, 2nd edn. Churchill Livingstone, Edinburgh

Woolf C J, Wall P D 1983 Endogenous opioid peptides and pain mechanisms: a complex relationship. Nature 306: 739–740

Wyke B 1979 Neurological mechanisms in the experience of pain. Acupuncture and Electro-therapeutics Research 4: 27–35

Wynn Parry C B 1980 Pain in avulsion lesions of the brachial plexus. Pain 9: 41–53

Yaksh T L, Rudy T A 1976 Analgesia mediated by a direct spinal action of narcotics. Science 192: 1357–1358

Zborowski M 1952 Cultural components in responses to pain. Journal of Social Issues 8: 16–30

7. Trigger points

INTRODUCTION

The development of neural hyperactivity at trigger points is one of the commonest causes of musculoskeletal pain, and yet, as Travell (1976) has said, trigger point activity is often poorly recognized and inadequately managed.

Undoubtedly a major reason why clinicians have been slow to bestow upon trigger points the importance they deserve is that, despite much having been written about them over the past 50 years, for most of that time their morphology and the manner in which they produce pain have remained decidedly enigmatic. The medical profession, however, can no longer continue to ignore them, as recent advances in knowledge concerning the neurophysiology of pain have at last shed considerable light on their pain-producing properties.

The structures in which trigger points may be found include the skeletal muscles and their tendons; the capsules and ligaments of joints; the periosteum; and the skin. Trigger points in the skin often occur in scar tissue and their distribution therefore varies from person to person. In other tissues, however, as already stated, they occur at much the same sites in everyone, where they may be recognized, long before they become activated, by being slightly tender to palpation. When, for reasons to be explained later, these potential trigger points undergo a process of activation, they become considerably more tender to touch because of a marked increase in the sensitivity of their nerve endings.

These exquisitely tender activated trigger points may be divided into those which are in a latent phase and those which are in a fully active phase.

Latent trigger points are those in which the degree of activation is not sufficient for them to cause pain, and they may therefore be discovered on routine examination of symptomless people. Sola et al (1955), in a survey of 200 fit young adults serving in the American Air Force (100 males, age range 17–27; and 100 females, age range 18–35), found that 54 of the females and 45 of the males had trigger points which, whilst exquisitely tender, were not causing pain and therefore were considered to be in the latent phase.

By contrast, an active trigger point is one in which the activation is of such intensity that impulses from it, by bombarding the central nervous system, cause pain to be referred locally in the vicinity of the point or at a site some distance away from it (the zone of pain referral).

The tendency for potential trigger points to undergo activation increases with age but, as Bates & Grunwaldt (1958) have shown, trigger point activation is at times the cause of musculoskeletal pain in children.

Active trigger points either develop de novo at potential trigger point sites or as a result of increased activity in latent ones.

MYOFASCIAL TRIGGER POINTS

Trigger points in muscle may become activated either as a primary or a secondary event. The parts of a muscle in which this most frequently occurs include its origin and its insertion; also any free border, and its belly, particularly in the region of its motor point.

Primary activation of myofascial trigger points

One of the most important reasons for the primary activation of myofascial trigger points is trauma inflicted upon a muscle, either in the form of a direct injury or sudden strain, or when the muscle is subjected to excessive or unusual exercise. The activation may at other times occur more gradually such as when a muscle is subjected to repeated episodes of minor trauma, or is repeatedly overloaded.

Trauma to muscle causes an inflammatory reaction to develop and the cellular damage associated with this results in the liberation of various chemical substances such as bradykinin, prostaglandins, histamine, serotonin and potassium ions capable of sensitizing A-delta (Group III) and C (Group IV) sensory nerve fibres.

The sensitization of A-delta fibres causes electrical impulses to be transmitted centripetally in the relatively fast conducting neospinothalamic pathway to reach the post-central gyrus of the parietal lobe (the somatosensory cortex). The result of this is the development of an immediate, short-lasting sharp type of pain — the 'first' pain.

The sensitization of C afferent fibres cause electrical impulses to be transmitted at a slower speed up the paleo-spino-reticulo-diencephalic pathway to reach firstly the limbic system and then the frontal lobe. The result of this is the development, after a short delay, of an persistent, ill-defined, dull, aching type of pain which is referred to a site near to or at times some distance from the activated trigger point itself. As stated in Chapter 6, a trigger point must contain various types of sensory nerve fibres but, as it is, the sensitization of its C afferent ones which causes it to become activated and give rise to this protracted, potentially disabling 'second' type of referred pain means that an activated trigger point is essentially a dense collection of sensitized C-polymodal nociceptors.

Trigger points may also become activated when muscles are kept in a state of persistent contraction by someone who is emotionally tense (see page 55). Other reasons for it include adverse environmental conditions such as excessive cold, excessive heat, damp or draughts. In addition, it may happen as a result of prolonged immobilization of muscles, such as may occur, for example, with protracted bed rest; with paralysis of a limb; and when part of the body is encased in a plaster cast. Also, it may occur during the course of febrile illnesses.

Finally, it has to be said that the factor(s) responsible for the activation of trigger/tender points in the generalized primary fibromyalgia syndrome are not known. There are good reasons for believing that this currently cryptogenic type of activation will ultimately turn out to be due to some as-yet unrecognized systemic biochemical disorder (see Ch. 5).

Secondary activation of myofascial trigger points

When pain develops in a muscle as a result of the primary activation of trigger points, trigger points are also liable to undergo the same process as a secondary event in synergistic muscles — if these should become overloaded as a result of compensating for the primarily affected one — and also in muscles which act as antagonists should they become strained counteracting the tension in the one primarily affected. In addition, trigger points are liable to become activated as a secondary event in any muscle which happens to be within an area to which pain has been referred. This not only occurs with pain which is referred from primary myofascial trigger points but also when it is referred from some visceral disease such as a myocardial infarction (see Ch. 12) or some somatic disorder such as disc or facet joint degeneration (see Chs 14 and 17).

Travell & Simons (1983) call trigger points which become secondarily activated in a zone of reference 'satellite trigger points'. Since these in turn may cause pain to be referred to some still more distant zone of reference, it is obvious that, by this knock-on effect, pain at times spreads for a considerable distance, with trigger points extending along a relatively straight line which intriguingly often corresponds closely to the course said to be taken by a traditional acupuncture tract. It is, for example, not uncommon for the primary activation of a trigger point in the lower part of the posterior chest wall to cause pain to be referred to the buttock, and for satellite trigger points in the gluteal muscles there to then cause pain to be referred down the iliotibial tract, and for this to be followed by the development of satellite trigger points along the length of that structure.

An activated myofascial trigger point may be located in an area of muscle which feels entirely normal, but often it occurs in a palpable taut band of muscle, or in a 'fibrositic' nodule.

Palpable taut bands

There has been much argument as to the nature of these very firm, rope-like structures in which trigger points are often to be found because, although the part of the muscle in which they are situated feels tense and resists stretching, this tension cannot be attributed to spasm, if for no other reason than that there is an absence of electromyographic activity (Kraft et al 1968). Also, there is no evidence to suggest that it is due either to a deposition of fibrous tissue, or to localized oedema, or to gelling of muscle colloids (myogelosis). Any hypothesis concerning the development of a palpable band has to take into account that it often disappears within seconds (or, at the most, minutes) of the muscle being subjected to stretch, or having a needle inserted into it. The most likely explanation, therefore, would seem to be that it occurs as a result of muscle fibres in a circumscribed area undergoing physiological contracture. Contracture in this sense does not imply the shortening of muscle fibres as a result of fibrosis, but rather, as pointed out by Travell & Simons (1983), a sustained intrinsic activation of the contractile mechanisms of the muscle fibres, in the absence of motor unit action potentials.

Before attempting to explain this concept further, it is first necessary to review some of the basic principles concerning the physiology of muscle contraction.

Every muscle fibre contains approximately 200 myofibrils, each of which is made up of serially-placed sarcomeres. It is these sarcomeres with their contained myosin and actin filaments which are the basic contractile units of skeletal muscle, and it is therefore the interaction between these filaments which is responsible for the contractile force. For such an interaction to take place, free ionized calcium has to be present and, in order to ensure this, the calcium energizer adenosine triphosphate (ATP) has to be available. Calcium is stored in the sarcoplasmic reticulum surrounding each myofibril, and the energy required for its release from this repository in order to allow a contraction to take place, and for it then to return to the repository following the contraction, in supplied by ATP.

Simons & Travell (1981), in attempting to explain the mechanism responsible for the formation of palpable bands around myofascial trigger points, have put forward the following ingenious hypothesis. They postulate that, when trauma activates a myofascial trigger point, it must often at the same time damage the sarcoplasmic reticulum — the calcium repository surrounding a myofibril — with the result that calcium ions are released. It is then likely that the development of a palpable band around the trigger point is due to this free ionized calcium, with energy provided by ATP, activating the actin-myosin contractile mechanism in the sarcomeres of a group of contiguous muscle fibres.

They further believe that the contractile activity responsible for the development of the tense band persists so long as the sarcoplasmic reticulum remains damaged and calcium ions together with ATP remain in the tissues. However, they realize that eventually the sarcoplasmic reticulum is bound to recover and that, even before this occurs, the calcium, by diffusing through the tissues, gradually loses its effectiveness. Therefore, although the mechanism proposed is certainly sufficient to explain the initial development of palpable bands, it does not explain their long-term persistence. This, they think, may be due to the circulation in the bands becoming impaired partly as a result of sustained contraction of the muscle fibres and partly because of an accumulation of metabolites causing a vasoconstrictor reflex response.

Support for this idea of an impaired circulation in trigger point-containing palpable bands comes from Fassbender (1975) observing changes in endothelial cells of capillaries in biopsy specimens of muscle around trigger points. Popelianskii et al

(1976) have also shown by means of radiosotope studies that there is a slowing of perfusion at trigger point sites.

Simon & Travell believe it might be as a result of this impaired circulation that the supply of ATP eventually becomes depleted, and that, even if by this time the sarcoplasmic reticulum has recovered its function, the lack of ATP and the energy it provides prevents the calcium from being returned to this repository. Consequently, the myosin heads do not release from the actin filaments, and therefore the shortening of the sarcomeres persists. They readily admit that this cannot be the complete explanation because even if calcium, in the absence of energy supplied by ATP, cannot return to the sarcoplasmic repository, it should nevertheless eventually disappear by a process of diffusion and cease to have its effect on the actin-myosin linkage. For this reason they feel that there must be a third mechanism, yet to be discovered, which maintains its concentration in the tissues.

The intriguing aspect of all this is that, is spite of the apparent complexity of the biochemical and physiological changes described, the abolition of a trigger point containing palpable band only requires the tension in the shortened sarcomeres to be reduced sufficiently to allow the linked actin and myosin filaments to separate. Sometimes this can be achieved simply by stretching the muscle, but more often by deactivating the trigger point in the band by means of stimulating A-delta nerve fibres with dry needles.

Fibrositic nodules

For years there was considerable confusion concerning the nature of fibrositic nodules and much uncertainty as to how they cause pain.

The first to examine fibrositic nodules microscopically was Ralph Stockman, Professor of Medical at the University of Glasgow, who, as discussed in Chapter 5, in 1904 reported that histologically there is evidence of patchy inflammatory hyperplasia of the connective tissue, and concluded that the pain results from sensory nerves being stretched or compressed by fibrous tissue proliferation and by inflamed connective tissue infiltrating the walls of nerves.

Subsequent early 20th-century investigators such as Schade (1919) failed to find any evidence of an inflammatory lesion. Schade carried out his studies in a German field hospital during the First World War. He located fibrositic nodules in the muscles of a number of soldiers and observed that these nodules continued to be palpable in a group of them who for, one reason or another, had to be deeply anaesthetized. He also noted that they continued to be palpable in another group which died, up to the time that rigor mortis set in. Furthermore, when this group came to a post-mortem examination, the muscles containing nodules were found to be histologically normal.

As a result of observing that the nodules continued to be palpable both under deep anaesthesia and after death he concluded that they could not have developed as a result of muscle going into spasm. Furthermore, he considered that the discovery of normal muscle tissue on histological examination ruled out any possibility that the nodules might have developed as a result of structural changes in the connective tissue. He therefore suggested that nodules develop as a result of a change in the colloidal state of muscle cytoplasm from sol to gel, and coined the term myogelose (muscle gelling or myogelosis) for this.

The first extensive, well-documented study of carefully selected material designed to demonstrate the histological changes associated with myogelosis was carried out by the German orthopaedic surgeon Glogowski and the pathologist Wallraff. In 1951 they reported the results of examining 24 biopsies of muscle hardening (muskelhärten), but despite the use of no less than 9 tissue stains, they were unable to demonstrate any significant abnormalities and concluded that myogelosis must occur at the sarcoplasmic level beyond reach of the light microscope.

In the meantime, in Britain, Copeman and Ackerman (1944) added to the confusion by erroneously concluding that nodules felt in the muscles of patients with low-back pain are nothing more than herniated fat lobules.

It was not until Brendstrup et al (1957) carried out the first controlled biopsy and biochemical study of fibrositic nodules that their true nature became apparent. In this study, the microscopic appearances of biopsies of paraspinal muscles containing palpable fibrositic nodules were compared with those of biopsies taken from normal contralateral paraspinal muscles in 12 patients undergoing operations for prolapsed intervertebral discs. They stressed that, as the subjects were fully anaesthetized and the muscle relaxed with curare, neither painfulness nor muscle spasm could have been factors in choosing the areas for biopsy, and that the selection of sites was done entirely by feeling for fibrostic nodules.

They found a striking difference between the microscopic appearances of the nodules, and those of the controls. By staining sections with toluidine blue, they were able to demonstrate in the 'fibrositic' specimens interstitial mucinous oedema containing acid mucopolysaccharides and an accumulation of mast cells. In addition, biochemical analysis of these specimens showed a much higher concentration of hexosamine and hyaluronic acid than in the controls. Hyaluronic acid has a strong water-binding capacity and therefore, not surprisingly, the extra-cellular fluid content of the 'fibrositic' specimens was considerably more than that of the control and constituted, in effect, an oedema of the connective tissue. At that time it was thought that oedema of this type, by distorting the peripheral nerve-endings, might be an important contributory factor in the development of pain (Wegelius & Absoe-Hansen 1956).

Knowledge concerning the structure of fibrositic nodules was advanced still further by Awad (1973) taking from 10 patients biopsies of muscle in which these nodules could be felt and examining them with the electron microscope. The skin overlying each nodule to be biopsied was carefully marked with an indelible pen. Muscle fasicles approximately 1 cm wide and 2 cm long were then dissected out at these sites after they had been grasped firmly between the opposing jaws of a modified chalazion clamp. The reason for doing this was partly to prevent the development of muscle contraction artifacts but also to ensure that the fluid content of the muscle remained trapped within the biopsy material.

When examined under the light microscope, the muscle fibres appeared normal except that in every case there seemed to be an increase in the number of interstitial nuclei. However, what was of much greater significance was the discovery in 8 of the 10 cases of a large amount of amorphous material in between the muscle fasicles which, when stained with toluidine blue, was shown to consist of acid mucopolysaccharides. This substance, which is known to have enormous water-binding properties, under normal conditions is only present in small amounts in muscle extra-cellular tissue.

On electron microscopic examination, it was noted that this amorphous material distended the spaces between muscle fibres which were themselves of normal appearance. In addition, large clusters of platelets were observed and mast cells were seen to be discharging mucopolysaccharide-containing granules into the intercellular space. The next most common finding of any significance was an increased amount of connective tissue (5 cases).

It was concluded that this water-retaining mucopolysaccharide amorphous substance in fibrositic nodules is what causes them to be space-occupying lesions which stretch the surrounding muscle tissue. It was also concluded that the accumulation of this substance in the extracellular tissues is what impairs the oxygen flow to muscle fibres and increases their acidity, and that it is this increased acidity which sensitizes muscle sensory nociceptors and converts them into pain-producing trigger points.

As Awad (1990) however has recently pointed out several questions remain to be answered, including, does the accumulation of mucopolysaccharides in fibrositic nodules occur as a result of an increased production of this normally occurring substance, or a decrease in its degradation, or a change in its quality?

Weakness and restriction of the movements of a muscle containing active trigger points

A muscle contaning active trigger points undergoes shortening and becomes somewhat weakened. Also, any attempt to extend it results in pain developing before its normal range is completed. Macdonald (1980) carried out a detailed study of painful movements in 10 patients with myofascial trigger points and concluded that:

When a particular muscle is affected the passive and active movements which stretch its length increase . . . awareness of pain; while the same modes of movement in a direction which shorten the affected muscle fibres do not increase the pain. Pain is increased when the affected muscle plays an agonist role in an active resisted manoeuvre (increasing its isometric tension); but when the muscle is not an agonist of such a manoeuvre no extra pain is produced.

Trigger points in skin, ligaments, and periosteum

Trigger points in seemingly healthy skin may become activated and cause pain to be referred either locally or at a distance (Sinclair 1949, Trommer & Gellman 1952) but in my experience this most commonly occurs in skin scars. It is therefore important to remember this possibility when investigating the cause of persistent post-operative pain.

A female (46) had a very badly infected appendix resected in April 1983. Five months later, because of chronic pelvic sepsis, she had to have the right ovary and fallopian tube removed, and one year later she underwent a hysterectomy. Soon after this latter operation she started to complain of intermittent but severe jabs of pain in the right lower part of the abdomen. As this continued for several months, she was extensively investigated, but when no visceral cause for her pain was found, she was referred to me to assess whether acupuncture might relieve it.

On examination, there were exquisitely tender trigger points in the midline scar and also one in the right iliac fossa. Deactivation of these with a dry needle on three occasions at weekly intervals resulted in the pain being brought under control.

Trigger points in the ligaments of joints are also a frequent cause of persistent pain, and yet these are often overlooked in spite of the fact that Leriche (1930), over 50 years ago, drew attention to the manner in which they develop in these structures following fractures and sprains. More recently Gorrell (1976) has described how to identify, and inject with procaine, ligamentous trigger points around the ankle joint. De Valera & Raftery (1976) have shown how pain, occurring as a result of pelvic ligaments becoming strained, may be relieved by injecting trigger points in these structures with a local anaesthetic. However, there are now good grounds for believing that such trigger points, like those in other structures, may be more readily deactivated by means of acupuncture, and this will therefore be discussed again in the chapters dealing with low-back pain, pelvic pain, and pain in and around joints.

It will be remembered that Kellgren (1939), by injecting hypertonic saline into the periosteum, and thereby artificially creating trigger points, was able to show that pain produced by this technique is felt either locally or referred at a distance, in a similar manner to that which occurs with muscle. Inman & Saunders (1944) confirmed this, and drew attention to the clinical importance of periosteal trigger points in various musculoskeletal pain disorders. More recently Mann (1974), recognizing that periosteal trigger points often become activated in the vicinity of joints, has evolved a method of deactivating them by means of what he calls 'periosteal pecking', a technique which will be referred to again in later chapters.

Increased electrical activity at trigger points

From various observations which have been made, it is reasonable to assume that all trigger points have increased electrical activity. For example, when Arroyo (1966) inserted a needle electrode into a fibrositic nodule, there was a continuous and prolonged burst of electrical activity similar to that produced by a normal muscular contraction of moderate degree.

Palpable myofascial bands, on the other hand, are electrically silent at rest (Kraft et al 1968). However when such a band is 'plucked' with a finger, in a similar manner to plucking a violin string, a transient burst of electrical activity with the same configuration as motor unit action potentials may be recorded electromyographically (Simons 1976a, Dexter & Simons 1981). It is undoubtedly this electrical hyperactivity of motor nerve and sensory nerve fibres at myofascial trigger points that is responsible for the so-called local twitch response, a transient contraction of muscle fibres which may either be seen or felt, or both, whenever a palpable band in a superficially placed muscle is 'plucked' by drawing a finger smartly across it.

It is also neural hyperirritability which causes both myofascial and non-myofascial trigger points to be exquisitely tender to touch, with pressure on them causing the patient to jump. The amount of pressure required to produce this is a measure of the degree of irritability present. Good (1949) was the first to draw attention to this involuntary jerking of the body but it has only been since 1968 when Kraft et al redescribed it that it has come to be known as the 'jump sign'.

This characteristic response is often accompanied by the utterance of some appropriate expletive such as 'ouch!' in the Western world, or 'ah shih!' amongst the Chinese. It is this particular utterance which has led the Chinese for centuries to refer to exquisitely tender acupuncture points as 'ah shih' (oh yes!) points.

SPECIFIC PATTERNS OF MYOFASCIAL PAIN REFERRAL

As stated in the last chapter, pain referred from myofascial trigger points does not follow a strictly dermatomal pattern or nerve root distribution (Travell & Bigelow 1946). It is no doubt because of this that many clinicians, when presented with a myofascial pain syndrome, fail to recognize it as being of organic origin (Bonica 1957). Yet it was over 40 years ago that Good in Britain, Kelly in Australia and Travell and her colleagues in America, all showed in numerous, profusely-illustrated reports (see Ch. 5) that each individual muscle in the body, when affected by trigger point activity, has its own specific pattern of pain referral.

The clinical picture naturally becomes somewhat confused when, as so often happens, there is a composite pain pattern due to more than one muscle being affected. However, knowledge of all the various individual patterns, each of which has to be learnt separately, reduces the chances of overlooking the myofascial origin of such pain and gives much needed guidance as to which muscles in particular should be examined in order to find the trigger points responsible for it.

In relationship to this, it should be noted that although trigger points are exquisitely tender to touch, patients themselves, somewhat surprisingly, are nearly always totally unaware of their presence, and therefore can be of no assistance in any search for them. It also has to be remembered that pain from any one point is often felt a considerable distance from it. For example, trigger point activity in the levator scapulae muscle not infrequently causes pain to spread down the whole length of the inner arm to the ring and little fingers. It is because a knowledge of the various specific patterns of pain referral is therefore so essential that, during the course of this book, each one will be described in detail.

Reproduction of specific myofascial pain patterns

It is often possible to reproduce a specific pattern of pain referral by applying sustained pressure to or by inserting a needle into the causative trigger point.

Myofascial pain pathways and their relationship to those taken by Chinese acu-tracts

When news first reached the Western world that the Chinese believed in the existence of structures now known as acu-tracts or meridians and had precisely defined the various courses taken by them around the body, the acu-tracts were immediately dismissed as figments of their imagination as it was impossible to demonstrate their presence anatomically. However, when one comes to study the paths taken by pain referred from activated trigger points, it is remarkable how often these coincide with those of Chinese acu-tracts. Macdonald (1982), for example, describes how he persuaded 52 consecutive patients with chronic musculoskeletal pain seen in his practice, to draw maps of their pain on diagrams of the human body. Somewhat to his surprise, he found that 85% of these patients drew thin lines linking one area of pain with another. And even more surprisingly, he found that 96% of these thin lines corresponded with that of the course taken by one or another of the Chinese meridians.

In particular, he describes one patient whose response to needle stimulation was quite remarkable in that whenever a needle was inserted into him he had a distinct feeling of 'warm water' flowing from it; and although the patient had no previous knowledge of Chinese acupuncture, when needles were inserted into various parts of his body, the paths taken by the 'warm water' coincided exactly with those taken by meridians. Figure 7.1 shows the drawing the patient made of the path taken by the 'warm water' flowing up his leg and back from a needle inserted into the heel, and, by comparing it with Figure 7.2, it will be seen that it is identical with that taken by the tract known to the Chinese as the 'urinary bladder' meridian. From the time that the Chinese first began to practise acupuncture they have described various sensations which may be elicited as a result of inserting a needle into an acupuncture point.

The eliciting of these is known as tê-chhi (pronounced derchi and meaning obtaining the chhi or vital energy). These sensations are of various types and include distension, aching, heaviness, tingling, soreness and warmth. Usually the sensation remains localized around the site where the needle is inserted, but occasionally it radiates some distance from it, and in rare instances it travels along the entire course taken by a traditional Chinese acupuncture channel or meridian. When this happens, it is known as Propagated Sensation along a Channel (PSC). The Cooperative Group of Investigation of PSC (1980) in China studied the distribution of needle sensations in 64,228 patients. It found that the needle sensation was localized in the majority, that about 20% of patients described sensations which radiated for short distances, and about 0.4% had sensations propagated along channels.

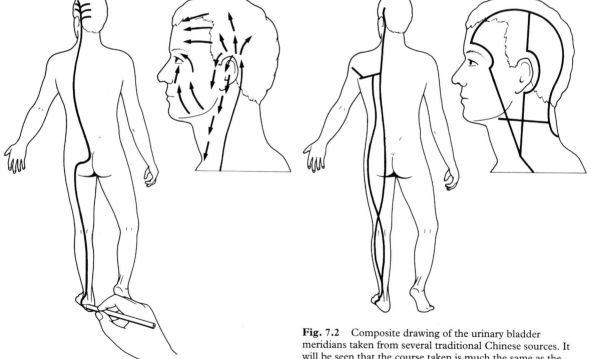

Fig. 7.1   The pattern of sensation drawn by a patient on an outline of the body following the insertion of a needle into his heel. Reproduced with permission from Alexander Macdonald's *Acupuncture from Ancient Art to Modern Medicine*, 1982.

Fig. 7.2   Composite drawing of the urinary bladder meridians taken from several traditional Chinese sources. It will be seen that the course taken is much the same as the pattern of sensation drawn by the patient in Figure 7.1. Reproduced with permission from Alexander Macdonald's *Acupuncture from Ancient Art to Modern Medicine*, 1982.

The Research Group of Acupuncture Anaesthesia at the Institute of Medicine and Pharmacology in the Fujian Province of China reported in 1986 that either mechanically compressing, or cooling, or locally anaesthetizing the soft tissues at some site along the course of such a sensation blocked its spread. Such an observation was somewhat surprising for it tended to support what is now generally accepted to be the untenable belief that acupuncture tracts or channels are peripherally situated anatomical structures. It is much more likely that these channels and the propagated sensation along them owe their existence to some as yet unidentified activity in the central nervous system.

In support of this idea are observations made by Xue (1986) which led him to the belief that PSC occurs as a result of activity in the parietal cortex. He came to this conclusion from descriptions of pain referral given to him by patients with a variety of different neurosurgical disorders. One of the most striking of these was that of a below-knee amputee who described propagation of sensation from a point on his stump not only upwards along the surface of his trunk but also downwards into his phantom limb.

It would seem likely that the ancient Chinese evolved their ideas concerning acu-tracts from similarly observing the pathways taken by pain arising both spontaneously and in response to needle stimulation. Although they were clearly wrong to believe that meridians are anatomical structures it may well be that such channels do exist as some form of electrical energy in the central nervous system (Becker et al 1976).

Examining for trigger points

The technique required in order to locate trigger points — whether they be in periosteum, skin or muscle, but particularly in the latter — requires much skill and practice. It is therefore regrettable that medical students are given no instruction in this, and yet much time is spent in teaching them other physical signs, some of which have not nearly as much everyday practical importance.

This is remarkable when one considers that, before the Second World War, Kellgren, by care-fully designed experiments and shrewd clinical observations, made fundamental contributions to our understanding of the mechanisms whereby musculoskeletal pain arises. The failure of most clinical teachers to recognize the importance of trigger points in the development of musculoskeletal pain is reflected in the fact that there is still little or no mention of them in any of the standard textbooks of general medicine, neurology, orthopaedics or rheumatology, in spite of the fact that in recent years various clinicians including Simons (1975, 1976b), Travell (1976), Reynolds (1981), Rubin (1981), Sola (1981) and Simons & Travell (1989), have given accounts of myofascial trigger point syndromes. Also, in 1983 Travell & Simons published an extensive and authoritative treatise on the subject, and in 1989 there was a comprehensive review of recent research at the first international conference to be held on the subject (Fricton & Awad 1990).

The reason for so little attention being paid to these myofascial pain syndromes in the teaching of undergraduates is that, until recently, as discussed in Chapter 5, they have been grouped together somewhat disparagingly under such ill-defined, non-specific and now unacceptable terms as muscular rheumatism or fibrositis (Ch. 5) with pain from a condition such as this being considered as no more than a self-limiting minor disability of no particular significance. The result of this has been that in any case of persistent and severe musculoskeletal pain, the muscles themselves are given no more than a perfunctory examination, whereas skeletal structures such as the joints, bones and intervertebral discs are subjected to close scrutiny with particular attention being paid to radiographic changes.

The potential danger of this is that if no abnormality is found radiographically, the pain is likely to be looked upon as being of little consequence. Furthermore, if, in spite of reassurance that nothing serious has been found, the patient should have the temerity to continue to complain about the pain, there is always the risk that it will be assumed to be of psychogenic origin, without the possibility of its persistence being due to the activation of trigger points in the muscles even being considered.

A secretary (42), who had complained of persistent low-back pain for 2 years, was referred to an orthopaedic specialist who, in view of X-rays of the lumbar spine and sacro-iliac joints showing no significant abnormality, informed her that there was nothing serious to worry about and gave no specific therapeutic advice. As the pain continued to be disabling she was next referred to a gynaecologist, who decided to carry out a dilation and curettage under a general anaesthetic. No abnormality was found, but 10 days later she had a pulmonary infarct! Her general practitioner, finding that she had marital problems, then decided that the low-back pain must be associated with these and referred her to a psychiatrist. The latter, however, to his credit came to the conclusion that her disability was physical in origin. As the patient by this time had lost much time off work, she asked whether she could try acupuncture, and 2 years after seeking medical advice she was finally referred to me.

On examining the back, exquisitely tender transversely placed rope-like bands could readily be identified in the muscles overlying the lumbar and sacral regions on both sides. After needles had been inserted into maximum points of tenderness in these on five occasions at weekly intervals she lost her pain.

Conversely, if a radiographic abnormality is detected, there is always the risk that it will immediately be assumed to be the cause of a pain, without consideration of the possibility that it might be nothing more than a chance finding in someone whose pain is primarily muscular in origin. This is a mistake which is particularly liable to be made when degenerative changes are found on X-rays of the spine, and it will be discussed at length in Chapters 14 and 17.

Another common mistake is to assume that, because pain radiates down a limb, or around the trunk, that it must inevitability be due to entrapment of a nerve root, even where there is objective neurological evidence for this. This mistake arises when the muscles have not been systematically examined to exclude the possibility that it might have occurred as a result of being referred from myofascial trigger points. This error will also be discussed in later chapters.

It therefore cannot be stressed too strongly that, in the assessment of musculoskeletal pain, not only is clinical and radiological examination of the bones and joints required, but also a systematic examination of the muscles for trigger points.

Guidance as to which muscles are likely to be affected by trigger point activity is obtained by paying careful attention to descriptions of referred pain patterns and by observing which movements of the body are restricted. Each muscle under suspicion should then be placed slightly on the stretch and systematically searched for trigger points by means of the application of firm digital pressure. The necessity for firm palpation has to be emphasized because trigger points are liable to be overlooked if the pressure exerted is too gentle. Firm pressure over a normal muscle causes no discomfort, but in the vicinity of a trigger point it is slightly uncomfortable, and over a trigger point itself, because it is a site where the nerve endings are in a state of supersensitivity, the discomfort is such as to cause the patient involuntarily to jerk and to utter an expletive (p. 85).

When a muscle overlies bone, as for example is the case with the supraspinatus muscle, the correct palpatory technique is to draw the fingers firmly across it with a motion similar to that employed in kneading dough (flat palpation).

When, with a muscle such as the triceps, it is possible to take a firm hold of its belly, the latter should be firmly squeezed between thumb and fingers which are then moved backwards and forwards with a rolling motion (pincer palpation).

When palpating a muscle for trigger points it is essential to have short finger nails, for the discomfort caused by allowing them to dig into the flesh is liable to be misinterpreted as trigger point tenderness.

Measurement of a trigger point's pressure threshold

As, by definition, a trigger point is a point of maximum tenderness, its presence may be determined objectively by measuring the pressure threshold over it and comparing it with that over a corresponding contralateral non-tender point. The pressure threshold is the minimum pressure or force which induces discomfort. The instrument used for measuring this, a pressure threshold meter (Fig. 7.3), is a force gauge fitted with a

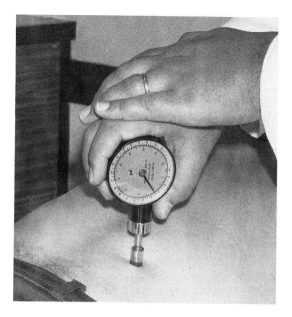

Fig. 7.3 Pressure threshold meter. Reproduced with the permission of Mr R J D'Souza.

disc-shaped rubber tip which has a surface area of exactly 1 cm². The gauge is calibrated in kg/cm² with a range of measurements up to 11 kg.

Before carrying out pressure threshold measurements on patients with myofascial trigger point pain, it is essential for them to be completely relaxed and for them to have been given a detailed explanation of the procedure. This involves locating a trigger point by means of manual palpation, and then, whilst the instrument is held against it at an angle of 90° exactly, steady pressure is applied until the patient reports the onset of discomfort. This should be done before and after the deactivation of a trigger point, for when this therapeutic procedure is successful the pressure threshold over the trigger point increases by about 4 kg (Fischer 1988a).

Although there is little or nothing to be gained by measuring pressure thresholds in everyday clinical practice, such measurements are of considerable help to those doctors and lawyers who have to make objectively-based decisions concerning compensation for post-accident myofascial trigger point pain. Pressure threshold measurements, before and after trigger point deactivation, are also of value in clinical trials (Fischer 1988b).

Thermography

Thermography, either of the infrared electrical type or the liquid crystal type, reflects the temperature of the skin in the form of a colour image. Fischer (1986) believes that this investigation is of value in the identification of myofascial trigger points, having found that the typical thermographic picture of the skin overlying such a point is a discoid 'hot spot' 5–10 cm in diameter produced as a result of the skin at that site being 0.5–1.0 °C warmer than adjacent skin. He feels that this is due to heat being conveyed to the skin surface from the deep tissues containing the trigger point as a result of an increase in flow of venous blood.

Swerdlow & Dieter (1992), however, have recently disputed Fischer's findings. Their reason for doing so is that when they investigated thermographically 365 patients with clinically demonstrable upper-back trigger points, although they found thermographic 'hot spots' to be present in the majority of these patients, the sites at which they were identified and the sites at which trigger points were located clinically did not correspond. They concluded from this that further research has to be done 'to determine the physiology responsible for these common and persistent thermal phenomena'. Their observations are of considerable importance because although the routine use of thermography for the identification of trigger points would never have been considered necessary, it initially looked as if this investigation might have been of value in providing objective evidence of their presence for medico-legal purposes.

Thermographic examination of the skin at a zone of trigger point pain referral shows the skin temperature to be raised in most cases (Hobbins 1989) but in some cases it is lowered. Simons (1987) attributes this to trigger points in different locations having different effects on the autonomic nervous system.

Autonomic concomitants of trigger point activity

Trigger point activity sufficient to cause the referral of pain may also cause disturbances of the autonomic system in its zone of referral

(Travell et al 1944). These include the pilomotor changes of goose flesh and localized sweating, either of which may appear both spontaneously and when pressure is applied to active trigger points. However, the one which often proves to be most troublesome is intense coldness of the distal part of a limb from localized vasoconstriction.

A female (35) who had been complaining of persistent intense coldness of the right foot for 3 years was referred by her general practitioner to a peripheral vascular surgeon for an opinion as to whether a sympathectomy might be helpful. No operation was advised but shortly after, as she had been complaining of pain around the right hip for the same period of time, she informed her doctor that she would like to try acupuncture for this, and was sent to see me.

On examination, she had exquisitely tender trigger points at the insertion of muscles into the greater trochanter, and also along the tensor fasciae latae. Once these had been deactivated by dry needle stimulation, the right foot became as warm as the left one.

As discussed in Chapter 6, active trigger points may also be present in cases of fully developed reflex sympathetic dystrophy.

The natural history of trauma-induced myofascial trigger point pain

With trauma-induced myofascial trigger point pain, the trigger point activation responsible for this type of pain, and the pain itself, both normally spontaneously disappear once the inflammatory reaction responsible for releasing trigger point-activating chemical substances has resolved.

Not infrequently, however, because of the development of a self-perpetuating circuit, the trigger points remain activated and the pain persists long after tissue healing has taken place. This post-traumatic persistent myofascial trigger point pain syndrome is a source of much diagnostic confusion because doctors not familiar with it are reluctant to accept that pain which persists for months or even years with no evidence of tissue damage to account for it can possibly be organic. Consequently, they all too often unjustly conclude that patients suffering from it are neurotic and at

times even refer them for psychiatric assessment. Moreover, because the cause of this pain so often goes unrecognized, it tends not to be treated appropriately, with the result that it is allowed to persist for unnecessarily long periods of time. Furthermore, because of all this, patients who seek compensation for post-accident pain of this type are liable to be considered to be exaggerating their symptoms for financial gain.

The following case history typifies this:

A man (27), whilst at work, fell from a ladder on to his back. This caused considerable bruising and pain in the lower lumbar and sacral regions. Radiographs of the spine showed no evidence of a fracture and all signs of soft-tissue damage disappeared fairly quickly. The pain, however, persisted and when 6 months later, it continued to be disabling in spite of intensive physiotherapy, an orthopaedic specialist expressed the opinion in his report that this might be due to the patient subconsciously exaggerating his symptoms in the hope of claiming industrial compensation. Nothing however could have been further from the truth for the patient, frustrated by his poor response to physiotherapy, asked his general practitioner if he thought acupuncture might be helpful, and as a consequence of this he was referred to me for assessment.

On examination, several well-defined exquisitely tender trigger points were found to be present in the muscles on both sides of the lower back, and after these had been deactivated with dry needles on four occasions at weekly intervals, the pain was alleviated and he was only too glad to get back to work with certainly no thought of claiming compensation.

The reason why this self-perpetuating circuit develops in some cases but not others is not certain. Fields (1987) postulates that in some cases this may occur as a result of motor efferent activity developing when the sensory input to the spinal cord from sensitized trigger point nociceptors activates motor neurons in the anterior horn. The muscle spasm brought about by this would then cause the trigger point nociceptors to remain activated and the vicious circle set up as a result would cause the pain to persist indefinitely (Fig. 7.4).

Another way in which a self-perpetuating circuit may be set up is by the development of efferent activity in the sympathetic system. This possibility was first put forward by Livingston (1943) to

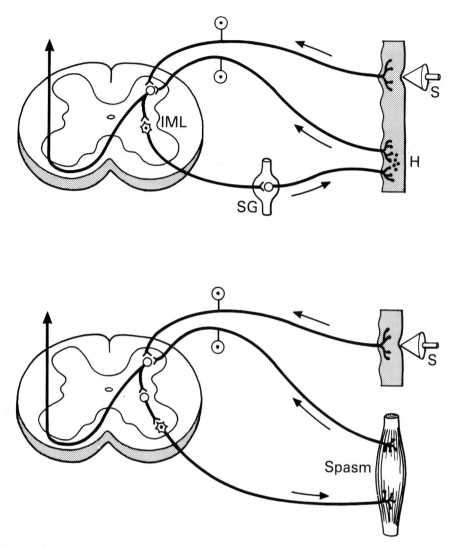

Fig. 7.4 Livingston's vicious circle. *Top*: A stimulus delivered at S activates a primary afferent nociceptor that, in turn, activates the sympathetic preganglionic neuron in the intermediolateral column (IML). The pregang lionic neuron activates the noradrenergic postganglionic neuron in the sympathetic ganglion (SG), which sensitizes, and can activate, primary afferent nociceptors (H) which, feed back to the spinal cord, maintaining the pain. *Bottom*: Nociceptive input may also set in motion another nociceptive input by activating motoneurons that cause muscle spasm. Prolonged muscle spasm activates muscle nociceptors which feed back to the spinal cord to sustain the spasm.

In both situations, the original noxious stimulus sets in motion a spreading and potentially self-sustaining process. In some cases the precipitating noxious input may be trivial and short lasting. In such cases, blocking the spasm or interruption of the reflex loops may provide long-lasting relief. Reproduced with permission from Howard Fields' *Pain*, McGraw Hill 1987.

account for a persistence of pain in his patients with sympathetic hyperactivity. With some of them this was of a primary type, but with others trigger points were also present.

The theory as to how sympathetic efferent activity may cause trigger point activation to persist is that the spinal cord input from a muscle nociceptor activates an intraspinally situated sympathetic preganglionic neuron. This activates a noradrenergic postganglionic neuron in the sympathetic ganglion. The sympathetic efferent activity created by this then keeps the intramuscular nociceptor in a state of hyper-activity. And the vicious circle which develops as a result of this causes the pain to persist indefinitely (Fig. 7.4).

It has to be said, however, that often there is no clinically obvious muscle spasm or sympathetic involvement and in such cases the underlying mechanism remains obscure. The following case is a good example of this.

A 65-year-old woman was referred to me with a pain in the lateral chest wall that had been present for 31 years! On examination there was no evidence of sympathetic involvement and no muscle spasm. There were however three well-defined trigger points in the serratus anterior muscle, and despite the exceptionally long history it only required the deactivation of these by means of dry needling on three occasions for the pain to disappear. She stated that the pain developed as a result of trauma to the chest wall incurred when 31 years previously she fell off her bicycle. She complained to doctors on many occasions about the pain but it was not until she eventually had to contact a physician about her heart that the trigger point origin of this long-standing pain in the lateral chest wall was recognized.

Characteristics of activated trigger points

From what has already been said it is now possible to summarize the various characteristics of activated trigger points.

1. Structures liable to contain trigger points include muscles, tendons, joint capsules, ligaments, the periosteum and the skin.

2. A trigger point, depending on the degree to which it is activated, may be either latent or active.
3. Neural hyperactivity causes both latent and active trigger points to be exquisitely tender. As a result of this, when such a point is palpated, the patient flinches in a manner which is out of proportion to the amount of pressure exerted on it by the examining finger. This is the so-called 'jump sign'.
4. Active trigger points are responsible for the referral of pain, either locally, or at some distant site, or both.
5. Each muscle has its own characteristic specific pattern of pain referral from trigger points contained in it.
6. The spontaneous pattern of pain complained of by a patient may sometimes be reproduced by exerting sustained pressure on, or inserting a needle into, an active trigger point.
7. Active trigger points are sometimes associated with autonomic disturbances in the zone of pain referral.
8. Active trigger points in a muscle cause it to become shortened and somewhat weakened.
9. A local twitch response may be observed when a palpable band in a superficially placed muscle is smartly 'plucked'.
10. A trigger point's neural hyperactivity may subside spontaneously or it may be maintained indefinitely as a result of motor or sympathetic efferent activity causing the development of a self-perpetuating circuit.

REFERENCES

Arroyo P 1966 Electromyography in the evaluation of reflex muscle spasm. Journal of the Florida Medical Association 53: 29–31
Awad E A 1973 Interstitial myofibrositis: hypothesis of the mechanism. Archives of Physical Medicine 54: 440–453
Awad 1990 Histopathological changes in fibrositis. In: Fricton J R, Awad E A (eds) Advances in Pain Research and Therapy. Raven Press, New York, vol 17, p 249–258
Bates T, Grunwaldt E 1958 Myofascial pain in childhood. Journal of Pediatrics 53: 198–209
Becker R O, Reichmanis M, Marino A A, Spadaro J A 1976 Electrophysiological correlates of acupuncture points and meridians. Psychoenergetic System 1: 105–112
Bonica J J 1957 Management of myofascial pain syndromes in general practice. Journal of the American Medical Association 165: 732–738
Brendstrup P, Jespersen K, Asboe-Hansen G 1957 Morphological and chemical connective tissue changes in fibrositic muscles. Annals of Rheumatic Diseases 16: 438–440
Cooperative Group of Investigation of PSC 1980 A survey of occurrence of the phenomenon of propagated sensation along channels (PSC). In: Advances in acupuncture and acupuncture anaesthesia: abstracts of papers presented at the National Symposium of Acupuncture, Moxibustion and Acupuncture Anaesthesia, Beijing 1979. The People's Medical Publishing House, Beijing, p 258–260
Copeman W S, Ackerman W L 1944 'Fibrositis' of the back. Quarterly Journal of Medicine 13: 37–51
de Valera E, Raftery H 1976 Lower abdominal and pelvic pain in women. In: Bonica J J, Albe-Fessard D (eds) Advances in pain research and therapy. Raven Press, New York, vol 1, p 935–936
Dexter J R, Simons D G 1981 Local twitch response in

human muscle evoked by palpation and needle penetration of a trigger point. Archives of Physical Medicine and Rehabilitation 62: 521–522

Fassbender H G 1975 Pathology of rheumatic diseases. Springer-Verlag, New York

Fields H H 1987 Pain. McGraw-Hill, New York, p 152

Fisher A A 1984 Diagnosis and management of chronic pain in physical medicine and rehabilitation. In: Ruskin A (ed) Current therapy in physiatry. W B Saunders, Philadelphia

Fischer A 1986 Temperature and pressure threshold measurements in trigger points. Thermology 1: 212–215

Fischer A 1988a Documentation of muscle pain and soft tissue pathology. In: Kraus H (ed) Diagnosis and treatment of muscle pain. Quintessence, Chicago

Fischer A 1988b Documentation of myofascial trigger points. Archives of Physical Medicine and Rehabilitation 69: 286–291

Fricton J R, Awad E A 1990 Myofascial pain and fibromyalgia. Advances in Pain Research and Therapy vol 17. Raven Press, New York

Glogowski G, Wallraff J 1951 Ein beitrag zur Klinik und Histologie der Muskelhärten (Myogelosen). Zeitschrift Orthópädie 80: 237–268

Good M G 1949 Acroparaesthesia — an idiopathic myalgia of elbow. Edinburgh Medical Journal 56: 336–368

Gorrell R L 1976 Troublesome ankle disorders and what to do about them. Consultant 16: 64–69

Hobbins W B 1989 Hot spots and trigger point correlation. Initial, Quarterly letter for thermal image analysis (Madison, Wisconsin) 10(1) 12–13

Inman V T, Saunders R B 1944 Referred pain from skeletal structures. Journal of Nervous and Mental Disease 99: 660–667

Kellgren H J 1939 The distribution of pain arising from deep somatic structures with charts of segmental pain areas. Clinical Science 4: 35–46

Kraft G H, Johnson E W, La Ban M M 1968 The fibrositis syndrome. Archives of Physical Medicine and Rehabilitation 49: 155–162

Leriche R 1930 Des effetes de l'anaesthésie à la novocaine des ligaments et des insertions tendinuses. Gazatte des Hospitaux 103: 1294

Livingston W K 1943 Pain mechanisms. Macmillan, New York

Macdonald A J R 1980 Abnormally tender muscle regions and associated painful movements. Pain 8: 197–205

Macdonald A J R 1982 Acupuncture from ancient art to modern medicine. George Allen & Unwin, London

Mann F 1974 The treatment of disease by acupuncture, 3rd edn. Heinemann Medical, London

Popelianskii I, Zaslavskii E S, Veselorskii V P 1976 Medicosocial significance, aetiology, pathogenesis and diagnosis of non-articular disease of soft tissues of the limbs and back (Russian). Voprosy Revmatizma 3: 38–43

Research Group of Acupuncture Anaesthesia, Institute of Medicine and Pharmacology of Fujian Province 1986 Studies of phenomenon of blocking activities of channels and collaterals. In: Zhang X (Chang H-T) ed. Research on acupuncture, moxibustion and acupuncture anaesthesia. Science Press, Beijing 653–667

Reynolds M D 1981 Myofascial trigger point syndromes in the practice of rheumatology. Archives of Physical Medicine and Rehabilitation 62: 111–114

Rubin D D 1981 Myofascial trigger point syndrome: an approach to management. Archives of Physical Medicine and Rehabilitation 62: 107–110

Schade 1919 Beiträge zur Umgrenzung and Klärung einer Lehre von der Erkältung. Zeitschrift Gesellschaft Experimentaler Medizin 7: 275–374

Simons D G 1975 Muscle pain syndromes — part I. American Journal of Physical Medicine 54: 289–311

Simons D G 1976a Electrogenic nature of palpable bands and 'jump' sign associated with myofascial trigger points. In: Bonica J J, Albe-Fessard D (eds) Advances in pain research and therapy. Raven Press, New York

Simons D G 1976b Muscle pain syndromes — Part II. American Journal of Physical Medicine 55: 15–42

Simons D G 1987 Myofascial pain syndrome due to trigger points. International Rehabilitation Medicine Association Monograph Series, no 1. Rademaker, OH: International Rehabilitation Medicine Association

Simons D G, Travell J G 1981 Myofascial trigger points, a possible explanation. Pain 10: 106–109

Simons D G, Travell J G 1989 Myofascial pain syndromes. In: Wall P, Melzack R (eds) Textbook of pain. Churchill Livingstone, Edinburgh, 2nd edn, p 368–385

Sinclair D C 1949 The remote reference of pain aroused in the skin. Brain 72: 364–372

Sola A E 1981 Myofascial trigger point therapy. Resident Staff Physician 38–45

Sola A E, Rodenberger M L, Gettys B B 1955 Incidence of hypersensitive areas in posterior shoulder muscles. American Journal of Physical Medicine 34: 585–590

Stockman R 1904 The causes, pathology and treatment of chronic rheumatism. Edinburgh Medical Journal 15: 107–116, 223–235

Swerdlow B, Dieter J N I 1992 An evaluation of the sensitivity and specificity of medical thermography for the documentation of myofascial trigger points. Pain 48: 205–213

Travell J G 1976 Myofascial trigger points: clinical view. In: Bonica J J, Albe-Fessard D (eds) Advances in pain research and therapy 1. Raven Press, New York, p 916–926

Travell J G, Berry C, Bigelow N 1944 Effects of referred somatic pain on structures in the reference zone. Federation Proceedings 4: 49

Travell J G, Bigelow N H 1946 Referred somatic pain does not follow a simple 'segmental' pattern. Federation Proceedings 5: 106

Travell J G, Simons D G 1983 Myofascial pain and dysfunction. The trigger point manual. Williams and Wilkins, Baltimore.

Trommer P R, Gellman M B 1952 Trigger point syndrome. Rheumatism 8: 67–72

Wegelius O, Asboe-Hansen G 1956 Mast cell and tissue water. Studies on living connective tissue in the hamster cheek pouch. Experimental Cell Research 11: 437–443

Xue 1986 The phenomenon of propagated sensation along channels (PSC) and the cerebral cortex. In: Zhang X (Chang H-T) (ed) Research in acupuncture, moxibustion and acupuncture anaesthesia. Science Press, Beijing, p 668–683

8. The deactivation of trigger points

INTRODUCTION

Although, as explained in Chapters 4 and 5, it is possible to deactivate trigger points by means of injecting a local anaesthetic into them, it has been shown that this may be done equally well by injecting any one of a number of different substances into these points, or even more simply and just as effectively by stimulating, with dry needles, nerve endings in the tissues overlying them. It is extremely fortunate that the injection of a local anaesthetic is not necessary, as occasionally and unpredictably it is associated with the development of serious adverse reactions. These include anaphylactic shock which may arise as a result of allergy to the local anaesthetic or to the preservative added to it, and various dose-related toxic effects.

The Committee on Safety of Medicines reported in 1986 (CSM update 1986) that, from 1964 onwards, anaesthetists had recorded on yellow cards a total of 561 adverse reactions to all the commonly-used local anaesthetics. These included syncope, palpitations, apnoea, cardiac arrest and convulsions. In the case of lignocaine, the currently most widely used local anaesthetic, the total number of reported reactions was 329 with 9 deaths.

It is therefore important to note that although Travell & Simons (1983) advocate the use of a local anaesthetic for the purpose of deactivating trigger points, they nevertheless admit that it only requires a minimal dose to bring on life-threatening anaphylactic shock in a susceptible person. Also that dose-related toxic effects may develop whenever a considerable quantity of a local anaesthetic has to be used for the deactivation of numerous trigger points. It is for these reasons that they recommend that, whenever this form of therapy is carried out, a tourniquet, intravenous diazepam, equipment for artificial respiration and a cardiac defibrillator should all be readily to hand.

In addition, the intramuscular injection of a local anaesthetic may cause muscle necrosis. This is particularly prevalent with long-acting anaesthetic agents. The risk is certainly less with shorter-acting ones and procaine is the least myotoxic of all those commonly in use. However, even with this, care has to be taken not to use it mixed with adrenaline as this increases the possibility of muscle damage (Benoit 1978). It should also be noted that procaine is made up as a solution in normal saline and, certainly, repeated intramuscular injections of isotonic sodium chloride have been shown to cause an inflammatory response (Pizzolato & Mannheimer 1961). Further, procaine, when injected into a muscle, is capable of producing a curare-like action (Harvey 1939), and for this reason occasionally causes a somewhat distressing, albeit temporary, loss of power. Also, when injected around a nerve it is liable to cause some transitory sensory loss.

Another disadvantage of using a local anaesthetic is that it is often necessary to identify and to deactivate a number of trigger points in the same area. However when such a substance is injected into a point it inevitably diffuses over a wide area and by suppressing the tenderness of neighbouring trigger points makes their identification difficult. In an attempt to avoid this complication, Travell advocates using only a 0.5% procaine solution. As this is not commercially available, she recommends diluting the standard 2% solution with isotonic saline by mixing three parts of saline with one part of procaine. It seems doubtful, however, whether even with such a dilute solution it is possible to ensure the anaesthetic effect remains localized, particularly as an experiment, conducted by herself to test the effectiveness of procaine in concentrations ranging from 0.1% to 2% in physiological saline, showed that a 0.5% solution produced as much anaesthesia as a 2% solution (Travell 1960).

A MULTIPLICITY OF METHODS OF DEACTIVATING TRIGGER POINTS

Travell & Rinzler in their classic contribution to the subject entitled 'The myofascial genesis of pain' published in 1952 stated that besides injecting a local anaesthetic into trigger points it is possible to deactivate them either by subjecting them to sustained pressure or by stretching the tissues and spraying the overlying skin with ethyl chloride. In passing, they mentioned that dry needling achieves the same effect!

Martin (1952), a specialist in physical medicine at the Royal Free Hospital, London, also that year reported satisfactorily alleviating myofascial pain (or what he called fibrositis) by injecting a rather curious mixture of benzyl salicylate and camphor in arachis oil into what, from his description of them, were clearly trigger points.

Sola & Kuitert (1955) then decided, in view of Martin's report, and because they were concerned about the potentially serious side effects of local anaesthetics, to see whether it would be possible to deactivate trigger points by injecting into them anything as simple as normal saline. They first tried this out in several individuals known to be sensitive to procaine and, on finding the results to be extremely promising, proceeded to use this method in 100 consecutive cases of myofascial trigger point pain in the neck and shoulder girdle treated by them at a United States Air Force Hospital in Texas. In their report of this trial, they concluded that 'the use of normal saline has none of the disadvantages often associated with the use of local anaesthetic but appears to have the same therapeutic value'.

A year later, Sola & Williams (1956) were able to confirm the usefulness of injecting saline into trigger points in a variety of myofascial pain syndromes occurring in over 1000 patients treated at the same hospital. In view of these encouraging reports, it is somewhat strange that little further interest appears to have been shown in this technique until 1980, when Frost et al reported the results of a double-blind comparison of the local anaesthetic mepivacaine and saline injected into trigger points. To their surprise, the group in which saline was used did better, with 80% of such patients reporting relief from pain as compared to 52% with mepivacaine.

That Sola and his colleagues were not the first to discover that the injection of substances other than local anaesthetics may be used for the alleviation of musculoskeletal pain is evident from the fact that when Joseph Needham, the distinguished sinological scholar, visited the medical historian, Charles Singer, at his home in Cornwall in 1947, Singer informed Needham that he was having injections of a local anaesthetic into his back to relieve his lumbago. He also told Needham that his physician had said that injections of distilled water or even the prick of a hypodermic needle without anything being injected sometimes did just as well. Needham (Lu Gwei Djen & Needham 1980a) states:

I therefore wrote to Singer's consultant, Gilbert Causey, saying that if this were really so it approximated to the ancient Chinese practice of acupuncture and asked for further details. Causey replied that his interest in such techniques had been awakened first by a member of the French school, J. J. Forestier, whom he had heard lecture in 1929. Causey's custom was to inject all types of fluid — Novocain, water, osteocalcin, camphrosalyl — with equally satisfactory results. Naturally he was uncertain how far these effects had a true physiological basis, but the proportion of subjects relieved or cured was much higher than could be expected on the basis of a placebo effect.

As stated in Chapter 3, it was during the first part of the 19th century that the English medical practitioner, Churchill, first drew Western trained doctors' attention to the effectiveness of dry needling in alleviating musculoskeletal pain. That it only had intermittent phases of popularity during the rest of the 19th century and the early part of the 20th century would seem to have been for no other reason than that nobody at that time could provide a credible explanation as to how it might work.

The situation now, however, is quite different for, as a result of recent advances in knowledge concerning the neurophysiology of pain, it is clear that the reason why it is possible to alleviate pain emanating from trigger points either by injecting, via needles, one or another of a wide range of different substances into these structures or, even more simply, by inserting needles into the tissues overlying them, is because these seemingly different types of therapy all have one factor in common, namely, needle stimulation of A-delta nerve fibres. As also discussed in Chapters 6 and 10, the effect of stimulating A-delta afferents with needles is to block the C afferent input to the spinal cord from trigger points as a result of stimulation of this type evoking activity in complex pain modulating mechanisms situated in the central nervous system.

One of the first physicians to use dry-needling extensively for the deactivation of trigger points during the latter part of this century was Karel Lewit of Czechoslovakia. Lewit (1979) reported favourably on the use of this technique in a series of 241 patients with a variety of different myofascial pain disorders treated during the years 1975–1976. Both he and, since then, Jaeger & Skootsky (1987) have stressed that in their opinion the effectiveness of dry needling for this purpose is related to the precision with which a needle is inserted into the trigger point. It is certainly essential to locate each trigger point accurately, but there are now grounds for believing that it is not necessary to insert the needle into the trigger point itself and that it is easier, safer and just as effective to insert it into the tissues overlying a trigger point.

My reasons for saying this are that some years ago, when attempting to deactivate a trigger point in the scalenus anterior muscle, it seemed prudent to me, in view of the proximity of the apex of the lung, only to insert the needle for a short distance under the skin, and found that this was sufficient to relieve the pain referred down the arm from this trigger point. Superficial needling at trigger point sites elsewhere in the

body was then tried and found to be equally effective. Not long after this Macdonald et al (1983) confirmed my findings by showing that it is possible to alleviate low-back pain by inserting needles to an approximate depth of only 4 mm at trigger point sites.

Bowsher (1990) has now explained why superficial needling is all that is required by pointing out that the A-delta sensory afferents, which are the ones stimulated whenever a needle is inserted into the body, are present mainly but not exclusively in the skin and just beneath it.

Superficial dry needling for the relief of musculoskeletal pain is not some recent innovation. In that part of the 1st-century book *Huang Ti Nei Ching* where it discusses the insertion of needles into certain points on the back along the so-called urinary bladder meridian, it clearly advocates the employment of shallow needling (Lu Gwei Djen & Needham 1980b).

Superficial dry needling at trigger point sites

When carrying out superficial needling for the relief of myofascial trigger point pain, each trigger point must be accurately located and then care must be taken to ensure that the needle is inserted into the tissues immediately overlying it. This is in order to make certain that the A-delta nerve fibres stimulated in this manner and the referred pain-producing C afferent fibres in the trigger point project to the same dorsal horn. The needle-induced A-delta afferent activity is then enabled to block the trigger point's C afferent input to the spinal cord by evoking activity in enkephalinergic inhibitory interneurons situated in the border of Lamina I and II of this dorsal horn by two separate means (Bowsher 1990).

One way in which this occurs is by the A-delta afferent fibres in the outer part of the dorsal horn having branches which project directly to these inhibitory interneurons (Fig. 8.1). The other is by these inhibitory interneurons undergoing excitation by the more indirect means of activity developing in the descending inhibitory system. This happens as a result of there being a pathway which links the neospinothalamic tract and the upper end of the descending inhibitory system in the periaqueductal grey area of the midbrain for,

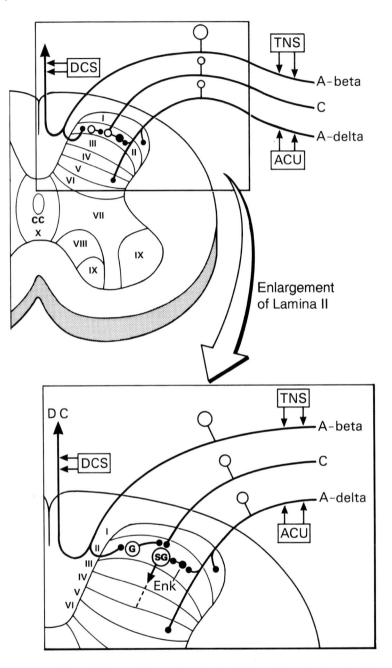

Fig. 8.1 Entry of primary afferents into the dorsal horn of the spinal cord, and circuits involved in TENS and acupuncture. Roman numerals refer to laminae numbers. SG = Substantia gelatinosa cell. G = GABAergic interneuron, presynaptically inhibiting primary afferent C fibre terminal. Enk = Enkephalinergic interneuron, postsynaptically inhibiting substantia gelatinosa neuron. The enkephalinergic interneuron is not only activated, as shown, by A-delta primary afferent terminals, but also by serotoninergic fibres descending from the brainstem (see Fig. 8.2). CC = Central canal. DC = Dorsal column. DCS = Dorsal column stimulation. TNS = Low-threshold, high frequency stimulation. ACU = High-threshold, low frequency stimulation. Dr David Bowsher's diagram in Journal of British Medical Acupuncture Society 1990. Reproduced with permission.

as explained in Chapter 6, this allows A-delta sensory afferent-generated electrical impulses in this ascending pathway to promote activity in the opioid peptide mediated serotinergic fibres situated in the descending dorsolateral funiculus (Fig. 8.2).

While this would seem to be how brief stimulation of A-delta nerve fibres with a dry needle brings about immediate nocigenic pain relief, it does not explain why such relief at times continues to last for weeks, months or even permanently. However, with respect to this, it has to be remembered that movements are often markedly restricted by pain and once the latter has been alleviated by acupuncture the consequent restoration of movements and associated stretching of the tissues stimulates activity in low-threshold mechanoreceptors and their attached A-beta nerve fibres. As discussed in Chapter 6, it has for long been known that activity in the branches of the A-beta fibres which reach Lamina II of the dorsal horn suppress the C afferent input to the cord.

This, however, is certainly not the whole answer and it is generally recognized that there is still much to be unravelled concerning the pain suppressing effects of acupuncture (see Ch. 10).

Acupuncture points

It has been suggested that those of us who practise acupuncture by inserting needles into the tissues overlying trigger points do not use traditional acupuncture points (Vincent 1989, Filshie & Abbott 1991). Before coming to such a conclusion however it is first necessary to ask, what is an acupuncture point?

In investigating this, Yang & Ren (1986) inserted needles into classical acupuncture sites in cadavers and then from careful anatomical dissection came to the conclusion that such points are invariably where peripheral nerves terminate. Pan & Zhao (1986), for the same reason, put needles into classical acupuncture sites in limbs about to be

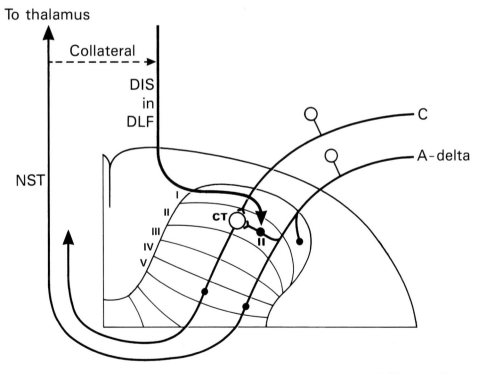

Fig. 8.2   Diagram of dorsal horn to show the local intraspinal connection between A-delta nerve fibres and enkephalinergic inhibitory interneuron (II), whose function it is to inhibit activity in C afferent terminal cell (CT). Also, to show the indirect A-delta link with inhibitory interneuron via the collateral connecting the A-delta afferent's ascending pathway — the neospinothalamic tract (NST) with the descending inhibitory system in the dorsolateral funiculus (DIS in DLF).

amputated and inserted them to whatever depth was necessary to cause patients to experience needle sensations (Ch. 7). Then, by an ingenious electrolytic process, they caused free ferric irons to be deposited in the tissues around the tip of each needle, and the iron then gave a Prussian blue reaction on injecting potassium ferrocyanide into the tissues. Following amputation, the blue stained tissue was fixed and impregnated with silver before being examined microscopically. By means of this method they found that the depth at which acupuncture points lie varies from 0.4–3.2 cm and that the sites where they are to be found include muscles, tendons, periosteum and the subcutaneous tissues. Like Yang & Ren, they found that each point contains free nerve endings. This, of course, is in keeping with Bowsher's observation (1987) that:

superimposition of a map of acupuncture points on an illustration of the course and *termination* of peripheral nerves taken from a standard textbook of anatomy show that they coincide more often than not — particularly the (anatomically) unnamed branchlets.

It is therefore apparent that a so-called acupuncture 'point' is a localized area of tissue containing a plentiful supply of nerve bundles and it is now known that these bundles are predominantly made up of A-delta afferents and sympathetic efferents. It is because of these sympathetic efferents and the sweat glands which they innervate that the skin overlying an acupuncture 'point' has a lower electrical resistance (impedance) than skin elsewhere.

Many attempts have been made to detect acupuncture points by searching for areas of lowered skin impedance with various types of electrical measuring devices. In general, however, such apparatus, when used for this purpose, has proved to be unreliable and this method of point detection cannot be recommended.

As myofascial trigger point pain is readily alleviated by needling the tissues directly overlying trigger points it would seem reasonable to conclude from what has been said that these must be sites where there is a plentiful supply of A-delta nerve fibres and that such sites therefore may be considered to be superficially placed acupuncture points.

With reference to this, it is of considerable interest to note that Melzack et al (1977) compared the spatial distribution of trigger points on maps compiled by Travell & Rinzler (1952), Sola & Kuitert (1955), Kennard & Haugen (1955) and Sola & Williams (1956), with that of traditional Chinese acupuncture points on maps compiled by Mann (1966). They also compared the pain syndrome said to be associated with each of these acupuncture points in two well-known traditional Chinese acupuncture textbooks (Mann 1967, Kao & Kao 1973) with that said to be associated with the trigger point closest to it.

This analysis revealed a 71% degree of correspondence both between the spatial distribution and the associated pain patterns of traditional acupuncture points and trigger points, findings which let Melzack and his colleagues to conclude that:

the close correlation between trigger points and acupuncture points for pain is remarkable since the distribution of both types of points are historically derived from such different concepts of medicine. Trigger points are firmly anchored in the anatomy of the neural and muscular systems, while acupuncture points are associated with an ancient conceptual but anatomically non-existent system of meridians which carry Yin (spirits) and Yang (blood). Despite the different origins, however, it is reasonable to assume that acupuncture points for pain relief, like trigger points, are derived from the same kind of empirical observation: that pressure at certain points is associated with particular pain patterns, and brief, intense stimulation of the points by needling sometimes produces prolonged relief of pain. These considerations suggest a hypothesis; that trigger points and acupuncture points for pain, though discovered independently and labelled differently, represent the same phenomenon.

Clearly from this it is evident that Melzack and his colleagues considered that trigger points and acupuncture points are one and the same. However, in the light of what has already been said concerning differences in their structural make-up, it would seem to be more likely that they are of two different types, and that their close spatial correlation is because there are A-delta afferent-innervated acupuncture points in the skin and subcutaneous tissues immediately above intramuscularly placed predominantly C afferent-innervated trigger points.

Manual acupuncture versus electroacupuncture

Acupuncture may be carried out manually or, alternatively, by the method first employed in the last century of passing an electric current through the needle (electroacupuncture). Electroacupuncture will be discussed further in the next chapter, but at this stage it should be said that at the present time there is a wide difference of opinion as to its therapeutic indications. Some authorities both in the East and in the Western world seem to use it as the method of choice in all cases. Others including Lewith (1985) and myself believe that it, together with the closely allied technique of transcutaneous electrical nerve stimulation (TENS), should be reserved for use in the alleviation of neurogenic pain; the suppression of operative and postoperative pain; the treatment of heroin addiction; and perhaps when manual stimulation of needles fails to relieve pain of musculoskeletal origin.

From clinical observations made by myself and others, it is my belief that in the routine treatment of myofascial trigger point pain disorders, from which incidentally the majority of chronic pain patients suffer, it is better to use manual acupuncture. A detailed description of how this should be carried out will therefore be given but firstly various matters relating to acupuncture needling in general will be considered.

Acupuncture needles

The standard acupuncture needle is made of stainless steel. There are some who advocate the use of gold and silver needles in the belief that they have special therapeutic properties but there is no scientific evidence for this.

Both reusable and disposable needles are available but in the present climate of concern about the spread of AIDS (Vittecoq et al 1989) and in view of the very real risk of transmitting the hepatitis B virus (Kent et al 1988) it is preferable to use disposable needles.

Acupuncture needles range from 7 mm to 125 mm in length and from 0.20 mm to 0.35 mm in diameter. However, for the superficial type of needling advocated in this book, a relatively short, moderately thin needle should be used and the one most commonly employed by me is 30 mm in length and 0.30 mm in diameter. Clearly this is longer than is necessary, as with shallow needling a needle is never inserted to a depth of more than 5–10 mm, but it is better to use a needle two or three times this length in order to avoid inserting it up to the hilt with the risk of breaking it. And the advantage of using a needle of this diameter is that it is thin enough to be readily inserted but not so thin as to buckle when it is pushed through the skin.

Wheal and flare response to needling

When a needle penetrates the skin, the resultant tissue injury may be associated with the development of erythema at the needle insertion site followed in some cases by the fairly rapid build up of some localized oedema (wheal) and spread of the erythema into the surrounding skin (flare). Lewis (1942) observed this sequence of events following any superficial injury to the skin and at the time thought that the vasodilation responsible for it was solely due to the release of histamine. However, it is now known that an injury of this type stimulates unmyelinated C sensory fibres and that, as a result of this, a number of powerful vasodilating substances are liberated into the tissues, including Substance P, neurokinins A and B, and other peptides (Melzack & Wall 1988).

Needle sensations

From the time that the ancient Chinese first started to use acupuncture it has been known that needling may give rise to the development of one or another of a number of characteristic sensations. These sensations are collectively known in Chinese as tê chhi (sometimes spelt teh chi and pronounced derchi). They include numbness, aching, soreness and tissue distension (see Ch. 7) and should not be confused with the initial pain produced by the needle pricking the skin.

Traditional Chinese acupuncturists believe that these sensations are only readily obtainable if needling is carried out at designated acupuncture points. Vincent et al (1989), however, failed to confirm this when, in a carefully conducted trial, they found that these sensations could equally well be elicited by needling either classical or non-classical (sham) acupuncture points.

Those whose practice it is to insert needles into designated points, also state that, for acupuncture to be successful, it is essential to obtain a needle sensation and for this reason advocate that manipulation of the needle should be continued until this happens. It is not, however, in my experience necessary to obtain tê chhi when carrying out superficial needling at trigger point sites for the relief of musculoskeletal pain. In accord with this, Macdonald (1989) has recently confirmed that when he and his colleagues (Macdonald et al 1983) showed that low-back pain may be alleviated successfully by means of inserting needles into the skin and subcutaneous tissues overlying trigger points and leaving them without any further form of manipulation for approximately 5 minutes, the eliciting of needle sensations was not found to be necessary.

Variable responsiveness to needle stimulation

The amount of needle stimulation required by individuals is widely variable. About 10% of the adult population and also most children are strong reactors and only need minimal needle stimulation to alleviate their pain. Another small group of adults are weak reactors and require exceptionally vigorous and prolonged stimulation. There are also a few people who do not respond at all.

Adult strong reactors

Felix Mann (1983a) believes he can recognize strong reactors by virtue of their having particularly sensitive, intuitive, lively personalities; in addition, many of them are so intolerant of pharmacological substances that they react adversely to the substances if given in anything more than very small doses. He admits, however, that in spite of many years' experience he is only right in his prediction as to whether or not a person will prove to be a strong reactor in about 3 out of 4 cases.

It therefore follows that the only certain way of assessing a person's responsiveness is by means of trial and error and as the effect of stimulating a strong reactor too vigorously is to cause a temporary but nevertheless distressing exacerbation of pain it is essential whenever treating a person for the first time to ensure that only the minimum amount of stimulation required to abolish the exquisite tenderness at a trigger point site is given.

It is remarkable how very little stimulation strong reactors require. In discussing this Mann (1983b) remarks:

I have many patients who respond best to only one or two shallow pricks with thin, sharp needles, with needles not left in place, and the treatment repeated only infrequently.

Strong reactors often experience a pleasantly relaxed feeling whilst being needled and following it may feel soporific and eventually may fall into a deep sleep. It is also in strong reactors that the phenomenon known as propagation along a channel (see Ch. 7) occurs.

Finally, as Mann (1974) has pointed out, it is only strong reactors who experience sufficient pain suppression from acupuncture anaesthesia (analgesia) for it to be used for major surgery (see Ch. 9).

Complications associated with dry needling

Providing that anyone practising acupuncture only uses needles which have been sterilized adequately and has a good knowledge of anatomy, the procedure is relatively safe. There are certainly far less harmful effects from it than from many of the drugs being prescribed currently for combating pain.

Vaso-vagal attacks

Some people faint at the sight of a needle let alone when it is inserted into them. People who are apprehensive about needles or have a past history of fainting when being inoculated should not be persuaded against their will to have treatment with acupuncture. As a liability to fainting is often unpredictable, it is important that at least on the first occasion treatment should be given lying down.

Convulsions

Very occasionally a person who has fainted in response to needle stimulation may proceed to have an epileptiform fit.

Post-treatment drowsiness

It is not uncommon for a patient to feel sleepy following acupuncture. The greater the amount of stimulation given, the more likely this is to occur, but in a strong reactor it may happen when this is only carried out quite lightly. Again, as such a reaction is impossible to predict, it is wise for a new patient to be accompanied by a friend who can if necessary drive the car on the journey home.

Damage to viscera

Viscera should not be damaged providing reasonable safeguards are taken. However, Peacher (1975), in reviewing the complications of acupuncture, reports cases where death has resulted from puncturing the heart. The spleen or liver may also be damaged but this usually occurs when such an organ is enlarged. A competent clinical examination before starting treatment should give warning of this hazard.

The one organ which can all too readily be punctured, however, is the lung. Many practitioners tend to forget how high up the in the neck the lung extends and how near to the chest wall it is, particularly when emphysematous. Needles in the neck and chest should never be inserted vertically but always at a shallow angle.

Haemorrhage

With acupuncture needles inserted relatively superficially as advocated in this book, bleeding is remarkably uncommon, and, when it does occur, is readily controllable by simple pressure. Occasionally a painful haematoma develops from bleeding under the skin. This is particularly liable to occur in the elderly and in those on steroids, due to abnormal capillary fragility.

THE TECHNIQUE OF DEACTIVATING TRIGGER POINTS

When one first starts to practise acupuncture, there is an instinctive feeling that to achieve any worthwhile effect it is necessary to apply a strong stimulus to A-delta nerve fibres. Certainly this may so when needling traditional acupuncture points not in the immediate vicinity of trigger points, for in *An Outline of Chinese Acupuncture* compiled by the Academy of Traditional Chinese Medicine (1975) various obviously very vigorous forms of stimulation are described including lifting, thrusting, rotating, vibrating, scraping, twirling, twisting, snapping and pounding the needle. However, when a needle is inserted superficially into the tissues overlying a trigger point at a site where the A-delta nerve fibres became chemically sensitized at the same time and for the same reason as the trigger point's C afferent fibres (see Ch. 7), the amount of stimulation required is surprisingly light.

It is my current practice when treating a patient for the first time to push a needle into the tissues overlying a trigger point to a depth of about 5–10 mm and to leave it there without any form of manipulation for 30 seconds.

The amount of stimulation required is the minimum necessary to abolish the exquisite tenderness which before needling made the patient wince involuntarily. Therefore, on withdrawing the needle, pressure as firm as before needling is applied to the trigger point site to see whether this has been achieved. One 30–second period of needling is sometimes all that is required but, when it is not, the needle should be replaced and left in situ for up to 2–3 minutes. Very occasionally this proves to be insufficient and the needle has to be re-introduced for an even longer period.

The purpose of adopting this step-by-step approach when determining a patient's individual responsiveness to acupuncture is to reduce the risk of causing a temporary but nevertheless distressing exacerbation of pain as a result of exceeding that person's optimum needle-stimulation requirement. As stated previously, with people who react very briskly to acupuncture, even a 30-second period of stimulation may prove to be too much. It is therefore necessary to inform every patient undergoing acupuncture for the first time that, for the reasons stated, the initial treatment may temporarily exacerbate their pain. It is important to do this for, should it happen without warning, it may be the cause of much unnecessary alarm or despondency. Admittedly any such flare-up usually only lasts for 12–24 hours, but occasionally it persists for several days. When this happens, great care must be taken to ensure that only light stimulation is applied on all subsequent occasions, and even then it is sometimes better to increase the intervals in between treatments.

In cases where there has not been a flare-up of pain following the first treatment, and this is in the majority of cases providing the graduated approach described above is followed, the time for which needles are left in situ at subsequent treatment sessions should either be kept the same as on the initial occasion or increased if the pain relief has not been as good as might be expected.

The number of treatment sessions

There seems to be general agreement amongst physicians in the Western World who use acupuncture for the relief of pain that, so far as chronic pain is concerned, treatment should not be carried out more often than once a week. This is because the full effects of this type of therapy often do not become apparent for several days and it may therefore be misleading to try to assess how much response there has been to it before the end of this time. At the end of 7 days, however, it is possible to determine whether or not any further treatment is required and, if so, depending on the response to whatever amount of stimulation was given the previous week, to decide whether this stimulation should be increased, decreased or kept the same. In cases where the pain is of a more acute type, it is often better to repeat the needling every 2–3 days.

It occasionally happens that the deactivation of trigger points on one occasion alone is sufficient to give lasting relief from long-standing pain.

This, however, is exceptional and normally several treatment sessions are required. Usually in a case where acupuncture is going to prove to be successful, there is a certain amount of relief following the first treatment, but this is short-lived and may last for no more than a few hours or, at the most, 1 or 2 days. Each time treatment is given, the period of relief from pain should increase so that after the third session any benefit should last for several days. If progressive improvement of this nature is not observed following the third time acupuncture is given, then this form of therapy should be discontinued as it is unlikely that the patient will obtain any lasting benefit from it. If, on the other hand, progress is satisfactory, then after the third session it may be possible to discontinue treatment or to increase the intervals between each one from once a week to once a fortnight and then to once a month. However, response to treatment follows no constant pattern, and each case has to be dealt with on an individual basis.

The number of sites to be needled

It is important for needling to be carried out at every active trigger point site. The failure of trigger point pain to respond to acupuncture is often because one or more trigger points have been overlooked. Trigger points, therefore, should be sought in a systematic manner (see Ch. 7).

There may be as many as 12–15 trigger points to be dealt with at any one time. Once all the obviously active trigger points have been deactivated, it is important for the patient to be reassessed in order to check that no trigger points have been missed. This should be done by testing the range of movements now possible, and by once again firmly palpating the areas likely to contain trigger points both at rest and whilst movements are carried out against resistance.

It is my usual practice when first treating a patient, and on all occasions with strong reactors, to deactivate each trigger point in turn with the same needle. However, in those cases when it is apparent that needles can be left in situ for an appreciable period without fear of exacerbating the pain there is no contraindication to needling a number of trigger points simultaneously.

Local steroid injections in the deactivation of myofascial trigger points

For many years now, the local injection of steroids into trigger points has been used widely in the treatment of a variety of painful musculo-skeletal disorders. There would seem to be certain situations in which this is the treatment of choice, but usually it is only necessary to deactivate the trigger points by means of acupuncture.

One of the advantages of injecting a steroid into trigger points over acupuncture is that the former has both a local and central effect. It is generally agreed that a steroid injected locally exerts a powerful anti-inflammatory effect by virtue of it having a variety of actions on the tissue. Some of the more important of these actions include inhibiting the production of collagen; decreasing the number of mast cells and fibroblasts; decreasing the permeability of connective tissue and the synthesis of hyaluronic acid; reducing the aminotripeptidase activity; and in addition stabilizing the lysosomal membranes. As Glyn (1971) pointed out 20 years ago, it is probably the latter which is the primary action, and that the other pharmacological mechanisms are secondary to it. Undoubtedly the pain-relieving effect of a locally-injected steroid is largely due to this local anti-inflammatory action. It is likely, however, that in addition it is partly due to a central action, for like dry needling over trigger points, it has a non-specific tissue irritant effect. Therefore, it is reasonable to suppose that when injected into a trigger point, it stimulates peripheral nerve endings and by so doing evokes activity in pain-modulating mechanisms in the nervous system in exactly the same manner as acupuncture achieves its analgesic effect.

A disadvantage of using a local steroid is that, because it has such a powerful irritant effect, there is often considerable post-injection pain for up to 24 hours. Also, there is always the risk that a steroid injection into a tendon may cause it to rupture. This is not of any particular consequence, e.g. with the long head of the biceps, but rupture of the Achilles tendon may be irreparable (Yates 1977). In addition, there is a limit to the number of times that a local steroid can be used, as repeated injections over a short period are liable to produce undesirable systemic effects, and locally to cause atrophy of the subdermal fat and some violaceous discolouration of the skin (Yates 1977). These local effects are particularly likely to occur when a long-acting agent is used, such as triamcinolone. It is, moreover, unwise and not particularly practicable, as well as usually quite unnecessary to inject a steroid into multiple trigger points such as are often present with musculo-skeletal disorders.

In my opinion, the only real indications for using a local steroid in preference to acupuncture in order to alleviate musculoskeletal pain is when this is associated with a marked inflammatory reaction such as so often occurs with disorders around the shoulder joint or at times with lesions of the epicondyles at the elbow. Its use may also occasionally prove necessary when, following the stimulation of a number of trigger points with dry needles, one or two of them prove resistant to this form of therapy.

Decisions, however, as to whether to use a local steroid or acupuncture are often far from easy and will be referred to again in greater detail when discussing individual disorders.

Laser therapy

The term laser is an acronym for 'light amplification by stimulated emission of radiation' and instruments used for laser therapy are either high, medium or low power emitters of radiation.

High-energy lasers which produce heat at infrared wavelengths are now widely used as cutting beams by surgeons.

Low-power instruments such as the helium-neon (He-Ne) laser which produces visible red light and the gallium-arsenide (Ga-As) laser are about 10,000 times weaker and because of this do not burn the tissues. It was hoped that this so-called athermic irradiation would have two therapeutic effects — the promotion of tissue healing and the alleviation of pain.

Seichert (1991), in a wide-ranging review of the subject, states that so far as the promotion of tissue healing is concerned, recent carefully conducted studies have failed to confirm low-power lasers' ability to influence this, as was originally suggested by results obtained from initial uncontrolled trials, and he is led to conclude that both for wound healing and the treatment of skin lesions lower-power laser irradiation of the skin is no better than irradiating it with naturally occurring 'normal' light.

It was also hoped that because laser therapy has such obvious practical advantages over dry needling that it would prove possible to use it instead of acupuncture for the relief of pain. Certainly some of the earlier uncontrolled trials suggested that this might be so (Walker 1983, Seitz & Kleinkort 1986).

It would seem reasonable to assume that any analgesic effect a low-energy laser might have would occur as a result of it stimulating nociceptive nerve endings in the same way as dry needling does, and for that reason laser analgesia therapy is often referred to as laser acupuncture. Apart from the fact that such a term is etymologically incorrect, Jarvis et al (1990), from electrophysiological studies on the cornea in rabbits, have shown that low energy He-Ne lasers have no appreciable stimulating effect on either A-delta or C nociceptors.

Further, Brockhaus & Elger (1990), in a controlled trial comparing the effects of needle acupuncture and laser acupuncture on the pain threshold of humans subjected to experimentally induced pain (cutaneous heat stimuli of 43°C), showed that the threshold remained uninfluenced by laser acupuncture but was significantly increased by needle acupuncture.

Recent clinical trials have similarly cast doubt on low-power lasers' ability to relieve pain.

Lundeberg et al (1987) carried out a study comparing the effects of a He-Ne laser, a Ga-As laser and a placebo laser in the treatment of lateral epicondylitis and found no significant difference in the results obtained with these three types of laser. Haker & Lundeberg (1990), believing that the dose of the Ga-As laser in the 1987 trial was too low, increased it in a trial comparing the effects of this type of laser and a placebo laser in two groups of patients with lateral epicondylitis and found no significant differences in their therapeutic effects.

Devor (1990), during the course of discussing these disappointing recent findings, points out that the red light emitted by He-Ne lasers used for pain relief is so weak that 'its beam packs about the same "radiation" punch as a small flashlight with a piece of red cellophane over the front', and that lasers of this type 'are not really very different from laser pointers used today in many lecture halls'. He then goes on to state that there is up to now no evidence to suggest that the pain relieving effect of a low-energy laser is any better than that of a placebo and ends up by asking, 'if a red flashlight with mystical labels is as effective as a $10,000 laser instruments, who wins when the laser is purchased?'

It is clear that further research has to be done in this field and the routine employment of a low-energy laser for the relief of myofascial trigger point pain cannot be recommended until such time as one is developed which is powerful enough to stimulate A-delta nerve fibres as effectively as, or even more effectively than, dry needling does.

REFERENCES

Academy of Traditional Chinese Medicine 1975 An outline of Chinese acupuncture. Foreign Language Press, Peking, p 10–13

Benoit P W 1978 Reversible skeletal muscle damage after administration of local anaesthetic with and without epinephrine. Journal of Oral Surgery 36: 198–201

Bowsher D 1987 The physiology of acupuncture. Intractable Pain Society 5: 15–18

Bowsher D 1990 Physiology and pathophysiology of pain. Journal of the British Medical Acupuncture Society 7: 17–20

Brockhaus A, Elger C E 1990 Hypalgesic efficacy of acupuncture on experimental pain in man. Comparison of laser acupuncture and needle acupuncture. Pain 43: 181–185

C S M Update 1986 Anaethetists and the reporting of adverse drug reactions. British Medical Journal 292: 949

Devor M 1990 What's in a laser beam for pain therapy? Pain 43: 139

Filshie J, Abbot P 1991 Acupuncture for chronic pain: A review. Journal of the British Medical Acupuncture Society 9: 4–14

Frost P A, Jessen B, Siggaard-Andersen J 1980 A controlled double-blind comparison of mepivacaine injection versus saline injection for myofascial pain. Lancet 1: 499–501

Glyn J H 1971 Rheumatic pains: some concepts and hypotheses. Proceedings of the Royal Society of Medicine 64: 354–360

Haker E, Lundeberg T 1990 Laser treatment applied to acupuncture points in lateral humeral epicondylalgia. A double-blind study. Pain 43: 243–247

Harvey A M 1939 The actions of procaine on neuromuscular

transmission. Bulletin of the Johns Hopkins Hospital 65: 223–238

Harvey A M 1939 The actions of procaine on neuromuscular transmission. Bulletin of the Johns Hopkins Hospital 65: 223–238

Jaeger B, Skootsky S A 1987 Double-blind, controlled study of different myofascial trigger point injection techniques. Pain suppl 4S 292

Jarvis D, MacIver M B, Tanelian D L 1990 Electrophysiologic recording and thermodynamic modeling demonstrate that helium-neon irradiation does not affect peripheral A-delta or C fiber nociceptors. Pain 43: 235–242

Kao F F, Kao J J 1973 Acupuncture therapeutics. Eastern Press, New Haven, Connecticut

Kennard M A, Haugen F P 1955 The relation of subcutaneous focal sensitivity to referred pain of cardiac origin. Anesthesiology 16: 297–311

Kent G P, Brondrum J, Kennylside R A, Lafazia L M, Scott H D 1988 A large outbreak of acupuncture-associated hepatitis B. American Journal of Epidemiology 127: 591–598

Lewis T 1942 Pain. Macmillan, New York.

Lewit K 1979 The needle effect in the relief of myofascial pain. Pain 6: 83–90

Lewith G T 1985 Acupuncture and transcutaneous nerve stimulation. In: Lewith G T (ed) Alternative therapies. Heinemann Medical, London

Lu Gwei Djen, Needham J 1980a Celestial Lancets, Cambridge University Press p 210, 1980b, p 209

Lundeberg T, Haker E, Thomas M 1987 Effect of laser versus placebo in tennis elbow. Scandinavian Journal of Rehabilitation Medicine 19: 135–138

Macdonald A J R 1989 Acupuncture analgesia and therapy. In: Wall P D, Melzack R (eds) Textbook of pain 2nd edn. Churchill Livingstone, Edinburgh, p 915

Macdonald A J R, Macrae K D, Master B R, Rubin A P 1983 Superficial acupuncture in the relief of chronic low-back pain. Annals of the Royal College of Surgeons of England 65: 44–46

Mann F 1966 Atlas of acupuncture. Heinemann Medical, London

Mann F 1967 The treatment of disease by acupuncture, 2nd edn. Heinemann Medical, London

Mann F 1974 Acupuncture analgesia. Report of 100 experiments. British Journal of Anaesthesia 46: 361–364

Mann F 1983a Scientific aspects of acupuncture, 2nd edn. Heinemann Medical, London, p 41–46 1983b p 32

Martin A J 1952 Nature and treatment of fibrositis. Archives of Physical Medicine 33: 409–413

Melzack R, Stillwell D M, Fox E J 1977 Trigger points and acupuncture points for pain: correlations and implications. Pain 3: 3–23

Melzack R, Wall P 1988 The challenge of pain, 2nd edn. Penguin Books, Harmondsworth p 100

Pan C, Zhao A 1986 Morphological study of sensations produced by needling different points. In: Zhang X (Chang H-T) (ed) Research on acupuncture, moxibustion and acupuncture anaesthesia. Science Press, Beijing, pp 618–625

Peacher W 1975 Adverse reactions, contraindications and complications of acupuncture and moxibustion. American Journal of Chinese Medicine 3: 35–46

Pizzolato P, Mannheimer W 1961 Histopathologic effects of local anaesthetic drugs and related substances. Charles C Thomas, Springfield, Illinois.

Seichert N 1991 Controlled trials of laser treatment. In: Schlapfach P, Gerber N J (eds) Physiotherapy: controlled trials and facts. Rheumatology. Karger, Basel, vol 14, p 205–217

Seitz L M, Kleinkort J A 1986 Low-power laser; its applications in physical therapy. In: Michlovitz S L (ed) Thermal agents in rehabilitation. Davis, Philadelphia, p 217–238

Sola A E, Kuitert J H 1955 Myofascial trigger point pain in the neck and shoulder girdle. North West Medicine 54: 980–984

Sola A E, Williams R L 1956 Myofascial pain syndromes. Neurology 6: 91–95

Travell J 1960 Temperomandibular joint pain referred from muscles of the head and neck. Journal of Prosthetic Dentistry 10: 745–763

Travell J, Rinzler S H 1952 The myofascial genesis of pain. Postgraduate Medicine 11: 425–434

Travell J G, Simons D G 1983 Myofascial pain and dysfunction. The trigger point manual. Williams & Wilkins, Baltimore, p 80

Vincent C A 1989 The methodology of controlled trials of acupuncture. Journal of the British Medical Acupuncture Society 6: 9–13

Vincent C A, Richardson P H, Black J J, Pither C E 1989 The significance of needle placement site in acupuncture. Journal of Psychosomatic Research 33(4) 489–496

Vittecoq D, Mettetal J F, Rouzioux C, Bach J F 1989 Acute HIV infection after acupuncture treatments. New England Journal of Medicine 320: 250–251

Walker J 1983 Relief from chronic pain by low power laser irradiation. Neuroscience Letters 43: 339–344

Yang F, Ren S 1986 Relative regularity between Jingluo points and spinal segmental innervation. In: Zhang X (Chang H-T) (ed) Research on acupuncture, moxibustion and acupuncture anaesthesia. Science Press, Beijing, pp 618–625

Yates D A H 1977 Use of local steroid injections. British Medical Journal 1: 495–496

9. Electrical stimulation of peripheral nerves

INTRODUCTION

The use of electricity for the relief of pain is not some recent innovation for the ancient Greeks employed the electrical discharge that emanates from the skate-like torpedo fish in attempting to alleviate persistent headaches and chronic arthralgias. Then, when in the middle of the 18th century Pieter van Musschenbroek discovered that it is possible to store electricity in what has come to be known as the Leyden jar, the possibility of using electricity in the treatment of disease was once again explored. And, as previously stated (Ch. 3), in 1825 the French physician Sarlandière became the first man to pass electricity through acupuncture needles. His contemporaries, however, viewed electroacupuncture with considerable suspicion as there was little or no understanding as to how it might work, and because by that time all forms of electrical treatment had been brought into disrepute by charlatans using them inappropriately (Kane & Taub 1975).

The situation today, however, is very different as during the latter part of this century the electrical stimulation of peripheral nerves for the relief of pain has been placed on a rational and scientific basis, and the events that have led to this will now be described.

ELECTROACUPUNCTURE

It was in 1958 that doctors at the First Shanghai People's Hospital decided to try to alleviate severe post-tonsillectomy throat pain in one of their patients by vigorously manipulating, by hand, a needle inserted into the first dorsal interosseous muscle. They chose this point, known in the tra-

ditional system of Chinese acupuncture as Ho-Ku (sometimes spelt Hegu), or Large Intestine 4, as needle stimulation of it had been used by the Chinese for centuries in the treatment of various painful disorders around the face, but this was the first time that any attempt had been made to suppress severe postoperative pain in this manner.

This procedure proved to be so effective that they next decided to use it on a patient immediately prior to the carrying out of a tonsillectomy in an attempt to suppress pain developing during the course of the operation. And once a report of this was published, acupuncture anaesthesia was soon being used throughout China (Macdonald 1982). It quickly became apparent, however, that in order to suppress operative pain, peripheral nerve endings have to be stimulated very strongly for at least 20 minutes, and that to achieve this by means of manipulating needles manually is a very laborious process. It was therefore in order to make this process easier that the Chinese turned to electroacupuncture, and before long were using it not only during operations but also for the treatment of various painful and non-painful conditions.

The Western world knew little or nothing about all this until 1972 when President Nixon visited China and saw demonstrations by doctors of the use of acupuncture as an anaesthetic and in the treatment of disease. Nixon's personal physician, Walter Tkach, was so impressed by what he saw that on his return to America he lost no time in publishing a report about it in the popular press entitled *I have seen Acupuncture work* (Tkach 1972). This was couched in such enthusiastic terms as to arouse much interest amongst the general public and it was not long before leaders of the medical profession, both in America (Bonica 1974) and in Britain (Smithers et al 1974) visited China to see the practice of acupuncture for themselves.

Any initial enthusiasm that there may have been in the Western world for adopting this technique for the purpose of controlling surgically-induced pain was seriously undermined when an article in the Daily Telegraph in 1980, under the title *China bursts acupuncture bubble* (Earnshaw 1980) sadly drew attention to a report that had recently appeared in the Shangai newspaper *Wen Hui Bao* revealing that during China's cultural revolution, doctors had been forced to use, and patients had been cajoled into receiving, acupuncture prior to undergoing major surgery as a matter of political expedience, regardless as to whether or not it was likely to be effective. Further, that when the procedure, as so often happens, failed to provide adequate pain control, the patient was ordered not to scream but instead to shout out political slogans! It also stated that any doctor who deliberately defied official policy by employing some alternative form of anaesthesia took the risk of being denounced as a counter-revolutionary and punished. This depressing state of affairs, according to the newspaper, was further compounded by those who wielded political power publishing misleading reports concerning the effectiveness of the method.

It is only right to stress, however, that subsequent to the revolution, doctors in China have done everything in their power to make amends for the shortcomings of their political masters by conducting research into the various aspects of acupuncture with the highest possible standards of integrity, and so far as the relief of pain is concerned have helped to place the technique on a sound scientific basis.

Electroacupuncture, whether it is being used for the suppression of operative or postoperative pain, or for the alleviation of neurogenic or musculoskeletal pain, involves the passing of a low frequency current of between 1–3 herz through needles inserted either into acupuncture points, or trigger points, or motor points, usually for about 20 minutes and with an intensity of current that is high enough to cause a sensation of discomfort just below the pain-threshold level

for the individual concerned. This is liable to be associated with powerful contractions of the muscle and considerable care therefore has to be taken to avoid this causing needles to become bent or broken (Academy of Traditional Chinese Medicine 1975). There certainly may be a place for it in the treatment of certain painful disorders but it is now generally agreed that it does not suppress surgically induced pain sufficiently to enable its use as an anaesthetic to be recommended (Mann 1974).

TRANSCUTANEOUS ELECTRICAL NERVE STIMULATION (TENS)

The next important advance in the use of electricity for the alleviation of pain was when, as a direct result of Melzack & Wall's spinal gate pain-control theory published in 1965, the technique of transcutaneous electrical stimulation of nerves was introduced. Melzack & Wall based their theory on the supposition that activity in large diameter myelinated primary afferent nerve fibres, by creating activity in inhibitory circuits present in the dorsal horn (the 'gate'), blocks the transmission of nociceptive impulses that pass along small diameter unmyelinated primary afferent fibres. They then argued that as large diameter fibres have a lower electrical resistance than small diameter fibres that it should be possible to suppress pain by preferentially stimulating large fibres in a peripheral nerve by means of passing an electric current through it.

It was as a direct consequence of this line of reasoning that Wall & Sweet (1967) set about stimulating electrically large fibres in peripheral nerves, first on themselves, and then on patients. They did this by three different methods including:

1. the stimulation of sensory roots entering the spinal cord (dorsal column stimulation)
2. the stimulation by electrodes surgically implanted around nerves and activated by subcutaneous radio-stimulators
3. the stimulation of peripheral nerve-endings by means of electrodes placed on the skin.

It is the third method, the transcutaneous electrical stimulation of nerves (TENS), that has proved to be so extremely useful in everyday clinical practice (Thompson 1984) and this one therefore that will be discussed in detail.

Conventional TENS

The manner in which TENS was carried out by Wall & Sweet and the one that, for reasons to be explained, should now be referred to as the conventional method, involves the placing of electrodes either over peripheral nerves; or over nerve-endings at trigger points or acupuncture points. The electrodes are connected to a portable battery-operated transistorized stimulator, and a high frequency current (10–300 herz or more) is passed through them at an intensity low enough to ensure that the sensation produced is only one of a comfortable buzzing or tingling feeling considerably below the pain threshold. For this form of electrical stimulus to be effective it has to be applied for at least 30 minutes and often much longer, and because of this the prolonged contact of the electrodes with the skin may give rise to a dermatitis (Long & Carolan 1974).

Thompson (1987) and Woolf (1989) have provided comprehensive accounts of the indications for conventional TENS. In addition Johnson et al (1991a) have recently reported a very useful in-depth study of a large number of patients who successfully used TENS on a long-term basis for relief of a wide variety of chronic pain conditions. Johnson et al (1991b) have also studied patients' individual pulse frequency and pulse pattern preferences.

Acupuncture-like TENS

The next stage in the development of methods for relieving pain by means of electrical stimulation was when Melzack (1975), because of the disadvantages associated with conventional TENS just mentioned, and because as he said 'the use of needles has an aura of the mysterious and unknown' decided to study the effects on severe chronic pain of applying a brief intense electrical stimulus via electrodes attached to the skin overlying the course of a major peripheral nerve, or over trigger points, or over acupuncture points, depending on which happened to be the most

convenient in any particular case. In this study carried out by Melzack on a number of patients suffering from either intractable neurogenic or musculoskeletal pain the transcutaneously applied stimulus was clearly similar to that used with electroacupuncture, for it was, as already stated, of relative brief duration, and the current employed was of low frequency (3 or 10 herz), but of high intensity, as may be seen from his statement that:

the stimulation was begun by raising the voltage slowly until the patient claimed that it hurt. The voltage was then decreased slightly and the patient was asked if he could tolerate that level of stimulation for 20 minutes. After a tolerable level was determined, the stimulation was maintained for 20 minutes at the same voltage... if the patient complained of excessive pain, the voltage was lowered slightly. An attempt was made, therefore, to maintain stimulation at an intense but tolerable level.

The results of this study led him to conclude that:

... the procedure proves a powerful method for the control of some forms of severe pathological pain. The average pain decrease during stimulation sessions was 75% for pain due to peripheral nerve injury; 66% for phantom limb pain; 62% for shoulder-arm pain; and 60% for low-back pain. The duration of relief frequently outlasted the period of stimulation by several hours, occasionally for days or weeks.

Differences between conventional TENS, acupuncture-like TENS, electroacupuncture and manual acupuncture

Melzack's method has since been widely adopted with the result that there are now two quite distinct forms of transcutaneous electrical stimulation in regular use. The one being conventional TENS in which a high frequency (10–300 herz or more) low intensity current is applied for several hours; and the other, acupuncture-like TENS in which a low frequency (1–10 herz) high intensity current is applied for a much shorter period of time (Eriksson et al 1979).

It is important to stress that the mechanisms of action of these two types of electrical stimulation would seem to be different in view of the fact that the analgesia from acupuncture-like TENS is reversed by naloxone, but that from conventional TENS is not (Sjölund & Eriksson 1979).

The explanation for this would seem to be that acupuncture-like TENS, in common with all other forms of acupuncture, stimulates A-delta nerve fibres and this in turn leads to the development of activity in opioid peptide mediated pain modulating mechanisms (Chs 7 & 10). In contrast to this, conventional TENS stimulates A-beta nerve fibres and the effect of this (Ch. 6) is to evoke not only naloxone reversible activity in the opioid peptide mediated descending inhibitory system (Bowsher 1991) but also non-naloxone reversible activity in gamma-aminobutyric acid mediated inhibitory interneurons (Thompson 1989).

It also should be noted that because high intensity low frequency transcutaneous electrical stimulation is liable to cause unpleasant muscle contractions (Melzack 1975, Andersson et al 1976), Eriksson et al (1979) have introduced yet a third technique using trains of high frequency stimuli repeated at a low frequency.

It therefore follows that as conventional TENS and acupuncture-like TENS have such different parameters and would seem to involve different pain modulating mechanisms in the central nervous system, it is essential, when discussing the use of transcutaneous electrical stimulation in the treatment of any particular condition, to make clear which of these two quite different types of TENS is being referred to; also in the title of any report. For example, Bates & Nathan (1980) in their report entitled *Transcutaneous electrical nerve stimulation for chronic pain*, are, from the parameters specified in the text quite obviously discussing the use of conventional type TENS, whereas Mannheimer & Carlsson (1979) in their report entitled *The analgesic effect of transcutaneous electrical nerve stimulation (TENS) in patients with rheumatoid arthritis* are conversely quite clearly discussing an acupuncture-like stimulus in all three of their groups of patients, for each patient was given 'a final stimulation level immediately below that causing pain' for a period of only 10 minutes, although the frequency used in the three groups was different. In the first group this was a classical acupuncture-like frequency of 3 herz; in the second group it was a much higher one of 70 herz; and in the third

group these two frequencies were used in an alternating sequence.

Wolf et al (1981) are therefore to be commended for specifically inserting conventional before transcutaneous electrical nerve stimulation (TENS) in the title of their report *Examination of electrode placements and stimulating parameters in treating chronic pain with conventional transcutaneous electrical nerve stimulation (TENS)*.

In the everyday clinical management of individual patients, however, it would seem wrong to employ either conventional TENS, or acupuncture-like TENS, using rigidly laid down parameters because the requirements vary from person to person with the optimum having to be found in every case by means of trial and error. Much trouble therefore has to be taken in explaining this to patients and much time has to be spent in determining by means of experimentation which particular electrode sites and which stimulation parameters are optimal for any particular individual (Long & Hagfors 1975), a task that sometimes is better accomplished by admitting the person to hospital for a short time (Wynn Parry 1980).

It therefore follows from what has been said that there are four methods of stimulating peripheral nerves in order to evoke activity in the central nervous system's various pain-modulating mechanisms:

— conventional TENS
— acupuncture-like TENS
— electroacupuncture
— manual stimulation of needles or what is usually simply referred to as acupuncture.

And there is still a considerable amount of work to be done in deciding upon the relative indications for their use.

There would seem to be general agreement that with regard to the suppression of acute postoperative pain, the pain of childbirth, and the alleviation of chronic neurogenic pain, one or other of the various forms of electrical stimulation is required. However it would be inappropriate to enter into any further discussion of this in a book that is primarily concerned with the treatment of musculoskeletal pain.

There is much less agreement however as to the best way of stimulating peripheral nerves when attempting to alleviate musculoskeletal pain, with some people using one or other form of electrical stimulation exclusively, others using manual stimulation of needles exclusively, whilst yet others, and probably the majority, employing the latter form of stimulation in the first instance, and some type of electrical stimulation for cases that fail to respond to this.

In any attempt to resolve the various differences of opinion it is essential to bear in mind that because with conventional TENS the stimulus is of a high frequency low intensity type, in contrast to acupuncture-like TENS where it is of low frequency and high intensity, it is likely, for reasons previously stated, that the pain-modulating mechanisms in the central nervous system evoked by these two methods are different. Similarly, when one comes to compare the manual stimulation of needles in what is usually referred to as acupuncture, with the electrical stimulation of needles in what is commonly termed electroacupuncture, it has to be remembered that although the stimulus with both techniques is of a low frequency, in the case of the former it is only applied for from a few seconds to a few minutes, whereas with the latter it is applied for a very much longer period of up to 20 minutes or more. And, because of this, there are good grounds for believing, as will be discussed in Chapter 10, that the endogenous pain-modulating systems evoked by these two procedures may also be different.

It is considerations such as these that make it essential when discussing needle stimulation to clearly distinguish between acupuncture and electroacupuncture and not, as so often happens, to use the two terms as if they are synonymous. It is, for example, perhaps unfortunate that Yuen et al (1976) in discussing the use of electroacupuncture with strong stimulation applied for 20–30 minutes do so in a paper entitled *The response to acupuncture in patients with chronic disabling pain*. Conversely Loy (1983) is to be commended for entitling his report *Treatment of cervical spondylosis — Electroacupuncture versus physiotherapy* as this has the virtue of making it clear as to exactly what form of stimulation was used, and with what it was being compared.

It is somewhat surprising considering the obvious differences between ordinary acupuncture, and the various forms of electrical stimulation including conventional TENS, acupuncture-like TENS, and electroacupuncture that there have been so few trials to compare their relative effectiveness in the alleviation of musculoskeletal pain. One such trial that has been carried out was that of Fox & Melzack (1976) in which they compared acupuncture-like TENS with manually-operated acupuncture in 12 patients suffering from chronic low-back pain. Analysis of the data failed to reveal any statistically significant differences between the two types of treatment but unfortunately the number of cases was small and the design of the trial is open to criticism. One group of patients received two treatments with acupuncture followed by two with TENS, and the other group received treatment in the reverse order, with each of the treatments being given at weekly intervals. The reason why this was unfortunate is that the effect of any form of peripheral nerve stimulation is liable to be delayed so that with a cross-over trial of this type, with only a week in between two separate forms of treatment, it is often difficult to distinguish between the effect of the first form of treatment and that of the second.

There is therefore much scope for further large-scale well-designed comparative trials, but, in the meantime, it has to be said that many experienced physicians consider that in the treatment of chronic musculoskeletal pain, the manual manipulation of needles for a few minutes or in some instances even for only a few seconds (Mann 1974) is usually all that is necessary. Moreover, many of us believe that for those trained in Western medicine it is more appropriate to carry this out at points of maximum tenderness or trigger points (Lewit 1979) rather than at preselected Chinese acupuncture points. And that it is only in those cases which prove resistant to this type of treatment that some form of electrical stimulation should be tried.

It is for these reasons that when discussing the use of acupuncture in various painful musculoskeletal disorders in Part Three of this book, emphasis will be placed on the manual manipulation of needles inserted into the tissues overlying trigger points.

REFERENCES

Academy of Traditional Chinese Medicine 1975 An outline
of Chinese acupuncture. Foreign Language Press, Peking,
p 26
Andersson S A, Hahsson G, Holmgren E 1976 Evaluation of
the pain suppressant effect of different frequencies of
peripheral electrical stimulation in chronic pain conditions.
Acta Orthopaedica Scandinavica 47: 149–157
Bates J A V, Nathan P W 1980 Transcutaneous electrical
nerve stimulation for chronic pain. Anaesthesia
35: 817–822
Bonica J J 1974 Therapeutic acupuncture in the People's
Republic of China. Journal of the American Medical
Association 228 (12): 1544–1551
Bowsher D 1991 The physiology of stimulation-produced
analgesia. Journal of the British Medical Acupuncture
Society IX(2): 58–62
Earnshaw G 1980 China bursts acupuncture bubble. Daily
Telegraph, London, 24 October, p 13
Eriksson M B E, Sjölund B H, Nielzen S 1979 Long term
results of peripheral conditioning stimulation as an
analgesic measure in chronic pain. Pain 6: 335–347
Fox E J, Melzack R 1976 Transcutaneous electrical
stimulation and acupuncture: comparison of treatment for
low-back pain. Pain 2: 141–148
Johnson M I, Ashton C H, Thompson J W 1991a An in-
depth study of long-term users of transcutaneous electrical
nerve stimulation (TENS). Implications for clinical use of
TENS. Pain 44: 221–229
Johnson M I, Ashton C H, Thompson J W 1991b The
consistency of pulse frequencies and pulse patterns of
transcutaneous nerve stimulation (TENS) used by chronic
pain patients. Pain 44: 231–234
Kane K, Taub A 1975 A history of local electrical analgesia.
Pain 1: 125–138
Lewit K 1979 The needle effect in the relief of myofascial
pain. Pain 6: 83–90
Long D M, Carolan M T 1974 Cutaneous afferent
stimulation in the treatment of chronic pain. In: Bonica J J
(ed) Advances in neurology 4, International Symposium on
Pain. Raven Press, New York, p 755–759
Long D M, Hagfors N 1975 Electrical stimulation in the
nervous system. The current status of electrical stimulation
of the nervous system for the relief of pain. Pain 1:
109–123
Loy T T 1983 Treatment of cervical spondylosis.
Electroacupuncture versus physiotherapy. The Medical
Journal of Australia 2: 32–34
Macdonald A 1982 Acupuncture from ancient art to modern
medicine. George Allen & Unwin, London, p 116
Mann F 1974 Acupuncture analgesia. Report of 100
experiments. British Journal of Anaesthesia 46: 361–364

Mannheimer C, Carlsson C A 1979 The analgesic effect of
transcutaneous electrical stimulation in patients with
rheumatoid arthritis. A comparative study of different pulse
patterns. Pain 6: 329–334
Melzack R 1975 Prolonged relief of pain by brief, intense
transcutaneous somatic stimulation. Pain 1: 357–373
Melzack R, Wall P D 1965 Pain mechanisms: a new theory.
Science 150: 971–979
Sjölund B H, Eriksson M B E 1979 Endorphins and analgesia
produced by peripheral conditioning stimulation. In:
Bonica J J, Albe-Fessard D Liebeskind (eds) Advances in
pain research and therapy 3. Raven Press, New York,
p 587–599
Smithers Sir David, Alexander P, Hamilton-Fairley G, Adey
E, Williams P O, Goodwin J F, Cleland W P, McDonald E
Lawson, Wall P D 1974. Report of the British Medical
Delegation to China April–May 1974. Unpublished
documents, Medical Research Council, London
Thompson J W 1984 Pain: Mechanisms and principles of
management. In: Grimley Evans J, Caird F I (eds)
Advanced geriatric medicine 4. Pitman, London
Thompson J W 1987 The role of transcutaneous electrical
nerve stimulation (TENS) for the control of pain. In: Doyle
D (ed) 1986 International Symposium on Pain Control,
Royal Society of Medicine Services International Congress
and Symposium Series No. 123. Royal Society of
Medicine, London
Thompson J W 1989 Pharmacology of transcutaneous
electrical nerve stimulation (TENS) Journal of the
Intractable Pain Society of Great Britain and Ireland
7(1): 33–40
Tkach W 1972 I have seen acupuncture work. Today's
Health, July 1972, p 50–56
Wall P D, Sweet W H 1967 Temporary abolition of pain.
Science 155: 108–109
Wolf S L, Gersh M R, Rao V R 1981 Examination of
electrode placements and stimulating parameters in treating
chronic pain with conventional transcutaneous electrical
nerve stimulation (TENS). Pain 11: 37–47
Woolf C J 1989 Segmental afferent fibre-induced analgesia:
transcutaneous electrical nerve stimulation (TENS) and
vibration. In: Wall P D, Melzack R (eds) Textbook of pain,
2nd edn. Churchill Livingstone, Edinburgh, p 884–896
Wynn Parry C B 1980 Pain in avulsion lesions of the brachial
plexus. Pain 9: 41–53
Yuen R W M, Vaughan R J, Dyer H, Giles K E 1976 The
response to acupuncture therapy in patients with chronic
disabling pain. Medical Journal of Australia 1: 826–865

10. Neurophysiological pain suppressing effects of acupuncture

A historical review of methods of combating pain by pain

It would seem that man has always instinctively realized that it is possible by applying painful stimuli to the body to dispel from it pain of a more persistent nature. As Melzack & Wall (1982) pointed out,

Every culture, it appears, has learned to fight pain with pain: in general, brief, moderate pain tends to abolish severe, prolonged pain.

Cupping, a procedure in which a glass cup is heated and then held with its rim against the skin; and scarification, a procedure in which the skin is cut, often in several places, by a sharp knife, or by rather less sophisticated instruments such as flints, thorns, or fish bones, have been methods which for centuries have been used to induce bleeding with the idea that this would release from the body the devil or evil spirit responsible for some particular malady. In addition, however, because these two procedures happen to be acutely painful, they have also for a long time been used in the combating a pain of a more chronic nature such as that which so commonly affects the head, the back and joints.

Cauterization, the procedure in which intense heat is applied by one means or another to an affected part of the body, has also since ancient times been employed for a variety of reasons including the alleviation of pain. At the present time it is of course mainly used for the control of haemorrhage but in some of the less advanced parts of the world it is still used for other purposes. In Tibet, for example, one of its main indications is in the treatment of lumbago. First of all, several blisters are produced on the skin of the back by applying a red-hot branding iron to it. Next, cones packed with a crude mixture of sulphur and saltpetre are placed on the blisters and then lit with a flaming torch. As Graham (1939) comments 'the result is a girdle of burns deep enough to banish any thought of afflictions as mild as lumbago'.

A less horrific method of blistering the skin for therapeutic purposes is the application of some irritant substance to it such as cantharides, a technique certainly well known to Hippocrates, and used extensively since then for centuries, with, for example, William Wells, a physician at St Thomas's Hospital in the early part of the 19th century, applying this substance to the skin of the chest wall for the relief of pericardial pain (Baldry 1971). A practice closely allied to this, and first used at least 3000 years ago in the Far East, is one in which moxa, a substance obtained from the leaves of the mugwort plant, is applied to the skin in the form of a cone, and the latter set alight and allowed to burn down to its base resting on the skin. This is a process which by its very nature must be inherently painful and, yet, one which has as its main use the alleviation of painful disorders (see Ch. 1).

Acupuncture, which has been in use in the Eastern world for much the same period of time for the treatment of a wide range of diseases, may also be associated with the production of a certain amount of discomfort and yet has always had as one of its main indications the alleviation of pain. All of these methods just alluded to in which over the centuries brief intense pain has been used to drive out more protracted and severe pain are known collectively as 'counter-irritants', and, as Wand-Tetley (1956) in an extensive historical review of their clinical application has pointed out, their main use has always been in the alleviation of rheumatic pains.

Originally it was thought that they owed their efficacy to their ability to cast out evil spirits, but when this was no longer believed in, it was considered that it might be due to either the power of suggestion or distraction of attention. It has only been since the neurophysiology of pain has become better understood during the last 20 years that it has become apparent that the analgesic effect of all these various procedures lies in their ability to impart a noxious stimulus to the central nervous system and by so doing to alleviate pain by evoking activity in complex endogenous pain-modulating mechanisms. Melzack (1973) has termed this effect 'hyper-stimulation analgesia'.

There is therefore nothing special about acupuncture other than it is a more convenient and more acceptable means of applying a noxious stimulus than any of the other techniques just mentioned. There can be no doubt that when treating musculoskeletal pain by means of the acupuncture technique of deactivating trigger points, the insertion of needles into super-sensitive nerve endings at these sites provides a brief but nevertheless quite intense noxious stimulus. The pain produced by this, however, is quickly replaced by one or another of a variety of sensations, with the commonest of these, in my experience, being a feeling of numbness. It is these sensations, occurring once the initial momentary needle pain has subsided, that collectively are called by the Chinese tê chhi, and which they have always insisted have to be produced for acupuncture to be effective (see Ch. 8).

The placing of acupuncture on a scientific basis in the 1970s

It is somewhat surprising that so many people continue to base their practice of acupuncture on archaic concepts formulated in China many centuries ago considering that since the early 1970s the use of this technique, at least so far as the alleviation of pain is concerned, has been placed on a scientific basis, and that many of the ingenious experiments that led to this were carried out by medical scientists in that country. In discussing present-day views concerning the manner in which the noxious stimulus provided by acupuncture is thought to influence pain-modulating mechanisms in the central nervous system, it is first necessary to review some of the pioneer work carried out on this subject in China.

Chiang et al (1973) provided scientific evidence that acupuncture causes analgesia by measuring the pain threshold in normal adults by means of electrical dolorimetry before and after the insertion of acupuncture needles. They showed that acupuncture causes a significant elevation of pain threshold all over the body but that this tends to be greatest in the segment in which the needle is inserted. They also showed that this widespread analgesic effect of needling is not due to some chemical agent being released locally and then transported around the body through the cardiovascular system by demonstrating that its production is not interfered with, by occluding the blood supply to a limb above the site of acupuncture.

Evidence for a neural mechanism of acupuncture analgesia came from the Peking Medical College's Research Group of Acupuncture Anaesthesia (1973) who showed that in man the pain threshold is not elevated by acupuncture if a needle is inserted into tissues affected by loss of sensation. It was also noted by Chang (1973) that the pain threshold is unaffected by acupuncture if a local anaesthetic is injected into the acupuncture point, and that, in experimental animals, section of the anterolateral tract of the spinal cord abolishes its analgesic effect. Even more sophisticated experiments carried out by Chang (1973) included experiments on rats and rabbits in which he recorded impulses from single neurons in thalamic nuclei developing as a result of applying a painful stimulus to an extremity or electrically stimulating a peripheral nerve. He was able to show that inhibition of these impulses could be obtained by squeezing the tendo Achilles, or by applying a weak electrical stimulus to cutaneous nerves, or by inserting acupuncture needles into the tissues, and that the most effective inhibition was obtained when this acupuncture stimulation was carried out in the same segment as the painful stimulus had been applied.

Following this the Research Group of Acupuncture Anaesthesia (1974) produced evidence to show that acupuncture analgesia may be associated with the release of chemical substances into the central nervous system by demonstrating that the pain threshold in rabbits could be increased by infusing into their brains cerebrospinal fluid obtained from other rabbits which had received acupuncture stimulation.

The role of endogenous opioid peptides (EOPS) in the production of acupuncture analgesia (AA)

As Clement-Jones & Besser (1983) have pointed out, ever since acupuncture was first used in the 1960s to suppress the pain induced by surgery, it has been known that in order to achieve this, it is necessary to apply intense stimulation for at least 20 minutes, and that it was this time delay before the induction of analgesia, together with the long duration of this analgesia after needle stimulation has ceased, which added additional support to the idea that the mechanism underlying the induction of acupuncture analgesia must depend on the release of some humoral factor. This awareness that acupuncture analgesia is likely to be associated with the production of neurochemical substances happened to coincide with the discovery of the endogenous opioids in the central nervous system, and it was immediately assumed that both the relief of established pain and the suppression of induced pain by acupuncture must depend on the release of these substances into the brain and spinal cord (Han & Terenius 1982). Although subsequent research has provided ample evidence for this occurring in certain circumstances, the situation is by no means as straightforward as might at first have been thought.

One of the first to study by means of animal experiments the mechanisms underlying the development of acupuncture analgesia was the Canadian physiologist, Pomeranz. He and his colleagues began their studies of this in 1974, and when shortly after this endogenous opioid receptors (EORs) were found to be present in the

central nervous system (CNS) together with EOPS, they decided to establish whether it is the release of the latter into the CNS that is responsible for the development of AA. To this end Pomeranz & Chiu (1976) induced AA in awake mice by means of a 20-minute application of low frequency (4 Hz), strong intensity, electroacupuncture (EA) delivered through needles inserted into the 1st dorsal interosseous muscle — the traditional Chinese large intestine 4 (Ho-Ku) point (Fig. 15.11). The AA was tested by measuring the latency to squeak after applying heat to the noses of these animals. In order to establish whether or not the AA induced was EOP mediated, the effect of systemically administering naloxone, a specific opiate antagonist, was observed. It was as a result of this experiment that they had the distinction of being the first to report that naloxone blocks the development of AA and to conclude that it would therefore seem reasonable to assume that this type of analgesia is EOP mediated.

This was clearly a very significant finding, but what was even more exciting was when Mayer et al (1977) one year later confirmed that what Pomeranz and his colleagues had found in mice also applied to humans. They did this by means of an experiment showing that the analgesic effect of acupuncture on electrically-induced tooth pulp pain in man is similarly reversed by naloxone.

Two years later, the first clue that opioid peptide mediation of AA depends on the type of stimulation applied was provided by Sjölund & Eriksson (1979) when they showed that whilst both high-frequency low-intensity and low-frequency high-intensity electrical nerve stimulation alleviate pain, it is only the analgesia provided by the latter type of stimulation which is naloxone reversible. The situation, however, became temporarily confused one year later when Chapman et al (1980) reported their inability, to reverse with naloxone, AA induced in healthy volunteers subjected to experimentally inflicted dental pain. When, three years after this, by which time it was known that stress alone is capable of bringing about the release of EOPs (Ch. 6), Chapman et al (1983) concluded that any rise in the CSF or plasma EOP levels observed when EA is used in either animal or human studies, does not occur as a direct result of the acupuncture but rather as a result of the stress associated with the carrying out of such experiments.

However, the following year, Professor Han, the chairman of the physiology department at Beijing Medical University in China — who also since the 1970s has been extensively investigating, by means of animal experiments, the neurochemical basis of AA — helped to clarify the situation. Han et al (1984a), in experiments on rats given EA at stimulation frequencies of either 2, 15 or 100 Hz through needles inserted bilaterally into traditional Chinese acupuncture points Stomach 36 (Fig. 19.1) and Spleen 6 (Fig. 16.1) found that naloxone (1 mg/kg) completely abolished the analgesic effect of 2 Hz EA, partially reversed 15 Hz EA, and had no effect on 100 Hz EA. They found, moreover, that the doses of naloxone needed for 50% reversal of 2, 15 and 100 Hz EAA were 0.5, 1.0 and 24 mg/kg respectively. These findings led them to conclude that different kinds of EOP are released into the CNS in response to stimulation with different EA frequencies (metenkephalin at 2 Hz, dynorphin A at 100 Hz and a mixture of enkephalins and dynorphins at 15 Hz). They also concluded that the dose of naloxone needed to block EAA depends on the type of EOP released and therefore on the stimulation frequency of the EA employed.

In a similar manner, Han et al (1984b) found, in the rats, that the dose of naloxone needed for 50% inhibition of analgesia produced by morphine was 0.7 mg/kg, but for dynorphins it was 9–10 mg/kg.

The basic reason for this variable ability of naloxone to block analgesia produced either by morphine or endogenous opioids is that naloxone, morphine and endogenous opioids have different binding affinities for the mu, delta and kappa opioid receptors in the CNS. Both morphine and naloxone attach themselves principally to mu receptors, whereas met- and leu-enkephalins bind predominately to delta receptors, and dynorphins adhere mainly to kappa receptors (Bowsher 1987).

The lesson to be learnt from all this, as Han

(1985) has pointed out, is that when attempting to interpret the results of experiments designed to show whether or not the development of AA is EOP mediated by means of observing whether or not naloxone blocks the analgesia, it is essential to take into consideration both the parameters of the EA stimulus employed and the dose of naloxone administered.

There have so far been 28 reports confirming naloxone blockade of AA, and 7 reports which failed to observe this effect (Stux & Pomeranz 1987), and in the light of Han's findings it is interesting to reflect upon the reasons for this disparity. It is now generally accepted that the AA-OP mediated mechanism in both human and animal studies operates best with low-frequency, high-intensity stimulation. This accounts for 4 of the failed experiments, as one of these (Chapman et al 1983) involved the use of low-frequency low-intensity EA, and three of them involved the use of high-frequency low-intensity EA. The reason for the other three failed experiments might be because naloxone seems to work best when given before the treatment begins and fails to reverse analgesia once it has already developed (Pomeranz 1989). The implication of this is that EOP mediated AA is not naloxone reversible, as is so often stated, but rather naloxone preventable.

The suggestion made by Chapman et al (1983) that EOP mediated AA under experimental conditions may be stress induced has been refuted by Peets & Pomeranz (1987) showing that the AA which develops in anaesthetized animals is similar to that obtained in awake ones.

There are other good reasons for believing that the analgesia induced by conventional low-frequency high-intensity EA is EOP mediated. One of these is that Peets & Pomeranz (1978) have shown that a particular strain of mice with a congenital deficiency of opiate receptors respond poorly to morphine and produce much less AA than normal mice do. It was this observation which led them to speculate that the reason why 30% of humans fail to develop any worthwhile amount of AA is possibly because they have a genetic deficiency in their endorphin system.

Another reason is that it is possible to enhance the development of AA by protecting EOPs from degradation brought about by various enzymes including carboxypeptidase and leucine amino-peptidase. It is because of this enzyme degradation that analgesia produced by endorphins is relatively short lasting but Cheng & Pomeranz (1980) have shown that the administration of the D-amino acids, D-leucine and D-phenylalamine, by blocking the action of these enzymes, enhances the development of AA, and that this enhanced AA may in turn be blocked by naloxone, and that, further, a combination of D-amino acids and EA produce a greater amount of analgesia than either of these alone. It was this latter observation which led them to wonder whether possibly a combination of EA and D-amino acids will prove to be a potent method of treating clinical pain.

Yet another reason is that a microinjection of naloxone into certain specific sites rich in opioid peptides and their receptors in the spinal cord (Peets & Pomeranz 1985) and the brain (Zhou et al 1981) blocks the development of AA. Zhou et al (1981) showed, in experiments on rabbits, that it only required an injection of 1 μg of naloxone into the periaqueductal grey area of the midbrain, or either the nucleus accumbens or the amygdala in the limbic system, or the habenular nucleus situated in the dorsomedial aspect of the thalamus, to block the effect of AA by more than 70%. Zhou et al (1984) have also shown that it only requires a microinjection (5–10 μg) of morphine into any one of these same four nuclei to produce marked analgesia. These sites therefore are of considerable importance with respect to EOP mediated AA and they will be referred to again when discussing the long-term analgesic effect of acupuncture, as Han and his colleagues believe that it might be sustained activity in the so-called meso-limbic neural loop formed by these nuclei and the arcuate nucleus of the hypothalamus which brings this about.

Changes in endogenous opioid peptide (EOP) cerebrospinal fluid (CSF) levels in response to acupuncture

Other recent evidence in support of EOPS having a role in AA has come from studies of EOP levels in the CSF of patients before and after acupuncture.

In the first such study, Sjölund et al (1977) collected CSF from lumbar punctures in patients with chronic pain treated with acupuncture-like TENS. They measured CSF endogenous OP levels before and immediately after treatment. When treating low-back pain by applying electrodes to the lumbar region, they observed a doubling of CSF levels of these peptides immediately after 30 minutes of treatment. It is of considerable interest, however, that when they treated face pain by stimulating the Large Intestine 4 (Ho-Ku) acupuncture point in the first dorsal interosseous muscle of the hand (Fig. 15.11), they observed no changes in lumbar CSF endogenous OP levels. It is suggested that the reason for this was that a local segmental release of peptides had occurred in the backache patients and that the hand stimulation did not elevate peptides in lumbar CSF as it was the C8 segment that was being stimulated rather than the L5 one. Unfortunately, in this study, the CSF opioid substances were measured by receptor-binding assays which did not reveal which peptides were involved.

Clement-Jones et al (1980) measured cerebrospinal concentrations of beta-endorphin and metenkephalin by radioimmunoassay in a group of patients with recurrent pain before and after 30 minutes of low-frequency EA, and found that although the concentrations of metenkephalin remained unchanged, those of betaendorphin rose after this type of stimulus had been applied.

Morley (1985) however has issued a warning that care has to be taken in drawing conclusions from measurements of CSF levels of EOPs, because the presence of these substances in the CSF is most likely to arise from overspill of neuronal activity and therefore they do not necessarily reflect the degree of activity of peptides within neurons. Nevertheless, such measurements before and after 20–30 minutes of acupuncture stimulation, and the results of most of the naloxone studies, make it reasonable to postulate that the analgesic effect of such a stimulus is associated with the activation of EOP mediated pain-modulating mechanisms in the CNS.

As space does not permit all the evidence in support of EOP involvement in AA to be discussed those who wish to know more about the subject should consult various recently published comprehensive reviews (He 1987, Cheng 1989, Han 1989, Pomeranz 1989).

The role of serotonin (5-hydroxytryptamine) in the development of acupuncture analgesia (AA)

As the brain stem structures which form the upper part of the descending pain inhibitory system are linked to the dorsal horns by axons in the dorsolateral funiculus which have serotonin as their neurotransmitter, and as it is this descending system which is brought into action when A-delta nerve fibres are stimulated with dry needles (see Chs 6 and 8), it is not surprising that the development of AA is influenced by alterations in the CNS serotonin levels.

The Research Group of Acupuncture Anaesthesia at the Peking Medical College reported in 1975 that para-chlorphenylalanine, a serotonin synthesis inhibitor, when injected into the lateral ventricle of the rabbit, inhibits acupuncture analgesia (Han & Terenius 1982). McLennan et al (1977) found that cyproheptadine, a serotonin receptor blocker, similarly impairs the development of AA in the rabbit. Kin et al (1979) demonstrated that cianserin, another serotonin receptor blocker, also impairs it in the cat. Conversely, Han et al (1979) found that, in rats, the intraventricular administration of 5-hydroxytryptophan, a serotonin precursor, enhances AA.

With regard to humans, Han and his colleagues reported in 1978 that in patients undergoing the removal of impacted molar teeth, the administration of clomipramine, which blocks the re-uptake of serotonin, or pargyline, which blocks its degradation, potentiates the effect of AA (Han & Terenius 1982).

It is also of considerable interest to note, in view of what has been said earlier with regard to the apparent importance of the nucleus accumbens, the amygdala, the habenula, and the periaqueductal grey in the development of AA, that during the early 1980s, Han and his col-

leagues published several papers showing that the analgesia produced by this means is significantly attenuated when cianserin, the serotonin receptor blocker, is microinjected into any of these four brain nuclei (Han 1989).

Furthermore, in view of the fact, as stated earlier, that Han and his colleagues found that the type of opioid peptide released varies according to the frequency of EA employed, it should be observed that Zhang & Han (1985) have shown that the release of serotonin and its effect on the production of AA is the same with EA of different frequencies and different intensities.

Finally, in view of what has been learnt from the various animal experiments quoted, it is hardly surprising to find that simultaneous interference with both the serotonin and opioid systems results in a dramatic decrease or even complete abolition of the analgesia induced by EA (Han et al 1980, Zhou et al 1982).

Possible differences in the mechanisms underlying brief and prolonged acupuncture stimulation

From the results of numerous animal experiments, it is now evident that when a low-frequency high-intensity electroacupuncture stimulus is applied for the relatively long period of 20–40 minutes to suppress, for example, the pain of a surgical operation or pain induced experimentally, the acupuncture-produced analgesia is opioid peptide mediated.

The question, however, that has to be addressed is whether the analgesia produced as a result of stimulating sensitized A-delta nerve fibres in tissues overlying trigger points by means of manual needling carried out for a relatively brief period of from a few seconds to a few minutes is also opioid peptide mediated. One reason for asking this question is because Lewis et al (1980), in experiments on rats, found that the stress-induced analgesia brought about by prolonged foot shock is blocked by the administration of naloxone, whereas analgesia produced by briefly applied foot shock is not (see Ch. 6). The suggestion has been made that the analgesia produced by this latter method may occur as a result of the activation of one or more of the as yet less well understood non-opioid systems.

The answer, however, would seem to be that the short-duration type of manual acupuncture used for the purpose of deactivating trigger points is opioid peptide mediated for, as Bowsher (1990) has pointed out, it only requires a brief pin prick type stimulus to be applied to A-delta nerve fibres to produce excitation in enkephalinergic inhibitory interneurons situated on the borders of Lamina I and II of the dorsal horn and for this in turn to have a modulating effect on the C afferent noxious input to the spinal cord. In passing, it is relevant to note in relationship to this that the analgesic effect of injecting trigger points with a local anaesthetic would also seem to be opioid peptide mediated as its development has recently been shown to be blocked by the administration of naloxone (Fine et al 1988).

Furthermore, although the stimulus delivered by briefly applied manual acupuncture is clearly not as powerful or prolonged as that provided by electroacupuncture applied (as it usually is) for about 20–40 minutes, it would seem reasonable to assume that it is nevertheless strong enough to bring into operation both supraspinal and spinal opioid peptide mediated pain modulating mechanisms, considering that it is possible to produce profound analgesia by injecting no more than a minute amount of morphine directly into the periaqueductal grey area (Herz et al 1970, Mayer & Watkins 1981, Yaksh & Aimone 1989), and bearing in mind that C fibre terminals in the dorsal horn are richly supplied with opiate receptors (Fields et al 1980), and that there is a concentration of enkephalin- and dynorphin-containing neurons in the substantia gelatinosa adjacent to these C terminals (Aronin et al 1981).

Comparative effectiveness of and indications for manual and electroacupuncture

Following on from this, it has to be asked whether electroacupuncture and manual acupuncture are equally effective in relieving pain, and, even if they are, whether some types of pain are better treated by one and some by the other.

There is certainly no argument that they are both equally effective in suppressing experimentally-induced pain provided that with either of these two methods a prolonged stimulus is applied.

Reichmanis & Becker (1977), from a review of 24 studies of acupuncture analgesia for the relief of experimentally-induced pain reported in the literature, found that 17 of them (71%) showed a significant analgesic effect using either manual or electrical stimulation but that many investigators noted that with either method the full analgesic effect could only be attained provided the stimulation was continued for at least 20 minutes.

From this it will be seen that, for the relief of experimentally-induced pain, equally good results may be obtained from the use of either manual or electrical stimulation, but with the proviso that with either method the stimulus has to be given for the relatively long period of 20 minutes or more. Certainly in research into the effects of acupuncture on experimentally induced dental pain, equally good results have been obtained using either electrical or manual stimulation but it is essential to note that the stimulus has always been given for a prolonged period. For example, Andersson & Holmgren (1975) used electrical stimulation for up to 75 minutes; Chapman et al (1976) used electrical stimulation for 20 minutes; Mayer et al (1977) used manual stimulation for 30 minutes; and Chapman et al (1980) also used manual stimulation for 30 minutes.

Similarly, when using acupuncture to stimulate the body's pain-modulating mechanisms sufficiently to suppress surgically-induced pain, the results of using manual or electrical stimulation are similar but it is essential with either to apply the stimulus for at least 20 minutes (Mann 1974).

It would seem that the only advantage of electrical stimulation over manual stimulation when using acupuncture for a prolonged period is that it is more convenient and less tiring for the person applying it. The effect of applying this type of low-frequency high-intensity acupuncture for 20–40 minutes to a few specially selected traditional Chinese acupuncture points for the purpose of suppressing surgically or experimentally induced pain is to raise the pain tolerance to this type of pain for approximately 90 minutes (Macdonald 1989).

When acupuncture is used for the relief of chronic pain, there are some conditions in which it is necessary to apply a stimulus for a prolonged period but with others it seems better only to stimulate for a brief period. Certainly in the alleviation of neurogenic pain, a fairly prolonged stimulus seems to be required and therefore electroacupuncture, acupuncture-like TENS or conventional TENS (see Ch. 9) has to be used, but for the relief of musculoskeletal pain the situation is not so clear cut.

Some physicians advocate applying the stimulus for a relatively long time and therefore employ electroacupuncture. For example, Rutkowski et al (1977) gave 15-minute sessions of low-frequency electroacupuncture in cases of chronic low-back pain. Also Loy (1983), in a study in which he compared acupuncture with physiotherapy in the treatment of cervical spondylosis, stimulated acupuncture points electrically for as long as 30–40 minutes. Such prolonged stimulation however is in marked contrast to that used by Fox & Melzack (1976) when they successfully alleviated low-back pain by strong manual rotation of needles inserted into acupuncture points for only one minute. Certainly in treating musculoskeletal pain by deactivating trigger points, an increasing number of physicians use the technique described in this book of manually stimulating the needles for only a brief period ranging from a few seconds up to, but not more than, 10 minutes, depending on the patient's individual speed of reaction to acupuncture. These physicians have found that if stimulation is carried out too enthusiastically, it is all too easy to exacerbate the pain. In fairness, it has to be said that it is not possible to state dogmatically that manual stimulation is superior to electroacupuncture in the alleviation of musculoskeletal pain as, up to now, adequate clinical trials designed to compare the two methods have not been conducted. However, there is no doubt that when one only wants to apply a brief intense stimulus to sensitized A-delta nerve fibres in the vicinity of trigger points, the manual method is simpler, with the amount of stimulation given being more readily adjustable to the patient's individual responsiveness, and with it

being easier to ensure that every trigger point contributing to the pain is deactivated.

Relative effectiveness of applying stimulation near to or at some distance from the painful area

In the traditional Chinese practice of acupuncture, stimulation of acupuncture points some distance from the painful area is sometimes recommended. However, several investigators including Andersson & Holmgren (1975), Chapman et al (1980), and Jeans (1979) have shown that stimulation of acupuncture points close to the area of pain is more effective.

The explanation for this would seem to be, as already discussed in Chs 6 and 8, that dry needle stimulation of A-delta nerve fibres in the same segment as that from which the pain is emanating (segmental acupuncture) achieves its pain-relieving effect by two means. One is by it having a direct excitatory effect on dorsal horn enkephalinergic inhibitory interneurons at the same level as the C afferent impulses responsible for the pain enter the cord, with the result that their onward transmission becomes blocked. The other is by it having an indirect excitatory effect on these inhibitory interneurons by virtue of the fact that the centripetal transmission of A-delta pinprick information in the anterolateral funiculus evokes activity in the descending inhibitory system situated in the dorsolateral funiculus. In contrast to this, dry needle stimulation of A-delta nerve fibres some distance away from the segment in which the pain is arising (extra-segmental acupuncture) clearly cannot be so effective as it is not able to have a direct influence on the spinal cord input of C afferent information responsible for the pain, and any pain relief it may give can only occur as a result of a somewhat non-specific evocation of activity in the descending inhibitory system. Shen et al (1978) have shown that section of either the central afferent limb (the anterolateral funiculus) or the central efferent limb of the descending inhibitory system (the dorsolateral funiculus) in the cat abolishes extrasegmental acupuncture.

Another factor which has to be taken into account when considering why segmental acupuncture for pain relief is more effective than that carried out extrasegmentally is that Soper & Melzack (1982) have shown that the periaqueductal grey area (PAG) at the upper end of the descending inhibitory system is somatotopically organized so that particular areas of the body project especially strongly to discrete regions of it (Groves et al 1973). The possible implication of this might be that the A-delta noxious input provided by inserting needles into acupuncture points in the vicinity of a painful area and the painful area itself project equally strongly to the same discrete region of the PAG, with the result that the descending inhibitory axons from this region of the PAG exert a particularly powerful modulating effect on the noxious spinal input responsible for the pain.

It has to be admitted, however, that the noxious stimulus of acupuncture does not necessarily have to be applied close to the site of pain for, as Melzack (1975) has shown, provided the stimulus is sufficiently intense, it is capable of having an analgesic effect whether it is applied to points near to or some distance from the pain. This is an observation which has been confirmed by experiments carried out by Le Bars et al (1979) on rats which showed that a stimulus applied anywhere in the body is capable of modifying pain perception, due to the effect of what they have called diffuse noxious inhibitory controls. These controls probably account for the action of a whole variety of counter-irritants used throughout history and which were briefly alluded to at the beginning of this chapter.

Is it necessary to carry out acupuncture stimulation at specific sites?

Following on from what has been said concerning diffuse noxious inhibitory controls, the question which has to be asked is whether it is necessary to insert needles into or apply electrodes over specific acupuncture points.

Practitioners of traditional Chinese acupuncture have over the centuries always taught that there are specific acupuncture points for the treatment of specific diseases and that pain is most readily alleviated if certain particular points are stimulated with the decision as to which ones to use depending on the area of the body affected by it. Such teaching, however, has recently been challenged. Taub et al (1977), for example, have shown that it is possible to achieve as much control over dental pain by stimulating an area between the fourth and fifth fingers as can be achieved by stimulating the point traditionally designated for this purpose in the Chinese system known as Ho-Ku (Hegu) or Large Intestine 4, situated in the first dorsal interosseous muscle.

When clinical trials of acupuncture were first embarked upon in the 1970s, mainly for the purpose off evaluating its ability to relieve pain, it was believed that for there to be any likelihood of success, specific acupuncture points had to be stimulated and that therefore the application of a stimulus at a random site some distance from a specific point could be used as a placebo in control groups. Such a belief, however, was to prove to be erroneous.

For example, in a trial carried out by Gaw et al (1975) for the purpose of assessing the effectiveness of acupuncture on osteoarthritic pain, and in another in which Co et al (1979) tested its effectiveness in relieving pain associated with sickle cell anaemia, the effect of needles inserted into 'real' traditional acupuncture points was tested against the effect of stimulating, by the same means, random points some distance from acupuncture points, referred to as 'sham points'. In these two trials, patients in both groups showed significant improvement but, as there was no difference between the two groups, this improvement was attributed to a placebo effect. However, such an interpretation is thought to be wrong (see Ch. 11), because, due to the effects of diffuse noxious inhibition, the use of sham points does produce an analgesic effect which is greater than that obtained in any group of patients 'treated' with a true placebo such as a nonfunctioning TENS machine (mock TENS). From a review of all randomized trials on acupuncture, Lewith & Machin (1983) have estimated that the response rates for real acupuncture, sham acupuncture and true placebos in these trials have on average been 70%, 50% and 30% respectively.

The results of these trials therefore serve to confirm that the random insertion of needles anywhere in the body produces a certain amount of analgesic effect but the degree of this is increased if needles are inserted into specific sites. Such sites include traditional Chinese acupuncture points discovered thousands of years ago, and points of extreme tenderness in the musculoskeletal system which the Chinese physician Sun Ssu-Mo was particularly enthusiastic about needling in the 7th century, and which in recent years have been rediscovered in the tissues overlying trigger points by physicians practising Western medicine.

The greater effectiveness of stimulating specific points as compared to sham points must largely be because the former have a richer supply of A-delta nerve fibres.

Traditional Chinese acupuncture points versus trigger points in the alleviation of musculoskeletal pain

It has to be admitted that at the present time there is no evidence to show that, for the alleviation of musculoskeletal pain, needle stimulation of A-delta nerve fibres in the tissues overlying trigger points gives any better results than carrying out this form of stimulation at traditional Chinese acupuncture points provided they are situated in the same segment as the area affected by pain.

Nevertheless, the considerable disadvantage of using traditional Chinese acupuncture points is that one has to come to decisions concerning the selection of points by the carrying out of diagnostic procedures designed to detect disturbances in tracts or meridians which are alien to the principles upon which the Western practice of medicine is based. Alternatively, one has to use a series of points in prescriptions, recipes or formulae to be found in textbooks and recommended for use in conditions diagnosed by the Western system of medicine but which nevertheless have their origins in the traditional Chinese approach to diagnosis.

One cogent reason for advocating the needling of A-delta nerve fibres in the tissues overlying trigger points for the alleviation of musculo-skeletal pain is because, as explained in earlier chapters, it is as a result of the sensitization of C afferent fibres at these points that this type of pain arises. Another reason is that these points can readily be located by the application of a palpatory technique routinely used in the clinical examination of patients by those trained in the Western system of medical practice.

Yet another reason for systematically locating trigger points and then deactivating each one in turn by means of dry needle stimulation of A-delta nerve fibres in the tissues overlying them is because it has become apparent from everyday clinical practice that when musculoskeletal pain emanates from a number of trigger points there is never any lasting relief from the pain if any one of the trigger points is overlooked and allowed to remain in a state of activation.

Possible mechanisms responsible for prolonged pain relief following acupuncture

Price et al (1984) made some fundamentally important observations in a group of patients with low-back pain and pain induced experimentally by repeatedly exposing, at 5-minute intervals, the backs and forearms of these patients to brief applications of noxious heat (43–51°C), when they attempted to alleviate these two types of pain by means of applying, bi-weekly, low-frequency high-intensity electroacupuncture to the lower back for a period of 25–30 minutes on each occasion.

They found that 60% of these patients experienced a raised tolerance to the experimentally-induced pain both in the lower part of the back and the forearm but, as might be expected from what has been said earlier, this only lasted for 90 minutes. In contrast to this, however, the 58% of patients who experienced relief from their chronic back pain found that, whilst this relief did not come on immediately, it increased gradually over some hours and persisted for several days. They were therefore able to demonstrate that electroacupuncture, when segmentally applied for the relief of musculoskeletal pain, is capable, as is briefly applied manual trigger point acupuncture, to relieve this type of pain for prolonged periods. From everyday clinical experience it is apparent that such relief may at times last for days, weeks, months or even longer.

The various acupuncture-induced pain-modulating mechanisms already identified would only be expected to alleviate pain for much shorter periods of time than this and therefore at present it is only possible to speculate as to the mechanisms responsible for this prolonged relief.

Han (1987) has suggested that this may occur following acupuncture, as a result of it causing a serotonin and metenkephalin mediated circuit to develop in a neuronal loop made up of the arcuate nucleus of the hypothalamus, the nucleus accumbens, the amygdala, and habenula, together with the periaqueductal grey and nucleus raphe magnus at the upper end of the descending inhibitory system (Fig. 10.1). His hypothesis is that it is because an ongoing circuit in this loop is set up that the descending inhibitory system is enabled to block any noxious input to the spinal cord for a long period of time.

Another very important matter to be taken into consideration when attempting to explain acupuncture's ability to provide prolonged pain relief is that movements are often markedly restricted by pain and once the latter has been alleviated by some form of peripheral nerve stimulation therapy, such as acupuncture or TENS, the consequent restoration of movements with stretching of the tissues leads to the activation of low-threshold mechanoreceptors and, as a result of this, to the evocation, of activity in the large diameter nerve fibre pain-modulating system, thus helping to ensure that the suppression of pain is maintained. It is for this reason that once pain has been relieved by acupuncture the patient should be encouraged to exercise the affected part whilst at the same time avoiding any overloading of the muscles.

The use of the term 'acupuncture'

From what has been said, it will be readily seen that it is a mistake when referring to acupuncture to use it as an all-embracing term for describing the therapeutic use of dry needles, as it is possible that its effects and its mode of action differ according to how it is applied. It is therefore essential when reporting the results of a clinical

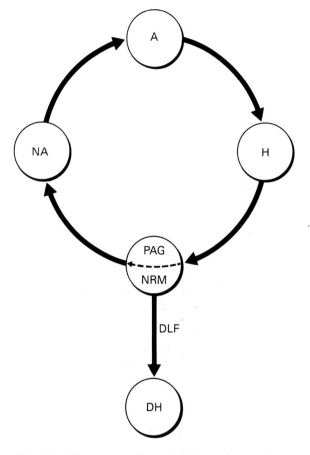

Fig. 10.1   Han's proposed mesolimbic loop of analgesia — A neuronal circuit involving the nucleus accumbens (NA), the amygdala (A), the habenula (H) and the upper parts of the descending inhibitory system, the periaqueductal grey (PAG) and nucleus raphe magnus (NRM), which are connected to the dorsal horn (DH) by the dorsolateral funiculus (DLF).

trial to state exactly which of several variables have been employed. These include the manner in which the stimulus is applied (i.e. by manual stimulation of needles, or electrical stimulation either of needles or via surface electrodes), the intensity of the stimulus, its duration, and (in the case of electroacupuncture) the current frequency. Also, a detailed description must be given as to the placing of the needles, including whether this is near the area affected by the pain or at a distance, and whether the points stimulated are of the traditional Chinese acupuncture type, or are at arbitrarily-selected, so-called sham sites, or are in the tissues overlying trigger points.

REFERENCES

Andersson A, Holmgren E 1975 On acupuncture analgesia and the mechanism of pain. American Journal of Chinese Medicine 3: 311–334

Aronin N, Difiglid M, Liotta A S, Martin J B 1981 Ultrastructural localization and biochemical features of immunoreactive leuenkephalin in monkey dorsal horn. Journal of Neuroscience 1: 561–577

Baldry P E 1971 The battle against heart disease. Cambridge University Press, Cambridge, p 46

Bowsher D 1987 Mechanisms of pain in man. ICI Pharmaceuticals Division

Bowsher D 1990 Physiology and pathophysiology of pain. Journal of British Medical Acupuncture Society 7: 17–20

Chang H T 1973 Integrative action of thalamus in the process of acupuncture for analgesia. Scientia Sinica 16: 25–60

Chapman C R, Beneditti C, Colpitts Y H, Gerlach R 1983 Naloxone fails to reverse pain thresholds elevated by acupuncture. Acupuncture analgesia reconsidered. Pain 16: 13–31

Chapman C R, Colpitts Y M, Benedetti C, Kitaeff R, Gehrig J D 1980 Evoked potential assessment of acupuncture analgesia: attempted reversal with naloxone. Pain 9: 183–197

Chapman C R, Wilson M E, Gehrig J D 1976 Comparative effects of acupuncture and transcutaneous stimulation in the perception of painful dental stimuli. Pain 2: 265–283

Cheng R S S 1989 Neurophysiology of electroacupuncture analgesia. In: Pomeranz B, Stux G (eds) Scientific bases of acupuncture. Springer-Verlag, Berlin p 119–136

Cheng B, Pomeranz B 1980 A combined treatment with D-amino acids and electroacupuncture produces a greater analgesia than either treatment alone: naloxone reverses these effects. Pain 8: 231–236

Chiang C Y, Chang C T, Chu H L, Yang I F 1973 Peripheral afferent pathway for acupuncture analgesia. Scientia Sinica 16: 210–217

Clement-Jones V, Besser G M 1983 Clinical perspectives in opioid peptides. British Medical Bulletin 39: 95–100

Clement-Jones V, Tomlin S, Rees L H, McLoughlin L, Besser G M, Wen H L 1980 Increased beta-endorphin but not met-enkephalin levels in human cerebrospinal fluid after acupuncture for recurrent pain. Lancet 2: 946–948

Co L L, Schmitz T H, Havdala H, Reyes A, Westerman M P P 1979 Acupuncture: an evaluation in the painful crises of sickle cell anaemia. Pain 7: 181–185

Fields H L, Emson P C, Leigh B K, Gilbert R F T, Iversen L 1980 Multiple opiate receptor sites on primary afferent fibres. Nature 184: 351–353

Fine P G, Milano R, Hare B D 1988 The effects of myofascial trigger point injections are naloxone reversible. Pain 32: 15–20

Fox E J, Melzack R 1976 Transcutaneous electrical stimulation and acupuncture: comparison of treatment for low back pain. Pain 2: 141–148

Gaw A C, Chang L W, Shaw L C 1975 Efficacy of acupuncture on osteoarthritic pain. New England Journal of Medicine 293: 375–378

Graham H 1939 Surgeons all. Rich & Cowan, London, p 24

Groves P M, Miller S W, Parker M V, Rebec G C 1973 Organisation by sensory modality in the reticular formation of the rat. Brain Research 54: 207–212

Han J S 1985 Acupuncture analgesia. Pain 21: 307–308

Han J S 1987 Mesolimbic neuronal loop of analgesia. In: Tiengo M, Eccles J, Cuello A C, Ottoson D (eds) Advances in Pain Research and Therapy Vol. 10. Raven Press, New York

Han J S 1989 Central neurotransmitters and acupuncture analgesia. In: Pomeranz B, Stux G (eds) Scientific bases of acupuncture. Springer-Verlag, Berlin p 7–33

Han J S, Chou P H, Luc C et al 1979 The role of central 5-hydroxytryptamine in acupuncture analgesia. Scientia Sinica 22: 91–104

Han J S, Tang J, Fan S G et al 1980 Central 5-hydroxtryptamine, opiate-like substances and acupuncture analgesia. In: Way E L (ed) Endogenous and exogenous opiate agonists and antagonists. Pergamon, New York p 395–398

Han J S, Terenius L 1982 Neurochemical basis of acupuncture analgesia. Annual Review of Pharmacology and Toxicology 22: 193–220

Han J S, Xie G X, Ding X G, Fan S G 1984a High and low frequency electroacupuncture analgesia are mediated by different opioid peptides. Pain, supplement 369: 543

Han J S, Xie G X, Goldstein A 1984b Analgesia induced by intrathecal injection of dynorphin B in the rat. Life Sciences 34: 1573–1579

He L 1987 Involvement of endogenous opioid peptides in acupuncture analgesia. Pain 31: 99–121

Herz A, Albus K, Metys J, Schubert P, Teschemacher H 1970 On the sites for the anti-nociceptive action of morphine and fentanyl. Neuropharmacology 9: 539–551

Jeans M E 1979 Relief of chronic pain by brief intense transcutaneous electrical stimulation — a double blind study. In: Bonica J J, Liebeskind J C, Albe-Fessard D G (eds) Advances in pain research and therapy 3. Raven Press, New York, p 601–606

Kin K C, Han Y F, Yu L P et al 1979 Role of brain serotonergic and catecholaminergic systems in acupuncture analgesia. Acta Physiologica Sinica 31: 121–132 (In Chinese, English abstract)

Le Bars S D, Dickenson A H, Besson J M 1979 Diffuse noxious inhibitory controls (DNIC) II. Lack of effect on non-convergent neurons, supraspinal involvement and theoretical implications. Pain 6: 305–327

Lewis J W, Cannon J T, Liebeskind J C 1980 Opioid and non-opioid mechanisms of stress analgesia. Science 208: 623–625

Lewith G T, Machin D 1983 On the evaluation of the clinical effects of acupuncture. Pain 6: 111–127

Loy T T 1983 Treatment of cervical spondylosis. Medical Journal of Australia 2: 32–34

Macdonald A J R 1989 Acupuncture analgesia and therapy. In: Wall P D Melzack R (eds) Textbook of pain, 2nd edn. Churchill Livingstone, Edinburgh p 906–919

McLennan H, Gilfillan K, Heap Y 1977 Some pharmacological observations on the analgesia induced by acupuncture in rabbits. Pain 3: 229–238

Mann F 1974 Acupuncture analgesia. British Journal of Anaesthesia 46: 361–364

Mayer D J, Price D D, Raffi A 1977 Antagonism of acupuncture analgesia in man by the narcotic antagonist naloxone. Brain Research 121: 368–372

Mayer D J, Watkins L R 1981 The role of endorphins in endogenous pain control systems. In: Emriett H M (ed) Modern problems in pharmacopsychiatry: the role of endorphins in neuropsychiatry. Karger, Basel

Melzack R 1973 The puzzle of pain. Basic Books, New York

Melzack R 1975 Prolonged relief of pain by brief intense transcutaneous somatic stimulation. Pain 1: 357–373

Melzack R, Wall P D 1982 The challenge of pain. Penguin, Harmondsworth, Middlesex, p 319

Morley J S 1985 Peptides in nociceptive pathways. In: Lipton S, Miles J (eds) Persistent pain. Grune & Stratton, New York. Vol 5 p 65–91

Peets J M, Pomeranz B 1978 CXBK mice deficient in opiate receptors show poor electroacupuncture analgesia. Nature 273: 675–676

Peets J M, Pomeranz B 1985 Acupuncture-like TENS analgesia is influenced by spinal cord endorphins but not serotonin: an intrathecal pharmacological study. In: Fields H L, Dutner R, Cervero F (eds) Advances in Pain Research and Therapy Vol 9. Raven Press, New York

Peets J M, Pomeranz B `1987 Studies of suppression of nocifensive reflexes using tail flick electromyograms and intrathecal drugs in barbiturate anesthetized rats. Brain Research 416: 301–307

Pomeranz B 1989 Acupuncture research related to pain, drug addiction and nerve regeneration. In: Pomeranz B, Stux G (eds) Scientific bases of acupuncture. Springer-Verlag, Berlin p 35–52

Pomeranz B, Chiu D 1976 Naloxone blockade of acupuncture analgesia: endorphin implicated. Life Sciences 19: 1757–1762

Price D D, Rafii A, Watkins L R, Buckingham B 1984 A psychophysical analysis of acupuncture analgesia. Pain 19: 27–42

Reichmanis M, Becker R O 1977 Relief of experimentally induced pain by stimulation of acupuncture loci. Comparative Medicine East and West 5: 281–288

Research Group of Acupuncture Anaesthesia, Peking Mecical College 1973 Effect of acupuncture on the pain threshold of human skin. National Medical Journal of China 3: 151–157 (in Chinese, English abstract)

Research Group of Acupuncture Anaesthesia, Peking Medical College 1974 The role of some neurotransmitters of brain in finger-acupuncture analgesia. Scientia Sinica (English translation) 17: 112–130

Rutkowski B, Niedzialkowska T, Otto J 1977 Electrical stimulation in chronic low-back pain. British Journal of Anaesthesia 49: 629–631

Shen E, Ma W H, Lan C 1978 Involvement of descending inhibition in the effect of acupuncture on the splanchnically-evoked potential in the orbital cortex of the cat. Scientia Sinica 21: 628–633

Sjölund B H, Eriksson M B E 1979 Endorphins and analgesia produced by peripheral conditioning stimulation. In: Bonica J J, Albe-Fessard D, Liebeskind (eds) Advances in pain research and therapy 3. Raven Press, New York, p 587–599

Sjölund B H, Terenius L, Eriksson M 1977 Increased cerebrospinal fluid levels of endorphins after electroacupuncture. Acta Physiologica Scandinavica 100: 382–384

Soper W Y, Melzack R 1982 Stimulation-produced analgesia. Evidence for somatotopic organization in the midbrain. Brain Research 251: 301–311

Stux G, Pomeranz B 1987 Acupuncture textbook and atlas. Springer-Verlag, Heidelberg

Taub H A, Beard M C, Eisenberg L, McCommack R K 1977 Studies of acupuncture for operative dentistry. Journal of the American Dental Association 95: 555–561

Wand-Tetley J I 1956 Historical methods of counter-irritation. Annals of Physical Medicine 3: 90–98

Yaksh T L, Aimone L D 1989 The central pharmacology of pain transmission. In: Wall P D, Melzack R (eds) Textbook of pain, 2nd edn. Churchill Livingstone, Edinburgh p 181–205

Zhang M, Han J S 1985 5-hydroxytryptamine is an important mediator for both high and low frequency electroacupuncture analgesia. Acupuncture Research 10: 212–215 (In Chinese, English abstract)

Zhou Z F, Du M Y, Wu W Y, Jian Y, Han J S 1981 Effect of intracerebral microinjection of naloxone in acupuncture and morphine analgesia in the rabbit. Scientia Sinica 24: 1166–1178

Zhou Z F, Xuan Y T, Han J S 1982 Blockade of acupuncture analgesia by intraventricular injection of naloxone or cianserin in the rabbit. Acupuncture Research 7: 91–94

Zhou Z F, Xuan Y T, Han J S 1984 Analgesic effect of morphine injected into habenula, nucleus accumbens and amygdala of rabbits (in Chinese, English abstract) Acta Pharmacologica Sinica 5: 150–153

11. Scientific evaluation of acupuncture

INTRODUCTION

Once advances in the neurophysiology of pain during the past 25 years had provided a certain measure of understanding as to how stimulating peripheral nerve endings with a dry needle, in the procedure known as acupuncture, is sometimes capable of alleviating pain by virtue of the ability of this form of stimulation to evoke activity in endogenous pain-modulating mechanisms, it soon became apparent that clinical trials would have to be carried out in order to evaluate in a scientific manner the effectiveness of this procedure's pain-relieving properties.

As Lewith (1984) pointed out, most trials so far carried out have been 'poorly designed with small numbers of patients, muddled entry criteria, short follow up, and no clear definition of success or failure'. Regrettably, a more recent meta-analysis of 51 controlled clinical studies has failed to reveal any improvement (Ter Riet et al 1990).

The purpose of this chapter therefore is to examine some of the shortcomings of studies already completed, and to discuss some of the difficulties inherent in conducting trials designed to assess the efficacy of acupuncture as a pain-relieving agent in order that with future trials some of the more obvious pitfalls may be avoided. This subject has also recently been discussed by Richardson & Vincent (1986), Vincent & Richardson (1986) and Zhang & Oetliker (1991).

The necessity for qualifying the term acupuncture

In evaluating the analgesic effects of acupuncture it is necessary to bear in mind that there are six different methods of carrying out this procedure depending on whether the needles are stimulated manually or electrically; also on whether the needles are inserted into the tissues overlying trigger points or into traditional acupuncture points; and if the latter, whether these points have been selected as a result of the time-honoured Chinese practice of diagnosing imbalances of energy-flow along meridians; or in accordance with recipes, prescriptions or formulae 'officially' recommended for disorders expressed in Western diagnostic terms, but which nevertheless stem from the traditional Chinese system of diagnosis. It therefore follows that as, at the present time, there are insufficient grounds for assuming that the effects of these different methods of carrying out acupuncture in attempting to alleviate various types of pain are necessarily comparable, it is essential when reporting the results of an acupuncture trial to state the particular method adopted in the title of the paper and to provide a detailed description of it in the text.

UNCONTROLLED TRIALS

In evaluating any recently introduced form of therapy it is not uncommon for preliminary uncontrolled studies of it to be carried out, and certainly since the medical profession in the Western world has become increasingly interested in acupuncture during the past 10–15 years, numerous reports of uncontrolled trials of this type of therapy in patients with musculoskeletal pain have appeared in the literature. Most of them have serious deficiencies and therefore brief reference will only be made to some of the more important ones including two large-scale studies carried out in mixed groups of chronic pain patients, and a few carried out on patients with specific types of pain, particularly migraine and low-back pain.

Spoerel (1976) studied the effect of administering a course of 10 daily acupuncture 'treatments' to 200 patients suffering from a variety of different types of pain, and showed that 61% experienced immediate improvement, and that 2 months later 42% still showed some improvement, Frost et al (1976) gave three sessions of acupuncture to acute and chronic pain patients and found that of those with chronic pain 70% obtained immediate relief and that this improvement was maintained in most of them at a 3 month follow-up.

There have been many uncontrolled studies of acupuncture in patients with migraine. The major shortcoming of most of them, as with the majority of all uncontrolled trials, is that the measurements used for assessing response to treatment have been inadequate. However, in those trials in which a reduction in medication was used as the 'yard-stick' of improvement, it was found that this ranged from 76% (Kim & Yount 1974a) down to 33% (Marcus 1979), and in studies where subjective measurements of pain relief were used, the proportions of patients deemed to show significant improvement were also extremely variable ranging from 92% (Laitinen 1975) to 54% (Cheng 1975). Several uncontrolled trials of acupuncture in patients with chronic low-back pain have also shown widely varying response rates ranging from 47% (Yuen et al 1976) to 83% (Pontinen 1979). Most of such trials have been of poor quality with assessments based on a small number of ill-defined outcome criteria. Two particular exceptions to this have been the study of Leung (1979)

and another carried out by Kim & Yount (1974b) in both of which a wide range of subjective and objective measures were employed.

The value of uncontrolled studies is clearly very limited as they give no indication as to how patients might have fared in the absence of treatment. Nevertheless the overall impression obtained from studying the results of those already carried out, and it cannot be any more than an impression with trials of this type, is that from 50–70% of patients with chronic musculoskeletal pain obtain worthwhile short-term relief from acupuncture.

CONTROLLED TRIALS

From what has just been said with respect to uncontrolled trials it is obvious that in order to assess adequately the effectiveness of acupuncture as a pain-relieving agent it is essential, as in the evaluation of any other form of treatment, for clinical trials to be carried out in a controlled manner. Such trials may take the form of assessing the response in one group of patients treated with acupuncture, and comparing this with any spontaneous improvement that may occur over a period of time in a control group receiving no treatment. Alternatively, and to be preferred, the response to acupuncture in one group can be compared with that in a control group receiving treatment either with a placebo or some other form of therapy used in routine clinical practice.

No-treatment controlled trials

There have been several no-treatment controlled trials of acupuncture reported in the literature, particularly on patients with back pain, and of these, two of the most notable because of their design and the quality of their assessment measures were those carried out by Coan et al (1980) on patients with chronic low-back pain and Coan et al (1982) on patients with chronic neck pain. In these two trials the acupuncture was of the traditional Chinese type with points selected for each patient on an individual basis as a result of information obtained from traditional Chinese diagnostic procedures.

In the low-back trial each patient in the treatment group was given 10 sessions of traditional acupuncture. On assessment immediately following this 70% of the patients were judged to have had significant pain relief, and at follow-up 40 weeks later it was still 58%. In contrast, the no-treatment group over a given period of time showed no improvement. In a similarly designed trial in patients with chronic neck pain, 80% in the treatment group showed immediate improvement, compared with only 2% in the control untreated group.

Any trial in which there is a no-treatment group at least has the merit that it is possible to assume with a certain degree of confidence that any improvement in the treatment group, over and above that observed in the control group, is due to the treatment itself, but it gives little or no information concerning specific as opposed to non-specific factors responsible for the treatment's effectiveness, or its comparative effectiveness with respect to other forms of therapy. For these purposes it is necessary to have as the control, either a group of patients treated with a placebo, or a group treated with some other established form of therapy.

Before discussing placebo-controlled trials and other treatment-controlled trials it is necessary to say something about the design of acupuncture trials in general.

Fixed or variable treatment parameters

In the carrying out of controlled clinical trials it is generally considered mandatory to standardize treatment parameters. This is certainly both essential and practicable in the elevation of drugs but so far as acupuncture trials are concerned it presents certain difficulties.

The selection of points

In trials on patients with some specific pain disorder it might be considered ideal for all those in the acupuncture treatment group to be stimulated at exactly the same sites. This is certainly practicable when traditional acupuncture points are selected from formulae, but clearly it is not, when such points are chosen on an individual basis as an essential part of the practice of pure traditional Chinese acupuncture, or when points in the tissues overlying trigger points are used, as with both of these methods the points requiring stimulation are liable to vary from person to person.

Type of stimulation

In any acupuncture trial the active treatment group should have the stimulus applied either electrically or manually but not, in my opinion, both at the same time. Edelist et al (1976) in the treatment of low-back pain firstly manipulated the needles manually until tê-chhi was elicited and then applied stimulation electrically. The combined use of manual and electroacupuncture in this manner clearly causes confusion, particularly when attempting to compare the outcome of such a trial with that obtained in trials using either one or the other of these two forms of stimulation.

Amount of stimulation at each treatment session

For the purposes of conducting acupuncture trials it might seem essential for the amount of dry needle stimulation given to each patient in the treatment group to be kept constant. In trials where manual stimulation is employed, this would mean keeping the needles in situ for the same length of time in everyone, and either not twirling them or twirling them, with in each case, this being carried out in exactly the same manner and to the same extent. It is however apparent from everyday clinical practice that with manual stimulation the optimum amount of stimulation for individuals is widely variable and can only be found for each person by a process of trial and error (Ch. 8). The insistence on a fixed amount of stimulation for every patient therefore is liable to result in some patients being overstimulated, with, as a consequence, their pain being exacerbated and in others being under-stimulated with the result that the treatment is not given a chance to exert its maximum effect.

Macdonald et al (1983) are therefore in my opinion much to be commended, for in their study on patients with low-back pain, they made provisions in their trial protocol for the manual stimulation of needles to be varied according to individual patients' requirements. They achieved this by laying down instructions that the needles had initially to be left in situ for 5 minutes, but that every time a treatment failed to produce a beneficial result, the length of time was to be doubled at the next treatment a week later until a maximum insertion time of 20 minutes had been reached.

A similar principle applies when using electro-acupuncture, acupuncture-like TENS, and conventional TENS (see Ch. 9). With all such methods, much time has to be spent in finding the optimum frequency and intensity of current for each individual (Wynn Parry 1984). And in order therefore to evaluate these treatment procedures accurately, clinical trial protocols should not insist on fixed parameters as at present but should, in my opinion, allow a certain amount of flexibility within laid down limits in order to allow for differences in individual requirements.

Number of treatment sessions

With acupuncture treatment it is rare for there to be any appreciable benefit after only one treatment and therefore it is not appropriate to attempt to evaluate the effectiveness of this type of treatment in a trial in which it is only given on one occasion as in that carried out by Jensen et al (1979) on patients with headache, or in Moore & Berk's (1976) trial in patients with chronic shoulder pain.

It usually requires 3–4 sessions before a decision can be made as to whether a patient is likely to respond to acupuncture (Lewith 1985) and often more than this before any long-term relief is obtained, with this varying according to the condition being treated and a person's individual response to acupuncture. It is often necessary to give up to 10 treatments. In acupuncture trials, therefore, it would not seem prudent to allow only a small fixed number of sessions to be given to every patient for fear that for some individuals this may not be sufficient to allow them to achieve their maximum response. At the same time it is difficult to evaluate the

results of a trial where the number of treatment sessions allowed is too widely variable as in Catton & Kim's trial (1975) where it ranged from 2–47. A realistic compromise would seem to be for a trial protocol to allow each patient to receive up to a maximum of 10 treatments depending on their individual requirements, as in the traditional Chinese acupuncture trial of Coan et al (1980) and the trigger point acupuncture trial of Macdonald et al (1983).

Double-blind or single-blind trials

For many years it has been widely accepted that for the evaluation of drugs it is essential to have a randomized placebo-controlled double-blind trial. In such trials, patients are randomly placed in either a treatment group or a placebo group and both the physician and the patients are kept in ignorance as to the distribution between the two groups. In addition, care is taken to ensure that the drug and the placebo substance are identical in appearance. These measures are of course adopted in order to avoid bias on the part of the physician or the patients influencing the outcome of the trial. It is now generally agreed that in evaluating acupuncture double-blind trials cannot readily be carried out. Weintraub et al (1975) attempted it in a study designed to assess the value of acupuncture in musculoskeletal pain. They did this by means of getting a Chinese acupuncturist to design two forms of treatment, the one utilizing traditional acupuncture points considered to be of specific value in the treatment of the painful disorders from which the patients suffered and the other utilizing traditional acupuncture points purported not to be of any therapeutic value in these conditions. Patients were allocated to one or other of these two types of treatment by means of an independent process of randomization. Then, an American physician, unaware of the patient's problem and of acupuncture theory but skilled in point localization and needle insertion, carried out the treatment.

It has to be admitted that by virtue of resorting to this highly contrived arrangement both the therapist and the patients were 'blind' as to whether, according to the beliefs of traditional Chinese acupuncture, specific or non-specific acupuncture points were being stimulated and thus whether 'real' or simulated acupuncture was being applied. Nevertheless, for reasons to be discussed at length when considering placebo-controlled trials, it would certainly require very large numbers before any difference in response between two such groups could be discerned, and it is not surprising that no differences were found between these two types of treatment 1 week after the second acupuncture session.

It is now generally agreed that for all practical purposes it is only really possible to employ a single 'blind' type of placebo trial in evaluating the pain-relieving properties of acupuncture, with the 'blind' person being an independent assessor. Even when this methodology is adopted it is imperative that the therapist, who is bound to know whether acupuncture or a placebo is being administered, is especially careful to avoid unwittingly making any comments that might influence the response of patients in either the acupuncture or the placebo groups.

The design of acupuncture trials

Of the various trials so far completed in which the effect of acupuncture has been compared either, with that of some other type of treatment in current use such as physiotherapy or, with that of some type of placebo treatment, the design of most of them has been one in which the comparison has been made between two groups, one receiving acupuncture and the other serving as a control. A few trials, however, have been of the cross-over type in which the treatments being compared have been given sequentially in random order to each patient in turn.

A cross-over design has certain disadvantages so far as acupuncture trials are concerned because the speed of response to acupuncture and the immediate duration of relief from it varies widely from person to person, with in some people there being a considerable delay before the full effect of this type of treatment manifests itself. It therefore follows that if acupuncture and then some other type of treatment are given with only a short interval in between, any delayed response from the acupuncture may interfere with an attempt to assess the effectiveness of the second treatment. Such a problem is not confined to acupuncture trials alone but applies to any trial in which some type of physical treatment is being evaluated. It is therefore apparent that if a cross-over design is used in trials of this kind it is essential for there to be a long interval of up to several months in between each type of treatment (Lewith & Machin 1983).

A further problem with a cross-over trial is that a person who seems to be doing well with the initial treatment may be reluctant or even unwilling to change from this to some other form of treatment. On balance, therefore, with acupuncture trials, group comparison would seem in general to be the more appropriate.

Numbers required in trials for the evaluation of acupuncture

The number of patients required in order to make an acupuncture trial statistically valid depends on several factors including the anticipated clinical differences between the treatments being compared, the level of statistical significance considered appropriate, and what are considered to be the chances of detecting such differences. This involves the application of considerable statistical expertise, and anyone requiring detailed knowledge of this should consult Machin's excellent contribution to the subject (Lewith & Machin 1983).

The assessment of results

Assessment of the results of an acupuncture trial should be made immediately at the end of a laid down course of treatment, and then at varying intervals after this, depending on the disorder being treated and in particular on its natural history.

Whilst agreeing with Richardson & Vincent (1986) in reference to trials already completed that 'the relative paucity of long-term follow-up data is especially disappointing with chronic pain patients where the need to demonstrate lasting benefits from a new treatment is of paramount importance', exception has to be taken to their view that 'temporary relief of pain in such a group may be of theoretical interest but will have little clinical significance' for it has to be remembered that even when the relief from chronic pain with acupuncture or for that matter any other form of treatment is found to be only short lasting, this is not necessarily a failure so far as the patient is concerned as the quality of life is often greatly improved by repeating the treatment at frequent intervals. And within this context, it has to be borne in mind that, whilst it may be possible to demonstrate that acupuncture, so far as the alleviation of chronic pain is concerned, is a valuable symptomatic form of treatment, the very nature of the condition makes it unlikely that it will often be shown to be a 'cure'.

Methods of measuring pain relief

Although, as previously stated, in the carrying out of acupuncture trials, a double-blind methodology would be ideal, it is really only practicable for these to be single-blind with the 'blind' person being an independent medical assessor. Unfortunately there are no objective means of measuring changes in the character and intensity of pain for as Scott & Huskisson (1976) have said 'measurement of pain must always be subjective since pain is a subjective phenomenon — only the patient can therefore measure its severity'.

Pain-measuring devices that have proved to be of value include the visual analogue scale, the graphic rating scale (Huskisson 1974a and b), and also the McGill Pain Questionnaire (Melzack 1975a). As patients find it extremely difficult to remember any changes that may occur in their perception of pain over a period of time, it is very helpful for them to be issued with diaries so that they can record details concerning pain levels, medication intake, and sleep on a daily basis (Lewith et al 1983). In addition to information provided by the patient, the assessor should take into account such factors as changes in mobility, and time off work as Gunn et al (1980) did in their trial on patients with chronic low-back pain. Finally, with certain disorders, such as, for example, shoulder-cuff lesions, use should be made of a goniometer for measuring joint movements (Fernandes et al 1980).

These subjective and objective methods of assessment clearly apply to pain trials in general

and as there is nothing particular about them in relation to acupuncture trials, they will not be discussed further but anyone who requires more detailed information should consult an extensive review of methods of measuring and assessing pain (Melzack 1983), a comprehensive summary of recent work on the subject (Reading 1989), and an account of how methods of measuring pain should be employed in the assessment of acupuncture treatment (Vincent & Chapman 1989).

Placebo-controlled trials

Before discussing placebo-controlled trials for the evaluation of the pain-relieving properties of acupuncture it is necessary to say something about placebos.

The term placebo, a word derived from the Latin work *placere* meaning to please, has an established ecclesiastical usage in the phrase Placebo Domino — I shall please the Lord — which appears in the opening antiphon of the vespers for the dead. According to the *Shorter Oxford Dictionary* it has, in addition, been used by the medical profession since 1811 to describe some medical substance given more to please than to benefit a patient. It has always seemed to me that it would have been more apposite for the word in the medical sense to have been derived from the Latin *placare* — to placate — because therapeutically it is given more to pacify or appease than it is to give pleasure to a patient!

A pure placebo is a pharmacologically inert substance which, if given with sufficient confidence by the physician and received with enough faith by the patient, is capable of relieving symptoms in a proportion of people. Beecher (1955) from a review of 15 reports in the literature concluded that a number of symptoms including nausea, anxiety, and various types of pain including postoperative pain, angina, and headache are relieved by a placebo such as a sugar or salt solution in about 35% of patients. People can therefore be divided into placebo responders and placebo non-responders, and as any drug depends for its action partly on its own individually specific therapeutic properties and partly on a non-specific placebo effect it follows that its overall effectiveness is dramatically enhanced in those people who are fortunate enough to be placebo responders (Melzack & Wall 1982a). This is why Lasagna et al (1954) found that a standard dose of morphine is only 54% effective in placebo non-reactors but 95% effective in placebo reactors.

Any chemical substance or physical procedure used as a form of therapy may have specific therapeutic properties of its own together with non-specific placebo ones common to all forms of treatment or it may simply be a non-specific placebo, and in order to establish whether a procedure such as acupuncture is either the first or the second, it is necessary to test it in clinical trials against some suitable known placebo.

Acupuncture might well be expected to have a powerful non-specific placebo effect considering that it is an esoteric form of therapy with an aura of mysticism, and a reputation for having apparently been used successfully in the Far East for centuries (Shapiro & Morris 1978); and therefore in order to assess whether it has specific effects over and above this, it is necessary to test it against some suitable equally powerful placebo.

Suitable placebos for use in acupuncture trials include simulated acupuncture and mock transcutaneous electrical nerve stimulation (TENS).

Mock TENS involves placing electrodes on the skin over acupuncture points and attaching them to a TENS machine that has been specially adjusted so as to make it appear to be working but with a switch left open so that no current reaches the patient.

Mock TENS has been found by Lewith & Machin (1981) and Thorsteinsson et al (1978) to be effective in about 30–35% of patients, but, more recently, Langley et al (1983, 1984) found that the placebo effect of any bogus form of treatment may be augmented by psychologically making it more impressive and that simply adding a distracting oscilloscope to a defunctioned TENS machine produced a 55% response rate in their series of patients.

The proportion of patients capable of responding to a physical placebo is therefore not constant, as it is in a double-blind drug trial in which the active drug and placebo are identical in appearance, but can be raised by the use of psychological devices including verbal suggestions and/or audio and visual signals. It should be noted with respect to this that Melzack (1975b) in studying the relief of pain with acupuncture-like TENS, reinforced the effectiveness of placebo mock TENS by keeping the oscilloscope wave form and the flashing lights on the defunctioned TENS machine used in the control group exactly the same as that on the normally functioning machine used on patients in the active treatment group. He also told the patients in the control group that they were being given a special high frequency Vanagas wave (Vanagas being the name of his department's engineer!). Macdonald et al (1983) in a trial of acupuncture in chronic low-back pain placed skin electrodes over trigger points and attached them by wires to an impressive but electrically non-functioning apparatus that had an 8-channel chart recorder covered with dials and lights and a cooling system that made a 'whirring' sound. Petrie & Langley (1983) in a study comparing the effects of acupuncture and mock TENS in chronic cervical pain described the mock TENS to patients as subliminal pulse therapy.

In addition to the trials just referred to, mock TENS has been used by Lewith et al (1983) in a study designed to compare its effect with that of acupuncture in post-herpetic neuralgia; and by Dowson et al (1985) in a trial to study the effects of acupuncture versus placebo in the treatment of headache. In both these trials the placebo response rate was of the usual order of 33%, and, as will be discussed later, there are arguments in favour of not having too impressive a TENS procedure because, by keeping the response rate down to this level, it only requires a relatively small number of cases in the acupuncture and control group to demonstrate which of the two is the more effective.

Of the various trials in which acupuncture has been compared with mock TENS in the alleviation of pain, most of them have shown acupuncture to be the more effective, but this might only mean that of the two it is a more powerful placebo! As Richardson & Vincent (1986) point out,

Where pharmacological research is concerned this problem hardly arises since the drug and its placebo counterpart are indistinguishable by the patient and doctor. Acupuncture and mock TENS however are palpably different and may arouse different expectations of improvement in the patient or may differ in other unspecified ways which could nonetheless affect their placebo power.

It is for this reason that, in a number of trials, the effect of acupuncture with needle stimulation carried out at acupuncture points has been compared with that of acupuncture with needle stimulation carried out at sites some distance away from acupuncture points. A patient is certainly less likely to be able to distinguish between these two types of acupuncture and therefore their non-specific placebo effect is more likely to be similar but the use of a control type of treatment of this kind as will be shown is certainly not without its problems.

Acupuncture at acupuncture points versus acupuncture at non-acupuncture points

There have been a large number of trials in which the pain relieving effectiveness of carrying out acupuncture with needles inserted into traditionally recognized specific points has been compared with the effectiveness of acupuncture performed in exactly the same manner, including the needles being inserted to a similar depth, but at non-acupuncture sites or what have come to be called sham points (Lewith & Machin 1983).

An excellently designed one was that of Co et al (1979) in patients with the pain associated with sickle cell anaemia. They found that pain relief was obtained in 15 of 16 painful episodes regardless of whether an acupuncture point or a sham site was treated. Of the trials to determine the value of acupuncture in the treatment of musculoskeletal pain that of Gaw et al (1975) in patients with osteoarthritis affecting various joints; of Yuen et al (1976) in patients with various types of chronic disabling pain; also of Edelist et al (1976), Godfrey & Morgan (1978), and Yue (1978) in patients with back pain, all showed that acupuncture in which traditional points were stimulated had a substantial pain-relieving effect but that there was no significant difference between this and that obtained by applying a similar type of acupuncture stimulation at non-specific points. Mendleson et al (1983) in a cross-over trial but with true and sham acupuncture treatment satisfactorily separated by a 4-week interval also found these two types of acupuncture to be equally effective but in a remarkably low percentage of patients ('true' acupuncture 26%, 'sham' acupuncture 21%). This low success rate, however, is probably accounted for by the patients having especially long-standing pain with a mean duration of 12 years. It should be noted in passing that in contrast to this well-planned cross-over trial just mentioned the one carried out by Lee et al (1976) is impossible to evaluate as the application of specific point acupuncture followed by non-specific point acupuncture, or vice versa, at very short intervals, made it impossible to distinguish the effect of one treatment from another.

In contrast to the trials already mentioned there have been two in patients with musculoskeletal pain where acupuncture carried out in the normal manner has been shown to be significantly more effective than acupuncture using non-specific sham points. There were Matsumoto et al's study (1974) in patients with shoulder pain and Man & Baragar's study (1974) in patients with rheumatoid arthritis.

Matsumoto et al divided 24 patients with shoulder pain into two main groups, but in order to give them, either manual or electroacupuncture at a trigger point, or simulated manual or electroacupuncture at a non-specific point, the patients had to be placed in 6 sub-groups so that only 4 patients received one of these various types of treatment, with the result that the numbers were too small for the comparative effectiveness of these different types of treatment to be adequately analysed.

Man & Baragar divided 20 patients, each with seropositive rheumatoid arthritis affecting both knees, into two groups. Hydrocortisone was injected intra-articularly into one knee in both groups. The other knee was treated either by electroacupuncture with needles inserted into what were considered to be correct traditional Chinese acupuncture points in one group, or by electroacupuncture with needles 'incorrectly placed because they have no known effects according to Chinese literature' in the other group. Pain was said to have been moderately decreased in 90% of patients in the classical acupuncture group and only very transiently in 10% of those having sham acupuncture.

The failure in the majority of trials to find significant differences between 'real' and 'sham' acupuncture may mean, either that both exert their effects through being equally strong non-specific placebos; or that because of factors such as diffuse noxious inhibitory control mechanisms (Le Bars et al 1979) both are equally effective specific forms of treatment; or that differences exist between them but, as Lewith & Machin (1983) have suggested, it needs very much larger numbers of patients in the 'real' and 'false' acupuncture groups, than have been used in any of the trials up to now, to demonstrate these.

In order to obviate the interpretative confusion created by employing sham acupuncture with needles inserted into non-specific points various ingenious methods have been devised of simulated acupuncture without the needles penetrating the tissues, but in order for such methods to fulfil a placebo role it is essential for them to be sufficiently akin to 'real' acupuncture as to be readily accepted by patients as being bona fide forms of this type of therapy. In this connection it is interesting to note that Borkovec & Nau (1973) have developed a treatment credibility rating method that is now used extensively in psychotherapy research and, as Richardson & Vincent (1986) suggest, it could be used with profit in future non-blind placebo-controlled acupuncture trials.

Moore & Berk (1976) have so far been the only ones to check with their patients at the completion of an acupuncture trial as to whether the type of placebo used was a convincing form of therapy. In their trial 42 patients with chronic shoulder pain were divided into two groups. One group received a traditional form of acupuncture in which needles were inserted into seven conventional acupuncture points and manually manipulated for three 3-minute periods, with two 4-minute rest periods in between, during the course of being kept in situ for a total of 17 minutes. In the other group the skin was simply pricked at each of the seven same points in order to simulate insertion, and following this the needle was tapped rapidly and lightly against the surface of the skin for similar three 3-minute periods separated by rest periods, with again the treatment lasting 17 minutes. Somewhat surprisingly 'the average percentage of improvement among those who had acupuncture was not, statistically, significantly different from those who had placebo', and even more surprisingly when patients in the two groups at the completion of the trial filled in a questionnaire asking them to speculate on whether they had received classic acupuncture or an imitation of it, all of them, except two subjects in each group (about 10%) thought they had received 'real' acupuncture. The placebo therefore was a convincing form of therapy.

Junnila (1982a) has also carried out a randomized comparison between acupuncture and pseudoacupuncture in cases of chronic musculoskeletal pain affecting one or another part of the body. In order that the patients could not see what was going on, they were placed in the prone position and acupuncture or simulated acupuncture was applied to the posterior aspects of their bodies. In the acupuncture groups needles were inserted into posteriorly situated traditional acupuncture points but before inserting these, and again 20 minutes later on withdrawing them, care was taken to show them to the patient. In the placebo pseudoacupuncture group, care was also taken to show the needles to each patient at the beginning of treatment, but instead of these being inserted, the skin on the patient's back about 1" away from each of the traditional acupuncture points was jabbed for 1 second with the nail of the little finger. Nothing further was then done until after 20 minutes had passed when removal of the needles was simulated including showing them to the patient 'with a flourish'!

On a horizontal pain scale, the reduction of pain in the treatment group was 80% and in the pseudo-acupuncture group 30%, thus supporting the idea that the procedure employed in this latter group was acting as a true placebo.

Jensen et al (1979) studied the treatment of headache in dental student volunteers by either applying acupuncture with a needle inserted into the traditional acupuncture point 'Liver' 3 between the 1st and 2nd metatarsal bones in the foot and twirling it for about 20 minutes, or by applying pseudo-acupuncture in which the needle, hidden from the patient's view, was placed against the skin without penetrating it, also for 20 minutes during which time the movements used in the 'real' acupuncture group were simulated.

Comparison of assessment questionnaires given to the students before and after acupuncture and pseudo-acupuncture showed a significant reduction in the number of days with headache following the former but not after the latter type of treatment. In this cross-over trial the grounds on which Jensen and his co-workers based their belief that the students did not know when they were receiving acupuncture and when they were receiving simulated acupuncture was to quote their words:

as the acupuncture needle is very thin and the insertion of the needle is practically painless in the region selected only 2 of the 29 participants reacted to the insertion. It therefore seems fairly reasonable that none of the experimental subjects were aware of the type of treatment they received either at the first or the second session.

It is clear from what has been said that when pseudo-acupuncture in a control group takes the form of needles inserted into sham points at exactly the same depth and manipulated in exactly the same manner as needles used in a 'real' acupuncture group, it is readily perceived by the patient as being a seemingly credible form of acupuncture and it therefore undoubtedly has a powerful non-specific placebo effect, but as in addition such a procedure would seem to have diffuse noxious inhibitory control effects, it is necessary as previously stated, to have large numbers of patients in the 'real' acupuncture group and in the 'sham' acupuncture group in order to give 'true' acupuncture a fair chance of demonstrating a greater degree of effectiveness. Dowson (1983) has estimated that the number required is more than a hundred in each group.

However, in order to avoid these difficulties, it is necessary to devise some form of simulated acupuncture in which needle penetration is avoided but this requires much subterfuge and there is always the very real risk that it may appear to patients to be so contrived and implausible and so unlike any bonafide form of acupuncture treatment as seriously to diminish its effectiveness as a placebo.

Mock TENS also has its disadvantages because its psychological impact is very different from that of any type of acupuncture which inevitably complicates the situation when attempting to assess their comparative effectiveness. Its advantage over using acupuncture with needles inserted into sham points as a placebo is that when its response rate is kept down to 33%, only about 40 patients are needed in each group (Dowson 1983).

It was in an attempt to avoid the disadvantages of the two types of placebo acupuncture already described and those of mock TENS that Vincent & Richardson (1986) suggested that perhaps some compromise form of sham acupuncture involving very shallow needle penetration at incorrect points might be better, as this would help to minimize any possible specific effects of needling whilst at the same time making the real and sham acupuncture seem almost identical to the patient.

This technique has already been adopted by Hansen & Hansen (1983) when they compared the effects of 'real' and 'sham' acupuncture in a cross-over trial in patients with chronic facial pain. The 'real' acupuncture was performed by inserting needles to a depth of 10–30 mm into traditional Chinese acupuncture points and with care being taken to elicit tê-chhi (the needle sensation) which many believe to be a sine qua non for true acupuncture. The 'sham' acupuncture was performed by inserting needles into non-specific points to a depth of only 2–4 mm and by carefully avoiding the production of needle stimulation.

They summarized their results by stating 'traditional Chinese acupuncture was found to be significantly more pain-relieving than placebo acupuncture according to the pain registration of the patients themselves and to their subjective preferences'.

Vincent (1989a) also used minimal acupuncture as the control, with needles inserted to a depth of only 2 mm at sham points situated 2–3 cm from standard acupuncture points, when assessing the effect of inserting needles to a depth of 1–2 cm at traditional sites in patients with migraine. Despite the fact that the intake to the trial was only fairly small (30 patients) he was able to show that true acupuncture was significantly more effective than the control procedure.

Vincent (1989b) has, however, recognized that because minimal acupuncture of this type has some physiological effect it might be better, in acupuncture trials involving the use of superficial needling at trigger point sites, to employ a completely inert placebo as a control.

Before bringing this discussion concerning placebo-controlled acupuncture trials to a close, it is necessary to point out that the question as to whether acupuncture is more than a placebo might no longer seem to be all that relevant (BMJ 1981) as Levine et al (1978) have now shown that both placebo-induced pain relief and acupuncture-induced pain relief can be blocked by naloxone, thus suggesting that both placebos and acupuncture alleviate pain by virtue of their ability to evoke activity in the body's endogenous opioid peptide-mediated pain modulating mechanisms.

However, as pointed out by Melzack & Wall (1982b) in favour of pain relief produced by acupuncture being more than a placebo effect is the fact that by the use of this procedure analgesia can be induced in animals such as rabbits (Chang 1973) and monkeys (Vierck et al 1971, Sandrew et al 1978).

Comparative trials

Trials so far carried out on patients with various painful musculoskeletal disorders for the purpose of comparing acupuncture with other types of treatment including physiotherapy, steroid injections, and non-steroidal anti-inflammatory drugs with respect to their relative efficacy, side-effects and patient acceptability, are listed in Table 11.1.

Detailed consideration will be given to each of these trials in turn when discussing the clinical applications of acupuncture in Part Three and therefore it is only necessary at this stage to make the general observation that most of them have serious shortcomings of one kind or another. The major criticism is that many of them were so small as to have been no more than pilot studies. Much caution therefore has to be exercised in interpreting their results and because of this there is much scope for further well-designed larger scale trials in order that the place for acupuncture relative to that for other forms of treatment in the relief of this type of pain may be more clearly defined; and in order to ascertain whether or not there are any particular clinical circumstances when the results from using acupuncture in

Table 11.1 Trials comparing either manual or electroacupuncture with another therapy in the alleviation of musculoskeletal pain

Author(s)	Clinical disorder	Alternative form of treatment
Ahonen et al (1983)	Tension headaches	Physiotherapy including ultrasound
Brattberg (1983)	Tennis elbow	Steroid injections
Fernandes et al (1980)	Shoulder cuff lesions	Physiotherapy; oral anti-inflammatory drugs; steroid injections
Gunn et al (1980)	Low-back pain	Medical treatment
Junnila (1982b)	Osteoarthritis	Piroxicam
Loh et al (1984)	Migraine and tension headaches	Medical treatment
Loy (1983)	Cervical spondylosis	Physiotherapy
Man & Barager (1974)	Rheumatoid arthritis	Steroid injections
Milligan et al (1981)	Osteoarthritis of knees	Physiotherapy

In all these trials groups were compared, with the exception of Loh et al's trial in which the design was a cross-over one.

combination with some other method of treatment are better than from using either of them by itself.

Manual stimulation versus electrical stimulation

In attempting to relieve musculoskeletal pain by means of some form of peripheral nerve stimulation there is a choice of four methods including manual acupuncture, electroacupuncture, acupuncture-like transcutaneous electrical nerve stimulation (TENS) and conventional TENS. Many physicians, including myself, believe that manual acupuncture is the treatment of choice for this type of pain and that any form of electrical stimulation should be kept in reserve for those cases that prove resistant to this. There are others, however, who use one or another method of electrical stimulation routinely in all cases. And up to now there have been few clinical trials comparing the efficacy of manual and electrical stimulation.

Both Laitenen (1976) and also Fox & Melzack (1976) have compared manual stimulation with transcutaneous electrical stimulation in the treatment or chronic low-back pain but, as Richardson & Vincent (1986) have pointed out, the results of these studies were somewhat inconclusive. Fox & Melzack only included 12 patients in an unsatisfactorily designed cross-over trial with the patients only being given each of the two types of treatment on two occasions. Laitinen's study was admittedly larger with 100 patients divided into two groups of 50, and with each group given an average of five sessions of one or other of the two types of treatment. Unfortunately however their 4-point rating scale method of assessing results was somewhat crude. Neither of these two trials showed any statistical differences between the two methods but it is possible that this was because of inadequacies in their designs and therefore further trials are required before differences of opinion concerning their comparative efficacy can be resolved.

Traditional Chinese acupuncture versus trigger point acupuncture

From the musculoskeletal pain trials so far conducted there is nothing to suggest that the results obtained with either traditional Chinese acupuncture or trigger point acupuncture are significantly different, but the one great virtue of the latter for those trained in the Western system of medicine is that it was developed from the application of principles rooted in that particular system. It is for this reason that Part Three will mainly be devoted to the clinical applications of trigger point acupuncture.

REFERENCES

Ahonen E, Hakumaki M, Mahlamaki S, Partanen J, Riekkinen P, Sivenius J 1983 Acupuncture and physiotherapy in the treatment of myogenic headache patients: Pain relief and EMG activity. Advances in Pain Research Therapy 5: 571–576

Beecher H K 1955 The powerful placebo. Journal of the American Medical Association 159: 1602–1606

Borkovec T D, Nau S D 1973 The role of expectancy and physiological feedback in fear research: a review with special reference to subject characteristics. Behaviour Therapy 4: 491–505

Brattberg G 1983 Acupuncture therapy for tennis elbow. Pain 16: 285–288

British Medical Journal Leading Article 1981 How does acupuncture work? 283: 746–748

Catton D V, Kim S 1975 Acupuncture for chronic pain — a small pilot project. American Journal of Chinese Medicine 3: 75–81

Chang H-T 1973 Integrative action of thalamus in the process of acupuncture for analgesia. Scientia Sinica 16: 25–60

Cheng A C K 1975 The treatment of headaches employing acupuncture. American Journal of Chinese Medicine 3: 181–185

Co L L, Schmitz T H, Havdala H, Reyes A, Westerman M P 1979 Acupuncture: An evaluation in the painful crises of sickle cell anaemia. Pain 7: 181–185

Coan R M, Wong G, Su L K, Yick C C, Wang L, Ozer F T, Coan P L 1980 The acupuncture treatment of low-back pain: a randomized controlled study. American Journal of Chinese Medicine 8: 181–189

Coan R M, Wong G, Coan P L 1982 The acupuncture treatment of neck pain. A randomized controlled study. American Journal of Chinese Medicine 9: 326–332

Dowson D 1983 Setting up a clinical trial. Journal of the British Medical Acupuncture Society May: 13

Dowson D I, Lewith G T, Machin D 1985 The effects of acupuncture versus placebo in the treatment of headache. Pain 21: 35–42

Edelist G, Gross A E, Langer F 1976 Treatment of low-back pain with acupuncture. Canadian Anaesthetists Society Journal 23: 303–306

Fernandes L, Berry H, Clark R J, Bloom B, Hamilton E B D 1980 Clinical study comparing acupuncture, physiotherapy, injection, and oral anti-inflammatory therapy in shoulder-cuff lesions. Lancet 1: 208–209

Fox E J, Melzack R 1976 Transcutaneous electrical stimulation and acupuncture: comparison of treatment for low-back pain. Pain: 2: 141–148

Frost E A M, Hsu C Y, Sadowsky D 1976 Acupuncture therapy. New York State Journal of Medicine 76: 695–697

Gaw A C, Chang L W, Shaw L C 1975 Efficacy of acupuncture on osteoarthritic pain. New England Journal of Medicine 21: 375–378

Godfrey C M, Morgan P A 1978 A controlled trial of the theory of acupuncture in musculoskeletal pain. Journal of Rheumatology 5: 121–124

Gunn C C, Milbrandt W E, Little A S, Mason K E 1980 Dry needling of muscle motor points for chronic low-back pain: a randomized clinical trial with long-term follow up. Spine 5: 279–291

Hansen P E, Hansen J H 1983 Acupuncture treatment of chronic facial pain — a controlled cross-over trial. Headache 23: 66–69

Huskisson E C 1974a Measurement of pain. Lancet 2: 1127–1131

Huskisson E C 1974b Pain mechanisms and measurements. In: The treatment of chronic pain. Medical and Technical Publishing, Lancaster

Jensen B L, Melsen B, Jensen S B 1979 The effects of acupuncture on headache measured by reduction in number of attacks and use of drugs. Scandinavian Journal of Dental Research 87: 373–380

Junnila S Y T 1982a Acupuncture therapy for chronic pain. A randomized comparison between acupuncture and pseudo-acupuncture with minimal peripheral stimulus. American Journal of Acupuncture 10(3): 259–262

Junnila S Y T 1982b Acupuncture superior to piroxicam in the treatment of osteoarthritis. American Journal of Acupuncture 10: 241–246

Kim K C, Yount R A 1974a The effect of acupuncture on migraine headaches. American Journal of Chinese Medicine 2: 407–411

Kim K C, Yount R A 1974b The effect of acupuncture on low-back pain. American Journal of Chinese Medicine 2: 421–428

Laitinen J 1975 Acupuncture for migraine prophylaxis: a prospective clinical study with six months' follow-up. American Journal of Chinese Medicine 3: 271–274

Laitinen J 1976 Acupuncture and transcutaneous electric stimulation in the treatment of chronic sacro-lumbalgia and ischialgia. American Journal of Chinese Medicine 4: 169–175

Langley G B, Sheppeard H, Johnson M, Wigley R D 1984 The analgesia effects of transcutaneous electrical nerve stimulation and placebo in chronic pain patients. Rheumatology International 2: 1–5

Langley G B, Sheppeard H, Wigley R D 1983 Placebo therapy in rheumatoid arthritis. Clinical and Experimental Rheumatology 1: 17–21

Lasagna L, Mosteller F, Von Felsinger J M, Beecher H K 1954 A study of the placebo response. American Journal of Medicine 16: 770–779

Le Bars D, Dickenson A, Besson J M 1979 Diffuse noxious inhibitory control parts I & II. Pain 6: 283–327

Lee P K, Modell J H, Andersen T W, Saga S A 1976 Incidence of prolonged pain relief following acupuncture. Anaesthesia & Analgesia: Current Researches 55: 229–231

Leung P C 1979 Treatment of low-back pain with acupuncture. American Journal of Chinese Medicine 7: 372–378

Levine J D, Gordon N C, Fields H L 1978 The mechanism of placebo analgesia. Lancet 2: 654–657

Lewith G T 1984 Can we assess the effects of acupuncture? British Medical Journal 288: 1475–1476

Lewith G T 1985 Acupuncture and transcutaneous nerve stimulation. In: Lewith G T (ed) Alternative therapies. Heinemann Medical, London, p 33

Lewith G T, Machin D 1981 A randomized trial to evaluate the effects of infrared stimulation of local trigger points versus placebo on the pain caused by cervical osteoarthrosis. Acupuncture & Electro-therapeutics Research 6: 277–284

Lewith G T, Machin D 1983 On the evaluation of the clinical effects of acupuncture. Pain 16: 111–127

Lewith G T, Field J, Machin D 1983 Acupuncture compared with placebo in post-herpetic pain. Pain 17: 361–368

Loh L, Nathan P W, Schott G D, Zilkha K J 1984 Acupuncture versus medical treatment for migraine and muscle tension headaches. Journal of Neurology and Psychiatry 47: 333–337

Loy T T 1983 Treatment of cervical spondylosis. Medical Journal of Australia 2: 32–34

Macdonald A J R, Macrae K D, Master B R, Rubin A P 1983 Superficial acupuncture in the relief of chronic low-back pain. Annals of the Royal College of Surgeons of England 65: 44–46

Man S C, Baragar F D 1974 Preliminary clinical study of acupuncture in rheumatoid arthritis. Journal of Rheumatology 1: 126–129

Marcus P 1979 Treatment of migraine by acupuncture. Acupuncture and Electro-therapeutics Research 4: 137–147

Matsumoto T, Levy B, Ambruso V 1974 Clinical evaluation of acupuncture. American Surgery 40: 400–405

Melzack R 1975a The McGill pain questionnaire: major properties and scoring methods. Pain: 1: 277–299

Melzack R 1975b Prolonged relief of pain by brief, intense transcutaneous somatic stimulation. Pain 1: 357–373

Melzack R (ed) 1983 Pain measurement and assessment. Raven Press, New York.

Melzack R, Wall P 1982a The challenge of pain. Penguin, Harmondsworth, p 43, 1982b: p 323

Mendleson G, Selwood T S, Kranz H, Kidson M A, Scott D S 1983 Acupuncture treatment of chronic back pain, a double-blind placebo-controlled trial. American Journal of Medicine 74: 49–55

Milligan J L, Glennie-Smith K, Dowson D I, Harris J 1981 Comparison of acupuncture with physiotherapy in the treatment of osteoarthritis of the knees. In: Conference proceedings of 15th International Congress of Rheumatology

Moore M E, Berk S N 1976 Acupuncture for chronic shoulder pain: an experimental study with attention to the role of placebo and hypnotic susceptibility. Annals of Internal Medicine 84: 381–384

Petrie J P, Langley G B 1983 Acupuncture in the treatment of chronic cervical pain. A pilot study. Clinical and Experimental Rheumatology 1: 333–335

Pontinen P J 1979 Acupuncture in the treatment of low-back pain and sciatica. Acupuncture & Electro-therapeutics Research 4: 53–57

Reading A E 1989 Testing pain mechanisms in persons in pain. In: Wall P D, Melzack R (eds) Textbook of pain, 2nd edn. Churchill Livingstone, Edinburgh, p 195–204

Richardson P H, Vincent C A 1986 Acupuncture for the treatment of pain: a review of evaluative research. Pain 24: 15–40

Sandrew B B, Yang R C C, Wang S C 1978 Electro-acupuncture analgesia in monkeys: a behavioral and neurophysiological assessment. Archives international de pharmacodynamie et de therapie 231: 274–284

Scott J, Huskisson E C 1976 Graphic representations of pain. Pain 2: 175–184

Shapiro A K, Morris L 1978 The placebo effect in medical and psychological therapies. In: Garfield S L, Bergin A E (eds) Handbook of psychotherapy and behaviour change. Wiley, New York, ch 10

Spoerel W 1976 Acupuncture in chronic pain. American Journal of Chinese Medicine 4: 267–279

Ter Reit G, Kleijnen J, Knipschild P 1990 Acupuncture and chronic pain: A criteria-based meta-analysis. Journal of Clinical Epidemiology 43(II): 1191–1199

Thorsteinsson G, Stonnington H H, Stilwell G K, Elveback L R 1978 The placebo effect of transcutaneous electrical stimulation. Pain 5: 31–41

Vierck C J, Hamilton D M, Thornby J I 1971 Pain reactivity of monkeys after lesions to the dorsal and lateral column of the spinal cord. Experimental Brain Research 13: 140–158

Vincent C A 1989a A controlled trial of the treatment of migraine by acupuncture. The Clinical Journal of Pain 5 (4): 305–312

Vincent C A 1989b The methodology of controlled trials of acupuncture. Journal of the British Medical Acupuncture Society. 6: 9–13

Vincent C A, Chapman C R 1989 Pain measurement and the assessment of acupuncture treatment. Journal of the British Medical Acupuncture Society 6: 14–19

Vincent C A, Richardson P H 1986 The evaluation of therapeutic acupuncture. Concepts and models. Pain 24: 1–13

Weintraub M, Petursson S, Schwartz M et al 1975 Acupuncture in musculoskeletal pain: methodology and results in a double-blind controlled clinical trial. Clinical Pharmacology and Therapeutics 17: 248

Wynn Parry C B 1984 Brachial plexus injuries. British Journal of Hospital Medicine 32: 130–139

Yue S J 1978 Acupuncture for chronic back and neck pain. Acupuncture & Electro-therapeutics Research 3: 323–324

Yuen R W M, Vaughan R J, Dyer H, Giles K E 1976 The response to acupuncture therapy in patients with chronic disabling pain. Medical Journal of Australia 1: 862–865

Zhang W, Oetliker H 1991 Acupuncture for pain control. A review of controlled clinical trials. In: Schlapbach P, Gerber N J (eds) Physiotherapy: Controlled Trials and Facts. Rheumatology. Basel, Karger, vol 14, p 171–188

PART THREE

The practical application of trigger point acupuncture

12. Chest pain

INTRODUCTION

In discussing the practical applications of trigger point acupuncture in Part Three of this book, the indications for its use in the alleviation of certain types of chest pain will firstly be considered because historically, some of the earliest clinical observations concerning the referral of pain from myofascial trigger points were made just before the Second World War on patients with trigger point activity in the muscles of the chest wall. Attention will mainly be directed to cardiac pain and to musculoskeletal pain because so far as chest pain is concerned it is in the alleviation of these two types of pain that acupuncture has its main application.

At the outset it has to be made clear that clinically there is often difficulty in distinguishing between cardiac and musculoskeletal chest pain because the pattern of distribution of pain, occurring as a result of the primary activation of trigger points in muscles of the chest wall, is often identical to that of pain of cardiac origin, and because these same chest wall muscles are liable to develop secondary trigger point activity in them as a result of lying within an area affected by cardiac pain.

Before discussing the differential diagnosis of these two trigger point pain syndromes it should be explained that attention was first drawn to the phenomenon of secondary trigger point activation in the muscles of the chest wall in patients with coronary heart disease by two University of Pennsylvania physicians, Joseph Edeiken and Charles Wolferth, when in 1936 they reviewed some cases of coronary thrombosis in which pain

in the shoulder had developed during the course of strict bed rest.

Edeiken & Wolferth reported that on examination of the muscles around the scapula in two of their patients, they found focal areas of exquisite tenderness, or what they called trigger zones in view of the fact that by applying pressure to these zones they were able to reproduce the spontaneously occurring pain in the shoulder. They further stated that one of their patients had noticed for himself that pressure over one of these so-called trigger zones caused pain to be referred to the left shoulder, up the left side of the neck and down the left arm.

The significance of such observations might readily have been overlooked had it not been that this report came to the attention of Janet Travell, the American physician who has since contributed so much to the subject of referred pain from trigger points, at a time when she herself was suffering from a painful shoulder, not following a coronary thrombosis, but after having strained some muscles during the course of her work. As she says in her autobiography, *Office Hours: Day and Night* (1968),

Poking around at night on the muscles over my shoulder blade, trying to give some 'do-it-yourself' massage, I was astonished to touch some spots that intensified, or reproduced my pain, as though I had turned on an electric switch. It was my first introduction to the enigmatic trigger area. No nerve existed, I knew, to connect those firing spots directly with my arm. I was baffled, but I did not discard the observation on the grounds that I could not explain it.

It was because Travell found that she could reproduce pain in herself in exactly the same manner as Edeiken & Wolferth had done in patients with myocardial infarction that prompted her to study the subject further. The opportunity to do this arose almost immediately when, in 1936, she was appointed to work under Dr Harry Gold in the Cardiac Consultation Clinic at Sea View Hospital on Staten Island, New York. At this hospital, with specialized in the treatment of tuberculosis, a large number of patients, having been kept in bed for long periods, suffered severe pain in their shoulders and arms. As she says in her autobiography,

When I examined them by systematic palpation of the scapula and chest muscles, I easily uncovered the presence of trigger areas. I knew what to look for . . . .

Her interest in the referral of pain from muscle having been aroused in this manner, she was prompted to read the various other important contributions to the subject published over the next few years including those of Kellgren (1938), Steindler & Luck (1938) and Steindler (1940). From these she learnt that such pain may be alleviated by injecting procaine into 'tender spots' (trigger zones) in the muscles.

As a result of reading these reports Travell decided in 1940 to persuade Dr Myron Herman, the medical resident at Sea View Hospital, to inject procaine into trigger areas in the chest walls of patients with painful shoulders at that hospital (Travell et al 1942). It was because the results of this treatment were so impressive that Travell and her cardiologist colleague, Seymour Rinzler, decided to investigate a number of other patients under their care in the general medical wards at the Beth Israel Hospital. The outcome of this was that in 1948 they published two outstanding papers. In the one they drew attention to the fact that trigger points may develop in the muscles of the chest wall as a secondary event in patients with cardiac pain and reported that it is possible to relieve the latter by injecting procaine into these trigger points, or by spraying the skin overlying them with ethyl chloride (Rinzler & Travell 1948). In the other they showed how closely the pattern of pain, occurring as a result of the primary activation of chest wall trigger points, may simulate that of ischaemic heart disease (Travell & Rinzler 1948).

They were not, however, the first to recognize this, as Gutstein (1938), Kelly (1944) and Mendlowitz (1945) had previously described how pain from 'tender spots' in the muscles of the chest wall may have a similar pattern of distribution to that of cardiac pain.

PRIMARY ACTIVATION OF TRIGGER POINTS IN MUSCLES OF THE CHEST WALL

The various factors responsible for the primary activation of trigger points in muscles of the chest wall include acute trauma, strain from any sustained activity particularly if this is of an unusual nature, nervous tension, and exposure to draughts.

CHEST WALL PAIN SIMULATING CARDIAC PAIN IN ITS PATTERN OF DISTRIBUTION

It is of course only pain from primarily activated trigger points in certain muscles on the left side of the neck and chest wall that is liable to have a similar pattern of distribution to that of cardiac pain.

Primary myofascial trigger point pain may simulate cardiac pain when there is trigger point activity in only one muscle. More often, however, it occurs as a result of such activity occurring in several muscles simultaneously, or when there is a chain reaction of trigger point activity from one muscle to another until ultimately several are involved.

As pointed out by Travell (1976), a good example of such a chain reaction is when trigger point activity arises in the sternal division of the sternocleidomastoid muscle causing pain to be referred down the length of the sternum. Pain in this distribution may then lead to the development of trigger point activity in the sternalis muscle, with as a result of this, pain being referred to the pectoral region and the development of secondary trigger point activity in the pectoralis major muscle. These trigger points may then be responsible for pain being referred to the left shoulder and down the left arm. This therefore is a good example as to how doing nothing more serious than straining a muscle in the neck may lead to the development of pain with a pattern of distribution exactly similar to that of coronary heart disease.

As it cannot be stressed too strongly it will be reiterated that what makes diagnosis difficult is that not only may the pattern of pain from a primary muscle disorder be similar to that of ischaemic heart disease, but that secondary trigger point activity may also develop in exactly the same muscles when they happen to lie within an area affected by pain from myocardial ischaemia.

The various muscles liable to be involved in these two separate trigger point pain syndromes include: in the neck, the sternal division of the sternocleidomastoid and the scaleni; in the chest, the sternalis, the subclavius, the pectoralis major, the pectoralis minor and the serratus anterior; and in the abdomen, the rectus abdominis and the external oblique muscles.

The clinical manifestations and treatment of trigger point activity in each of these muscles will now be considered in turn.

Sternocleidomastoid muscle

Trigger point activity in the lower end of the sternal division of the muscle may cause pain to be referred over the upper part of the sternum (Fig. 16.6). As trigger points elsewhere in this muscle refer pain to the face and scalp any discussion concerning the activation and deactivation of trigger points in this muscle will be deferred until Chapter 16.

Scalene muscles

Activation of trigger points

Trigger point activity in any of the three scalene muscles may occur as a primary event by straining the neck such as when pulling with the hands against a strongly resistant force, or when lifting or carrying awkwardly some heavy object; also, as a result of the strain of severe bouts of coughing; or by holding the neck in some awkward position, either when lying or standing. As a secondary event activity may occur when trigger points develop in the sternocleidomastoid muscle.

Specific pattern of pain referral

Pain from trigger points in either the scalenus anterior, medius, or posterior (Fig. 12.1) is liable to be referred anteriorly over the pectoral region; posteriorly along the medial border of the

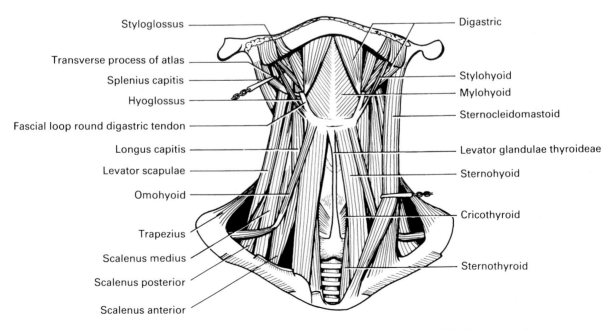

Fig. 12.1   Muscles of the front of the neck. On the right the sternocleidomastoid has been removed.

scapula; and laterally across the front of the shoulder and down the arm. When the latter occurs, it is felt both in the front and back at the arm and extends to the thumb and index finger (Fig. 12.2).

Pain from trigger point activity in one or other of these muscles on the left side may closely simulate that associated with coronary heart disease, because of its distribution and because sometimes it only comes on with exertion.

In making a diagnosis, it is helpful to remember that referred pain from the scalenus anterior is relieved when both the arm and clavicle are elevated by placing the forearm on the affected side across the forehead (Ochsner et al 1935); and it is aggravated by contracting the muscle by rotating the head as far as possible to the side of the pain whilst pulling the chin down into the supraclavicular fossa.

With regard to the effect the position of the arm has on this type of pain, it is of interest to note that a man under my care, with pain in the chest and down the right arm from trigger point activity in the right scalenus anterior muscle, found that although the pain was always aggravated by carrying heavy loads with the arm hanging down at the side of the body, it was never present when, with the arm held high, he carried the British Legion banner at ex-Servicemen's parades.

Trigger point examination

Trigger points in the scalenus anterior are found by palpating the muscle where it lies behind the posterior border of the sternocleidomastoid muscle. It is useful to distend the external jugular vein by putting pressure on it at the base of the neck, as the vein crosses the scalenus anterior muscle usually just about the level where trigger point activity in this muscle occurs.

As the scalenus medius lies lateral to the scalenus anterior and at a much deeper level against the transverse processes of the vertebrae,

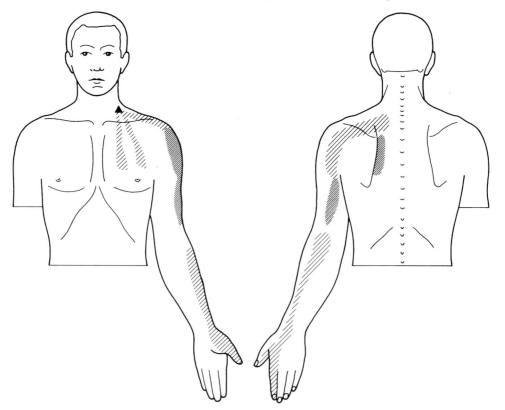

Fig. 12.2   The pattern of pain referral from a trigger point or points (▲) in a scalene muscle.

trigger points in the muscle may be readily identified by pressing against these structures. The scalenus posterior is far more difficult to palpate but fortunately trigger point activity in this muscle seems to be much less common than in the other two.

Associated trigger points

The scalenus anterior and medius muscles are often involved together.

Trigger points may develop in several muscles in areas to which pain from trigger point activity in the scalene muscles is referred. The anteriorly referred pain may cause trigger points to become activated in the pectoralis major. Pain down the back of the arm may cause trigger points to become activated in the triceps; and pain down the front of the arm may cause similar activity to develop in the brachioradialis and the extensor carpi radialis. Trigger point activity in the scalene muscles may also occur in association with it developing in the levator scapulae muscle (see Ch. 14).

Deactivation of trigger points

Deactivation of trigger points in the scalenus anterior and medius should be carried out with the patient in the supine position, with the head supported by a pillow and turned towards the opposite side. In deactivating trigger points in the scalenus anterior, care has to be taken not to puncture the external jugular vein, or to damage the cervical spinal nerve roots and part of the brachial plexus where they emerge in the groove between the scalenus anterior and medius. It must, however, be remembered that needling a scalene trigger point itself often cause momentary intense pain to shoot down the arm and that therefore this alone does not necessarily imply that a nerve root has been irritated.

Thoracic outlet entrapment syndrome

The possible part played by myofascial trigger point activity in the scalene muscles giving rise to compression of the brachial plexus and subclavian artery will be discussed in Chapter 15.

Sternalis muscle

Activation of trigger points

Trigger point activity arises in the muscle either as a primary event, usually as a result of trauma to the front of the chest, or as a secondary event when pain is referred to the region of the sternum, either as a result of coronary heart disease, or from trigger point activity in the lower end of the sternocleidomastoid muscle, or in a scalene muscle.

Specific pattern of pain referral

This muscle is only present in about 1 in 20 people, but when it does exist, the development of trigger points in it is liable to lead to the development of deep substernal pain with, at times, radiation of this across the left or right pectoral region and down the inner side of the arm to the elbow (Fig. 10.3).

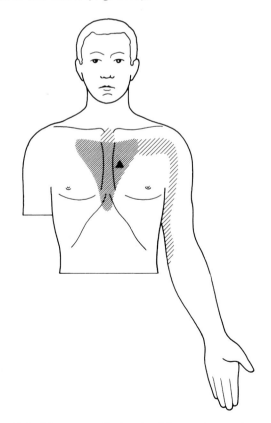

Fig. 12.3   The pattern of pain referral from a trigger point or points (▲) in the sternalis muscle.

Trigger point examination

Trigger points occur anywhere along the length of this muscle and are found by systematically palpating the muscle against both borders of the underlying sternum. Firm pressure on a trigger point causes considerable local tenderness and at times the referral of pain in a lateral direction.

Associated trigger points

Trigger point activity in this muscle is rarely an isolated event. It usually occurs in conjunction with trigger points in the pectoralis major muscle. And, as stated earlier, pain from trigger point activity in the sternal division of the sterno-cleidomastoid muscle may be referred downwards over the sternum and cause trigger points in the sternalis muscle to become activated.

Trigger point deactivation

A trigger point in this muscle is readily located by flat palpation. A needle is then inserted into the tissues overlying it after it has first been trapped between two fingers.

Subclavius muscle

Activation of trigger points

Trigger points in this muscle are liable to become activated for the same reasons as, and often in conjunction with, points in the pectoralis major muscle.

Specific pattern of pain referral

Trigger point activity in this muscle causes pain to be referred across the front of the shoulder, down the front of the arm in the midline, the front of the forearm on the radial side, and the radial side of the palmar surface of the hand and fingers. As Travell & Simons (1983) point out, pain for some curious reason is not felt at either the elbow or the wrist (Fig. 12.4).

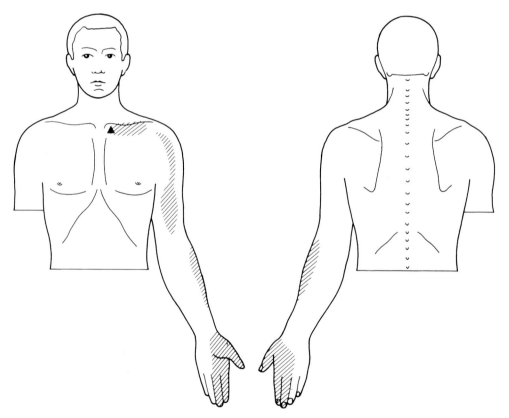

Fig. 12.4   The pattern of pain referral from a trigger point or points (▲) in the subclavius muscle.

Trigger point examination

Trigger points are usually to be found in this muscle at its medial end around the site of its insertion into the 1st rib (Fig. 12.4).

Associated trigger points

Trigger points in this muscle invariably occur in association with trigger point activity in the pectoralis major muscle.

Deactivation of trigger points

A needle should be inserted superficially into the point of maximum tenderness just below the clavicle.

Pectoralis major

Activation of trigger points

The factors which may cause primary trigger point activity in this muscle include lifting a heavy weight, or holding it for a sustained period; any task involving repeated adduction of the arm, such as when cutting a hedge with manually operated shears, or sustained adduction, such as when the arm is placed in a sling for any length of time; exposure of the muscle to draughts or damp; persistent contraction of the muscle from chronic anxiety; and in particular when a faulty slouching posture is adopted when reading, writing or carrying out some task at a work bench.

Secondary activity of trigger points may occur when pain from coronary heart disease is referred to the left side of the chest anteriorly.

Specific patterns of pain referral

This muscle is divided according to its various attachments into a clavicular section, a sternal section, and a costo-abdominal section. These merge together to be inserted by means of a tendon into the lateral lip of the bicipital groove of the humerus (Fig. 12.5). The specific patterns

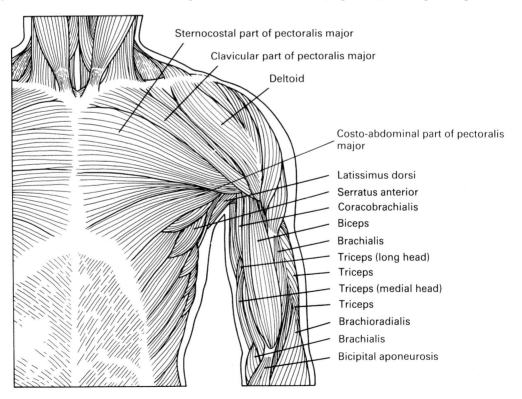

Fig. 12.5 Superficial muscles of the front of the chest and upper arm. Left side.

of pain referral vary according to the particular section affected.

Trigger point activity in the clavicular section of the muscle refers pain locally and in addition even more markedly over the shoulder as far as the anterior part of the deltoid muscle (Fig. 12.6).

Trigger point activity in the sternal section is found mainly along the parasternal and mid-clavicular lines, with trigger points along the parasternal line referring pain locally, and over the sternum. Trigger points in the mid-clavicular line give rise to severe pain over the anterior part of the chest and thus, on the left side, over the praecordium. From these it often spreads down the inner aspect of the arm, being felt particularly strongly over the medial epicondyle and terminates in the ring and little fingers (Fig. 12.7).

Trigger point activity along the lateral free margin of the muscle, where it forms the anterior axillary fold, gives rise to pain and tenderness in

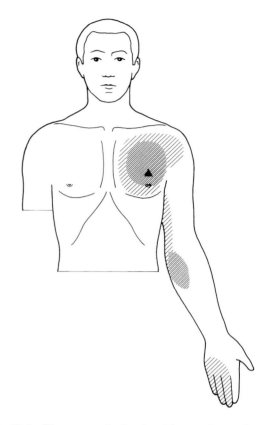

Fig. 12.7 The pattern of pain referral from a trigger point or points (▲) in the sternal section of the pectoralis major muscle.

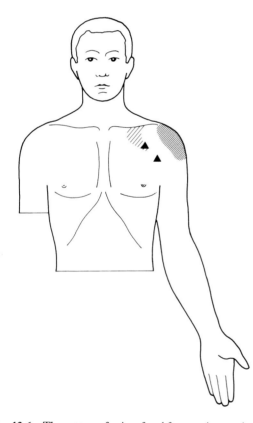

Fig. 12.6 The pattern of pain referral from a trigger point or points (▲) in the clavicular section of the pectoralis major muscle.

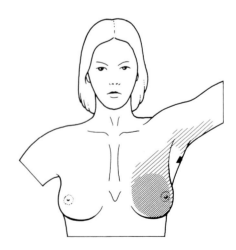

Fig. 12.8 The pattern of pain referral from a trigger point or points (▲) in the lateral free margin of the pectoralis major muscle.

the breast, as well as tenderness of the nipple. In women this not infrequently leads to an erroneous diagnosis of mastitis in spite of the texture of the breast being normal (Fig. 12.8).

Trigger point examination

Trigger points in the clavicular section and in the parasternal part of the sternal section should be located by flat palpation. Trigger points situated more laterally in the sternal part, and those in the anterior axillary fold should be located by grasping the muscle between the thumb and fingers, the arm having been abducted to about 90°, so as to put the muscle under moderate tension and thereby making it easier to find the points and to observe any local twitch response.

Associated trigger points

Trigger points in the pectoralis major may occur in conjunction with trigger points in the sternalis, sternocleidomastoid, and scalene muscles. The anterior deltoid may also develop them as it lies within this muscle's pain referral zone.

Deactivation of trigger points

When deactivating trigger points in the pectoralis major, or for that matter any muscle covering the chest wall, needles should never be inserted vertically for fear of penetrating the pleura and producing a pneumothorax, but should always be inserted in an oblique direction.

Bilateral trigger point activity

When trigger point activity occurs in both the right and left pectoralis major simultaneously the pain may be said by the patient to be 'across the chest', a description immediately raising the possibility of underlying coronary heart disease. However, the circumstances prevailing prior to the development of the pain may be of diagnostic help as shown by the following case history.

A maintenance fitter (47) sent for his general practitioner in the middle of the night because of pain across the chest and shortness of breath. The latter, in retrospect, almost certainly being due to the pain restricting normal chest movements. A pain relieving injection was given. Blood specimens were taken that night and the next 2 days for cardiac enzyme studies. These proved to be normal as did a subsequent ECG both at rest and after exercise.

However, as he continued to get episodes of pain across his chest most days he was at first given nifedipine (Adalat) but when it became obvious it was not angina, he was put on to naproxen (Naprosyn) and when this did not prove particularly helpful, he was placed on to clomipramine (Anafranil) as it was thought the persistence of the pain might be associated with nervous tension and depression. After 7 months he was referred to me for further assessment. On going back over the history it became apparent that the initial attack of pain had started after lifting a particularly heavy piece of machinery. The subsequent episodes of pain which he described as stabbing in character were not brought on by walking but usually came on after having exerted himself at work, and were particularly troublesome on lying in certain positions in bed.

From the history, therefore, it was most likely that the pain was myofascial in origin. On examination, trigger points were found in the sternal section of the pectoralis major, along the parasternal line on the right side and mid-clavicular line on the left side, also along the free edge of the costo-abdominal section of the muscle on the left side.

These trigger points had to be deactivated with a dry needle on three occasions at weekly intervals, and one further time 2 weeks later before lasting relief from the pain was obtained.

Pectoralis minor

Activation of trigger points

The factors responsible for trigger point activation in this muscle (Fig. 12.9) are similar to those responsible for this in the pectoralis major muscle. Trigger points usually only arise in this muscle when they are also present in the pectoralis major.

Specific pattern of pain referral

Pain from trigger point activity in this muscle is referred widely over the front of the chest so that, on the left side, this is over the praecordium; also over the front of the shoulder, and at times down the ulnar side of the arm to terminate in the middle, ring and little fingers (Fig. 12.10).

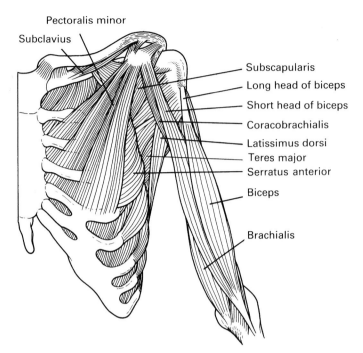

Fig. 12.9   The deep muscles of the front of the chest and arm. Left side.

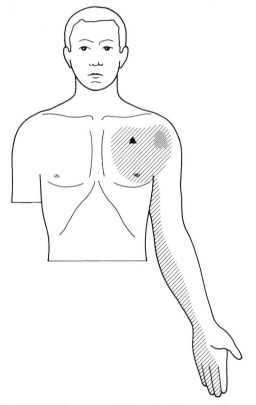

Fig. 12.10   The pattern of pain referral from a trigger point or points (▲) in the pectoralis minor muscle.

Trigger point examination

When locating trigger points in this muscle the patient may either be seated or lying in the supine position. In either case the pectoralis major is slackened by having the patient's arm lying comfortably to the side with the forearm across the abdomen. The pectoralis minor is then put on the stretch by getting the patient to brace the shoulder backwards. Trigger points are usually to be found in the lower part of the muscle where it is attached to the ribs, or in the upper part close to its attachment to the coracoid process.

Deactivation of trigger points

This is the same as for the pectoralis major muscle.

Serratus anterior muscle

Activation of trigger points

Trigger point activity may arise in this muscle (Fig. 12.9) when it is strained during the course of athletic pursuits or physical training; also, when the muscle is strained as a result of severe coughing; or when due to anxiety, the muscles of the chest wall are held tense.

Specific pattern of pain referral

Pain from trigger point activity in this muscle which wraps itself closely around the rib cage is referred to the side and back of the chest, and at times down the ulnar aspect of the arm (Fig. 12.11). The patient may also complain that it is painful to take a deep breath — the so-called stitch in the side.

Trigger point examination

With the patient lying down and turned so that the affected side is uppermost, the muscle is put on the stretch by pulling the arm backwards. Trigger points in palpable bands within this muscle are usually located in the mid-axillary line at about the level of the 5th and 6th ribs in line with the nipple (Fig. 12.11). A local twitch

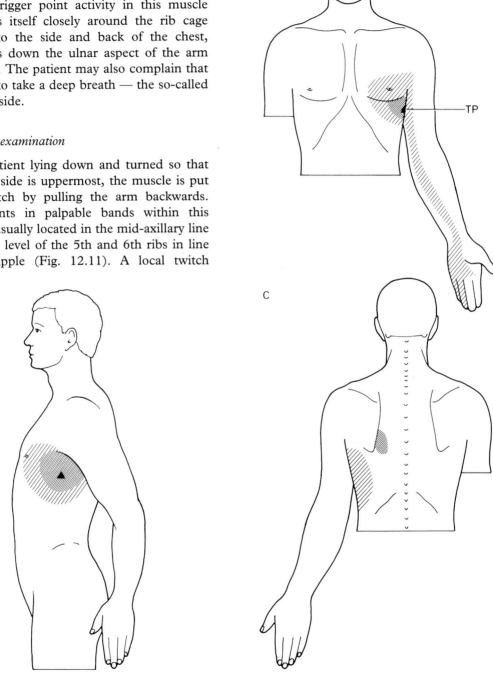

Fig. 12.11 A, B and C The pattern of pain referral from a trigger point or points (▲) in the serratus anterior muscle.

response may sometimes be elicited by sharply plucking these bands with the finger.

Associated trigger points

Trigger point activation in this muscle is often an isolated event. After a time trigger points in its main antagonist, the latissimus dorsi, may also become activated.

Deactivation of trigger points

The trigger points are deactivated by dry needle stimulation with the patient lying with the affected side uppermost, the needle being directed at a shallow angle almost parallel to the chest wall towards an underlying rib so as to avoid entering the pleural space.

Rectus abdominis and external oblique muscles

The effects of trigger point activity in these two muscles will be discussed in detail when considering abdominal pain in Chapter 20. It is necessary to state here, however, that trigger point activity in the upper part of the rectus abdominis muscle and in the upper part of the external oblique muscle may cause pain to be referred upwards over the lower part of the chest anteriorly. When this occurs, either on the left or right side, it is liable to be misdiagnosed as being pleural in origin in spite of the absence either of a pleural rub or any signs of intrapulmonary disease, and on the left side it may closely mimic the pain of coronary heart disease (Kelly 1944).

Activation of trigger points

This commonly occurs either as a result of acute trauma or chronic strain, the latter often having an occupational basis.

Trigger point examination

The patient should be placed in the supine position and instructed to stretch the muscles by holding the breath in deep inspiration. The trigger points in the upper part of the rectus abdominis are usually to be found in the angle

between the costal margin and the xiphisternum. In the upper part of the external oblique muscles trigger points are either long or under the lower border of the rib cage (Figs 20.3 and 20.4).

Deactivation of trigger points

Each trigger point should be trapped between two fingers prior to inserting a needle into the tissues overlying it.

THE DIFFERENTIAL DIAGNOSIS BETWEEN CARDIAC PAIN, AND PAIN ARISING FROM A PRIMARY DISORDER OF MUSCLE IN THE ANTERIOR CHEST WALL

As has already been stated, muscles in the chest wall when subjected to trauma of one kind or another may develop trigger point activity with the pattern of pain resulting from this being identical with that seen in coronary heart disease. Also, the same chest wall muscles may develop satellite trigger point activity as a result of being within the area affected by pain from coronary heart disease.

It is therefore easy to see that diagnostic confusion may readily occur and whilst it is obviously important not to overlook angina when present, it is equally essential not to diagnose chest pain as being anginal when it is only muscular in origin. This is a mistake as frequently made today as when Allison in 1950 wrote in reference to non-cardiac chest pain:

... the frequency with which such patients are seen in routine out-patient work emphasizes the need for a re-orientation towards pain in the chest, and suggests that in clinical teaching pride of place is too often given to angina pectoris in explanation of the pain, and too little regard is paid to local structural causes.

One particular circumstance when primary chest wall pain may be overlooked is when it occurs in someone known to have a history of coronary heart disease. Chest pain arising soon after recovery from a myocardial infarction, if accompanied by fever and a pericardial rub, is readily recognized to be part of the post-infarction syndrome (Dressler 1959), but if, however, it occurs by itself, there is a tendency to assume it must be anginal, and to overlook the possibility of it having arisen from muscles of the chest wall. Similarly, chest wall pain may erroneously be assumed to be anginal when it occurs at some time following coronary by-pass surgery.

The relevance of all this to the practice of acupuncture is that whilst, primarily occurring chest wall pain is readily alleviated by dry needle stimulation of trigger points, and whilst, as will be explained later, this may also have a limited place in the overall management of coronary heart disease, clearly before using such a method for the alleviation of any type of chest pain, it is essential to have made an exact diagnosis as to its cause. For this reason the various problems that arise in differentiating between cardiac pain and musculoskeletal pain will now be discussed.

In attempting to make this distinction, careful history-taking is clearly of prime importance but this by itself may be inconclusive.

As is well known, with ischaemic heart disease there is usually substernal tightness, with at times radiation of pain up into the neck, across the chest to the shoulder and down the left arm. Pain originating in the muscles of the chest wall, however, may have an exactly similar pattern, except that substernal tightness is unusual, it more frequently arising in the parasternal or praecordial region.

Although characteristically, angina is brought on by exertion, chest wall muscle pain also may be aggravated by this. The difference is that whereas with angina the amount of effort required to produce the pain is fairly constant, with skeletal muscle pain it is liable to vary widely from day to day. Also skeletal muscle pain is often aggravated by stretching and twisting movements of the chest wall.

Angina, on occasions, may also occur at rest. When this is due to the heart rate increasing in response to some emotional upset, it usually lasts for a relatively brief period. In contrast, when chest wall pain occurs at rest it is liable to persist for a long time.

Both types of pain may disturb sleep. With ischaemic heart disease this is sometimes because of a tachycardia brought on by dreaming, and with non-cardiac pain because of the adoption of some posture which puts the muscles on the stretch.

Physical examination also is only of limited value in view of the fact that trigger points may be present both with cardiac and non-cardiac pain. It is true, however, that the absence of them excludes the latter.

The response to a therapeutic trial of sub-lingual glyceryl trinitrate may also be misleading since the placebo effect of this ensures that up to 30% of patients with chest pain from any cause may be improved.

Electrocardiography, too, has its limitations, as it is not uncommon for a patient with widespread coronary heart disease to have a normal tracing. Conversely, any abnormal changes seen may only be a reflection of what has happened in the past and have no relevance to the pain under investigation. An ECG taken after exercise testing may also occasionally be misleading.

It therefore follows that there are times when in order to distinguish between cardiac and non-cardiac chest wall pain, either a coronary arteriogram, or assessment of left ventricular function by the more recently introduced technique of radionuclide technetium angiography performed at rest and during exercise (Borer et al 1977, Petch 1986), may be necessary. Epstein et al (1979) have reported the value of this non-invasive technique in distinguishing between musculoskeletal chest wall pain or what they term the chest wall syndrome, and the pain of coronary heart disease because as they stated 'one of the most important services the physician can perform for patients with the chest wall syndrome is to help them avoid the emotional and financial burdens often associated with an erroneous diagnosis of organic heart disease'. However, what they did not say, because they failed to recognize the importance of trigger points in the aetiology of chest wall pain, is how readily this type of pain can be alleviated by means of the acupuncture technique of deactivating these trigger points with dry needles.

INDICATIONS FOR TRIGGER POINT ACUPUNCTURE IN CORONARY HEART DISEASE

Angina

With the various highly effective anti-anginal agents now available, the place for acupuncture in the routine management of this disorder must be strictly limited. If, however, superimposed upon episodes of anginal pain, a more persistent type of pain develops with tenderness of the chest wall, then trigger points should be sought and, if found, deactivated by dry needle stimulation.

Myocardial infarction

The pain of myocardial infarction, although severe, is generally of relatively limited duration and usually satisfactorily controlled by analgesics. However, at times, in spite of a patient's general condition improving, the pain persists for an unusually long time, and when this occurs it may be due to the development of trigger points in the muscles of the chest wall (Rinzler & Travell 1948, Kennard & Haugen 1955). Such pain may readily be alleviated by deactivating these trigger points by inserting dry needles into them.

Coronary by-pass surgery

When chest pain recurs soon after a coronary by-pass operation, there is an instinctive tendency, particularly on the part of the patient, to assume it must be anginal and that the operation has been a failure. It has to be remembered, however, that trauma to the chest wall muscles whenever a thoracotomy is performed for any purpose is very liable to activate trigger points in these muscles and for this to be the cause of such pain. In such circumstances therefore a search for these should always be made and, if found, deactivated by dry needle stimulation.

MUSCLES OF THE POSTERIOR CHEST WALL

Myofascial pain in the upper part of the back, probably because it is not nearly so common as similar pain in the lower back, is frequently not recognized as such, and even when it is, is often inadequately treated.

Before discussing this further it should be noted that trigger point activity in certain muscles of the posterior chest wall such as the supraspinatus and infraspinatus cause pain to be referred mainly to the shoulder region and down the arm. These muscles will therefore be discussed in Chapter 13. And trigger point activity in others such as the levator scapulae, trapezius, and rhomboids causes pain to be felt predominantly in the neck, shoulder girdle and down the arm; a detailed account of these muscles will therefore be given in Chapter 14.

The two muscles in the posterior part of the chest in which trigger point activity causes pain to be felt in the upper part of the back itself as well as down the arm are the serratus posterior superior and the latissimus dorsi. It is to these two muscles therefore that attention will now be directed.

Serratus posterior superior

Activation of trigger points

Primary activation of trigger points in this muscle may occur as a result of protracted bouts of coughing. This may also happen when the scapula is pressed hard against it by the shoulders being persistently elevated and rotated forwards such as may occur when sitting for long periods at a desk or working surface that is too high. Also, satellite trigger points may develop in this muscle when trigger point activity in the scalene muscles causes pain to be referred to the posterior chest wall around the inner part of the scapula (Fig. 12.2).

Specific pattern of pain referral

This thin quadrilateral muscle, situated beneath the trapezius and the rhomboids, and attached medially to the spines of the 7th cervical vertebra and the first three dorsal vertebrae; and infero-laterally by four fleshy digitations to the 2nd, 3rd, 4th and 5th ribs near to their angles behind the upper part of the scapula, is liable to develop trigger point activity at various sites near to this inferolateral insertion (Fig. 12.12). When this occurs, pain is felt as a dull ache around the insertion of the muscle into the ribs behind the scapula. From there it radiates to the back of the shoulder and down the back of the arm to be felt particularly around the medial epicondyle. Occasionally it is felt down the inner side of the forearm and hand as far as the little finger (Fig. 12.13). This pain pattern is similar to that produced by compression of the 8th cervical nerve root (Reynolds 1981). It is distinguished from this by there being no objective neurological signs, and by the presence of exquisitely tender palpable bands (trigger points) in the muscle, with pressure on these reproducing the characteristic pain pattern.

Trigger point examination

The patient sits forwards with the arm stretched across the front of the chest in order to bring the scapula out of the way so that the muscle can be palpated where it lies behind the upper part of this bone deep to the trapezius and rhomboid muscles. The muscle is then examined by rolling a finger over it against an underlying rib. A trigger point will be felt as a firm band with pressure on this evoking the characteristic pain pattern. Associated trigger points may also be found in the rhomboids (p. 190) and in some of the nearby paraspinal muscles (p. 157).

Associated trigger points

Trigger points in this muscle are often associated with trigger point activity in the synergistic

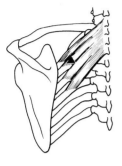

Fig. 12.12 With the arm to the side, a trigger point in the inferolateral part of the serratus posterior superior cannot be palpated as it lies behind the upper inner part of the scapula. To palpate a trigger point at this site, therefore, the scapula has to be pulled forwards as shown.

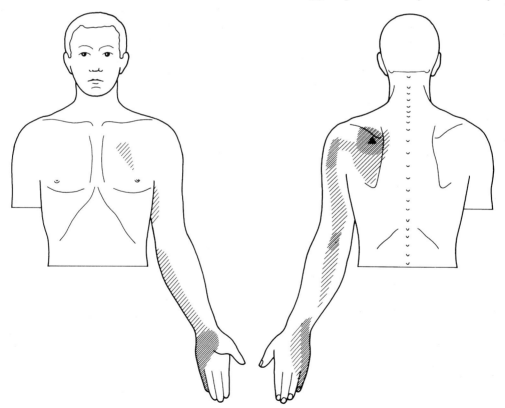

Fig. 12.13 The pattern of pain referral from a trigger point or points (▲) in the serratus posterior superior muscle.

inspiratory scalene muscles in the neck, the nearby erector spinae muscles, and overlying rhomboids.

Deactivation of trigger points

With the patient lying on the opposite side and with the scapula brought well forwards a needle is injected at an angle of 45ª into the tissues overlying a trigger point whilst fixing this between two fingers over a rib. Care must be taken not to insert the needle perpendicularly into an intercostal space as this may result in the pleura being penetrated.

Latissimus dorsi muscle

Latissimus dorsi, which translated from the Latin means 'widest of the back', is an appropriate name for this muscle with its extensive fan shaped attachment to the trunk stretching from the spinous processes of the lower six thoracic and all the lumbar vertebrae and sacrum in the midline, to the crest of the ilium, and to the last four ribs; and from where it sweeps upwards into

the axilla, to form with the teres major muscle, the posterior axillary fold prior to the tendons of these two muscles then joining together to be inserted into the bicipital groove of the humerus (Fig. 12.14). However, although this muscle covers such a large area of the back, trigger points usually only become activated in the part of it that is situated in the posterior axillary fold.

Activation of trigger points

These trigger points in the posterior axillary fold become activated when the upper part of the muscle at its insertion into the humerus, is subjected to strain. Examples of when this may occur include reaching forwards and upwards with the arm whilst carrying some heavy object; stretching the arm such as when hanging on to a rope; or straining the arm whilst engaging in some unusually heavy task such as digging or weeding.

Specific pattern of pain referral

From trigger points in the posterior axillary fold, pain of a dull aching type is referred to the

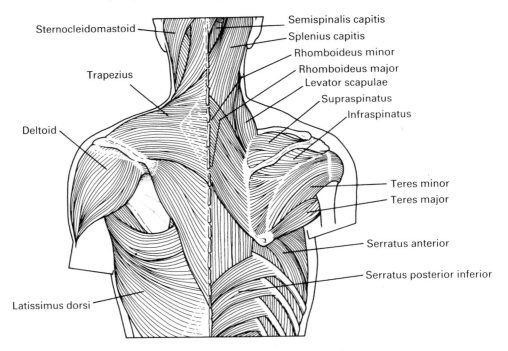

Fig. 12.14   Superficial muscles of the back of the neck and upper part of the trunk. On the left, the skin, superficial and deep fasciae have been removed. On the right, the sternocleidomastoid, trapezius, latissimus dorsi and deltoid have been dissected away.

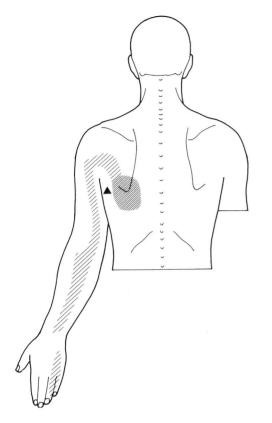

Fig. 12.15   The pattern of pain referral from a trigger point or points (▲) in the latissimus dorsi muscle where this muscle together with the teres major muscle forms the posterior axillary fold.

inferior angle of the scapula and the part of the back immediately around this; it may also extend to the posterior aspect of the shoulder, and down the inner side of the arm, forearm and hand, to terminate in the ring and little fingers (Fig. 12.15).

The pain is persistent and is neither aggravated nor relieved by any type of movements. It is because of this lack of relationship to movements and the fact that the trigger points responsible for it are tucked away in the posterior axillary fold which probably accounts for its myofascial origin being so easily and so often overlooked.

Trigger point examination

The trigger points are most readily found by placing the patient in the supine position, and putting the muscle on the stretch by abducting the arm and placing the hand behind the head. The muscle in the posterior axillary fold is then grasped between fingers and thumb, and with a rolling movement any firm bands present are identified and their points of maximal tenderness (trigger points) located.

Both the superficial and deep parts of the muscle in the posterior axillary fold should be examined, because when Simons & Travell (1976) inserted 7.5% saline into the muscle at this site, an injection into the deep fibres referred pain to the back around the lower part of the scapula, whilst an injection into the superficial ones referred pain down the arm.

Associated of trigger points

Trigger points are likely to develop at the same time in the anatomically closely related teres major (p. 178) and the long head of the triceps (p. 201).

Deactivation of trigger points

Once a trigger point is located it is held between the thumb and fingers whilst a needle is inserted into the tissues overlying it. As trigger points in this muscle tend to be grouped together, both in its superficial and deep parts, this procedure may have to be repeated several times. A strong twitch response is often elicited should the needle penetrate a trigger point in this muscle.

Paraspinal muscles

Myofascial pain in the posterior chest wall may also arise from trigger point activity in superficial paraspinal muscles (erector spinae) such as the iliocostalis thoracis and in deep paraspinal muscles such as the multifidus.

The pain from trigger point activity in the iliocostalis thoracis muscle at the mid-thoracic level is concentrated around the inferior angle of the scapula, but it also spreads upwards and downwards (Fig. 12.16).

The pain from trigger point activity in the multifidus at the mid-thoracic level remains localized around a trigger point usually to be found deep in the paravertebral region (Fig. 12.17).

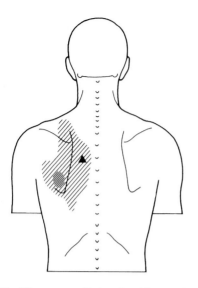

Fig. 12.16 The pattern of pain referral from a trigger point (▲) in the iliocostalis thoracis muscle.

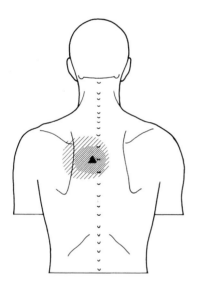

Fig. 12.17 The pattern of pain referral from a trigger point (▲) situated deep in the paravertebral gutter in the multifidus muscle at the mid-thoracic level.

Rectus abdominis muscle

Myofascial pain spreading transversely across the lower part of the posterior chest wall may arise surprisingly enough from trigger point activity in the upper part of the rectus abdominis where the muscle becomes inserted into the rib cage at the junction of the costal margin and xiphisternum (Fig. 20.3).

INTERCOSTAL NEURALGIA

Pain radiating from the back to the front of the chest, in a direction parallel with the ribs, and in the lower part of the chest continuing on to the anterior abdominal wall, may be due to irritation of an intercostal nerve root such as may occur with disease affecting one or more vertebrae. In all such cases, radiographs of the dorsal spine are mandatory. It should be remembered, however, that in the early stages of metastatic involvement of vertebrae the radiological appearances may remain normal and therefore there are times when a bone scan is also required. The possibility of the pain being the precursor of the rash of herpes zoster also has to be considered.

Alternatively, and what for long has been known, but somehow lost sight of, is that such pain may be due to a primary lesion in muscles. Kellgren in 1938 demonstrated this by experimentally injecting saline into paravertebral and intercostal muscles. And Kelly in 1944 confirmed it by clinically observing in patients under his care with pain around the chest that it emanated from foci of exquisite tenderness, now known as trigger points, in exactly the same way as it did from Kellgren's artificially-induced foci of hyper-irritability.

The following case illustrates how such trigger points may be overlooked unless specifically looked for:

A farmer (36) developed severe pain radiating from the back to the front of the right side of the chest in the 5th intercostal space. When after 2 years he continued to complain of this in spite of having been given analgesics for most of this time his general practitioner referred him to a pain clinic in order to exclude the possibility of nerve root entrapment. There were no objective neurological signs; also, chest and spine X-rays were normal. In spite of this an intercostal nerve block was carried out but with no significant improvement. When subsequently he was seen by me there were two foci of exquisite tenderness to be found, one in the multifidus muscle at the level of the 5th thoracic vertebra, and one in an intercostal muscle in the posterior axillary line. Deactivation of these two trigger points by dry needle stimulation resulted in temporary relief for a few days and after repeating this on two subsequent occasions at weekly intervals permanent relief was obtained.

SKELETAL PAIN

Ribs

Pain associated with traumatic bruising of a rib or rib fracture often persists for a surprisingly long time. Periosteal pecking of the rib with a dry needle at the site of the pain is surprisingly helpful in reducing both the severity and the duration of such pain.

Costal cartilages

Tietzes syndrome. This is an obscure but not uncommon condition in which there is pain and swelling of one or more costal cartilages, usually the second and third. Although a benign condition, the pain may persist for several months and is not always responsive to simple analgesics. Local infiltration with a corticosteroid is the standard recommended treatment, but this usually only gives temporary relief and there is a limit to how many times it can repeated. Pecking the costal cartilage with a dry needle in exactly the same manner as with periosteal pecking is therefore preferable as it gives equally good temporary relief and it is a procedure that can readily be repeated as often as is necessary.

POSTOPERATIVE PAIN

There is undoubtedly an important place for electroacupuncture and transcutaneous electrical nerve stimulation (TENS) in the control of pain immediately following a thoracotomy and surgical operations elsewhere in the body, but as this is outside the ambit of this book it will not be discussed further. However, pain persisting long after a thoracotomy may be due to the activation of trigger points in the surgical scar or in the muscles of the chest wall. It may also occur as a result of the division of an intercostal nerve.

Thoracotomy scar pain

It is not uncommon for persistent pain to develop in and around a thoracotomy scar and often for it to extend from there on to the anterior abdominal wall. Points of exquisite tenderness (trigger points) will be found in the scar, and there are often in addition satellite trigger points in that part of the anterior abdominal wall affected by the pain.

It often requires deactivation of these trigger points by dry-needle stimulation to be repeated several times before such pain is brought under control as is shown in the following case.

A man (56), discovered to have an opacity in the right lung on a routine chest radiograph, was submitted to a thoracotomy. Histological examination of the lesion proved it to be benign. One month later he began to complain of pain along the scar. He was reassured that there was no evidence of a stitch abscess but was offered no specific treatment. The pain persisted and eventually he was given Distalgesic to take as and when required. In spite of this the pain gradually became worse and by the time he was referred to me 12 months later, in addition to the chest pain, he was getting severe attacks of cramplike pain in the upper part of the anterior abdominal wall.

On examination four trigger points were found in the scar, two in the external oblique and one in the lateral border of the rectus muscle.

Deactivation of these trigger points had to be carried out on six occasions before any lasting relief was obtained. There is no doubt that the response would hve been quicker had such treatment been started earlier.

Section of an intercostal nerve

Persistent post-thoracotomy pain may also occur as a result of the division of an intercostal nerve. This is often associated with a severe burning and marked hyperaesthesia of the chest wall. This does not in my experience respond to acupuncture. Transcutaneous electrical nerve stimulation (TENS), however, is sometimes helpful.

REFERENCES

Allison D R 1950 Pain in the chest wall simulating heart disease. British Medical Journal 1: 332–336

Borer J S, Bacharach S L, Greer M V, Kent K M, Epstein S E, Johnston G S 1977 Real-time radionuclide cineangiography in non-invasive evaluation of global and regional left ventricular function at rest and during exercise in patients with coronary artery disease. New England Journal of Medicine 286: 839–844

Dressler W 1959 Flare-up of pericarditis complicating myocardial infarction after two years of steroid therapy. American Heart Journal 57: 501

Edeiken J, Wolferth C 1936 Persistent pain in the shoulder region following myocardial infarction. American Journal of Medical Science 191: 201–210

Epstein S E, Gerber L H, Borer J S 1979 Chest wall syndrome: A common cause of unexplained cardiac pain. Journal of the American Medical Association 241: 2793–2797

Gutstein M 1938 Diagnosis and treatment of muscular rheumatism. British Journal of Physical Medicine 1: 302–321

Kellgren J H 1938 A preliminary account of referred pain arising from muscle. British Medical Journal 1: 325–327

Kelly M 1944 Pain in the chest: Observations on the use of local anaesthesia in its investigation and treatment. Medical Journal of Australia 1: 4–7

Kennard M A, Haugen F 1955 The relation of subcutaneous focal sensitivity to referred pain of cardiac origin. Anesthesiology 16: 297–311

Mendlowitz M 1945 Strain of the pectoralis minor, an important cause of praecordial pain in soldiers. American Heart Journal 30: 123–125

Ochsner A, Gage M, Debakey M 1935 Scalenus anticus (Naffziger) syndrome. American Journal of Surgery 28: 669–695

Petch M C 1986 Investigation of coronary artery disease. Journal of the Royal College of Physicians of London 20 (1): 21–24

Reynolds M 1981 Myofascial trigger point syndromes in the practice of rheumatology. Archives of Physical Medicine and Rehabilitation 62: 111–114

Rinzler S, Travell J 1948 Therapy directed at the somatic component of cardiac pain. American Heart Journal 35: 248–268

Simons D G, Travell J 1976 The latissimus dorsi syndrome. A source of mid-back pain. Archives of Physical Medicine and Rehabilitation 57: 561

Steindler A 1940 The interpretation of sciatic radiation and the syndrome of low-back pain. Journal of the American Medical Association 110: 106–113

Steindler A, Luck J V 1938 Differential diagnosis of pain low in the back. Journal of the American Medical Association 110: 106–113

Travell J 1968 Office hours: day and night. World Publishing Company, New York

Travell J 1976 Myofascial trigger points: clinical view. In: Bonica J J, Albe-Fessard D (eds) Advances in Pain Research and Therapy, vol: 1. Raven Press, New York.

Travell J, Rinzler S 1948 Pain syndromes of the chest muscles. Resemblance to effort angina and myocardial infarction, and relief by local block. Canadian Medical Association Journal 59: 333–338

Travell J, Rinzler S, Herman M 1942 Pain and disability of the shoulder and arm: treatment by intramuscular infiltration with procaine hydrochloride. Journal of the American Medical Association 120: 417–422

Travell J, Simons D 1983 Pectoralis major muscle (subclavius muscle) in myofascial pain and dysfunction. The trigger point manual. Williams & Wilkins, Baltimore, p 577

13. The painful shoulder

INTRODUCTION

When presented with a case of persistent pain in the shoulder region, rheumatoid arthritis, other inflammatory arthritides, crystal arthropathy and haemarthrosis of the glenohumeral joint; osteo-arthritis of the acromioclavicular joint, and occasionally of the glenohumeral joint; and diseases of bone all have to be included in the differential diagnosis. Most commonly, however, such pain occurs either as a result of a lesion in the soft tissues in and around the glenohumeral joint, or because it is referred to the shoulder region from a disorder in the musculoskeletal system some distance from it. This chapter, therefore, will be devoted to discussing the place of acupuncture relative to that of other types of treatment including local corticosteroid injections in alleviating the pain associated with these two latter groups of conditions, but, before doing so, it is first necessary to say something about their clinical manifestations.

SOFT TISSUE LESIONS IN AND AROUND THE GLENOHUMERAL JOINT

These lesions include a tendinitis affecting one or other of the rotator cuff muscles; a subacromial bursitis; a bicipital tendinitis; and a capsulitis.

Rotator cuff tendinitis

It will be remembered that the musculotendinous cuff muscles, the supraspinatus, the infra-spinatus, the teres minor, and the subscapularis have a conjoined tendinous insertion into the humerus; the supraspinatus tendon being attached to the laterally placed greater tuberosity; the infraspinatus and teres minor tendons attached immediately below this; and the sub-scapularis tendon attached to the medially placed lesser tuberosity. As a result of these attachments to the humerus, they act as rotators of the joint and in addition, by combining with the deltoid muscle, abduct the arm.

A tendinitis is liable to develop in any of these rotator cuff muscles but the one most commonly affected is the supraspinatus muscle.

Tendinitis is a degenerative avascular necrosis of one or other parts of the rotator cuff. It is often a spontaneously occurring non-traumatic lesion but, at times, symptoms seem to develop when the shoulder has been subjected to some unusual strain such as may occur with house decorating or gardening. It affects adults of all ages but its highest incidence is in the 40–50s age group. Tendinitis in any part of the cuff is usually only associated with a nagging ache at rest but the pain is made worse by certain movements depending on which tendon or tendons in particular are involved.

With supraspinatus tendinitis, active abduction of the arm is painful through the intermediate range (60–120°). The painful arc is probably due to the inflamed tendon rubbing against the acromion because it is abolished by externally rotating the arm, thus placing the greater tuberosity behind the acromion, before carrying out abduction. The pain is also aggravated by resisted abduction. Tenderness is maximal over the tendon where it blends with the anterior part of the capsule of the shoulder joint.

The clinical presentation with infraspinatus and teres minor tendinitis is similar. In both conditions the pain is also localized around the greater tuberosity but it is resisted external rotation that makes it worse. Pain from subscapularis tendinitis is experienced over the lesser tuberosity and is aggravated by resisted medial rotation.

Natural history of tendinitis

When attempting to assess the effectiveness of any form of treatment, including acupuncture, in relieving the pain of tendinitis, it is important to realize that the natural history of the condition is usually for a mild ache at rest and pain brought on by certain movements to persist for weeks or months and then eventually to undergo spontaneous resolution. On occasions, however, the pain may suddenly become more intense due to the development of an acute inflammatory reaction in the tendon and the tissues adjacent to it, including those in the wall of the subacromial bursa. Calcium becomes deposited in a degenerative tendon and when, in the case of the supraspinatus tendon, this suddenly bursts into the subacromial bursa, there is very severe pain and marked restriction of movements, with abduction and external rotation in particular aggravating the pain.

Sudden severe pain may also occur as a result of a tendon becoming torn.

Subacromial bursitis

Subacromial (subdeltoid) bursitis used to be included amongst the primary causes of shoulder pain but it is now generally recognized that inflammatory changes in the bursa do not occur as a primary event but are always secondary to an inflammatory lesion in an adjacent tendon. As Cailliet (1981a) says 'any adjacent inflammation of the tendon causes inflammation of the bursa. It is inconceivable that bursitis could exist without tendinitis and vice versa'.

Cuff tears

It is generally agreed that cuff tears are far commoner than previously supposed. It is now being recognized that it only requires some minor injury to cause partial or complete tear of a tendon that has already been weakened by degenerative changes. The patient who is often in the 40–70 age range experiences a tearing sensation in the shoulder followed immediately by severe pain which often increases in intensity until it reaches a peak about 2 days later. It then remains very acutely painful for a further 4–7 days. On examination there is usually exquisite tenderness on palpation over the greater tuberosity. There is marked aggravation of pain on resisted abduction, and most significant of all, once the patient has raised the arm, there is an inability to control the lowering of it to the side. This, however, does not occur exclusively with a rotator cuff tear but may also be observed with a 5th cervical nerve root lesion.

It is essential to confirm the diagnosis and assess the extent of a tear by contrast radiography. Minor tears usually heal spontaneously within 2 months and require only symptomatic treatment. Extensive tears may need to be repaired surgically.

Bicipital tendinitis

The tendon of the long head of the biceps, attached above to the superior rim of the glenoid fossa, passes downwards enclosed in a sheath of synovium through the glenohumeral joint to emerge from it through an opening in the capsule close to the latter's humeral attachment. The tendon then descends in the bicipital groove situated between the greater and lesser tuberosities (Fig. 12.9). This structure is liable to develop a degenerative tendinitis that clinically presents with pain, and tenderness to pressure, over the bicipital groove. Moreover, the pain is characteristically aggravated by attempting to supinate the arm against resistance.

Acromioclavicular joint strain

As mentioned at the beginning of the chapter, the acromioclavicular joint is liable to develop osteoarthritis, but also when considering soft tissue lesions in the shoulder region, it has to be remembered that the joint may become mechanically strained. When this occurs, pain develops, which although limited to the tip of the shoulder, is aggravated by full passive adduction of the arm across the chest.

Treatment of soft tissue lesions around the glenohumeral joint

The principal object of treatment both for acute and chronic tendinitis and bursitis around the glenohumeral joint is to relieve pain for its own sake and to ensure that full movements of the joint are restored as quickly as possible, for the longer they remain restricted, the more likely it is that a disabling capsulitis or so-called frozen shoulder may develop. There is certainly little evidence that any form of treatment currently available significantly alters the natural history of such lesions.

The main purpose of this discussion is to consider the relative place of acupuncture in the treatment of tendinitis and bursitis. And it has to be said at the outset that, in my opinion, there would seem to be no place for it in the treatment of an acute lesion with very severe pain, such, for example, as may occur with an acute calcific supraspinatus tendinitis with or without an acute subacromial bursitis. With such a lesion, as Cailliet (1981b) states, the arm should be rested in a sling for the first few days. In addition, ice packs should be applied to the shoulder. Ice decreases the muscle spasm and has a powerful analgesic action. Immobilization, however, should never be prolonged for fear that it may lead to the development of a frozen shoulder (capsulitis). Within about 4 days, therefore, mobilization should be encouraged and this can be greatly assisted by controlling the pain with a non-steroidal anti-inflammatory drug and by injecting hydrocortisone (mixed with a local anaesthetic) into points of maximum tenderness.

There is, in my opinion, a place for acupuncture in the treatment of chronic tendinitis in spite of the fact that the only two controlled studies so far conducted would not seem to support this view. The first of these was carried out by Moore & Berk (1976). In their study on 42 patients with chronic tendinitis they compared the effects of traditional Chinese acupuncture with those of a placebo procedure in which needles did not penetrate the skin. As both treatments produced significant reduction in subjective discomfort, it was concluded that they must have achieved their effects through placebo-related factors already discussed in Chapter 11. The main criticism of this trial, however, is that only one treatment session was given, which as Richardson & Vincent (1986) have pointed out, can in no way be considered to be an adequate test of acupuncture.

The second was a study carried out by Fernandes et al (1980). The results of this study were somewhat confusingly published in two separate journals with Berry's name appearing first in one report (Berry et al 1980) and Fernandes' name appearing first in the other (Fernandes et al 1980)!

In this study on patients with rotator cuff lesions, patients were allocated at random to five treatment groups:

1. traditional Chinese acupuncture given once a week for 4 weeks
2. a single injection of a steroid plus a local anaesthetic
3. a steroid injection plus a course of a non-steroidal anti-inflammatory drug
4. 8 sessions of ultrasound
5. a placebo non-steroidal anti-inflammatory drug plus placebo ultrasound.

The trial was carefully conducted utilizing a large number of subjective and objective assessment measures before treatment, and again at 2 weeks and 4 weeks. No differences between the treatments were detected with most of the patients in each of the groups improving significantly. It was therefore suggested that the lesions being treated were of a self-limiting nature and that any beneficial effects were really due to a natural recovery. As quite rightly stated in the report, with the small numbers in each group, this cannot be considered to be any more than a pilot study. Furthermore without a 'no treatment' control group there is no way of telling whether the improvements were due to the treatments themselves or due to a natural recovery process.

It would seem unrealistic to suppose that acupuncture could influence the natural course of tendinitis. Further larger scale trials are required in order to determine objectively whether or not, as my experience leads me to believe, this type of therapy, repeatedly carried out during the course of this condition, does provide worthwhile symptomatic analgesia.

At the present time there is a general preference amongst rheumatologists for the use of local steroid injections in the treatment of rotator cuff lesions, and, as will be discussed later, also of capsulitis, in spite of the fact that the appropriateness and value of using them in these conditions has recently been questioned (Anon 1976). Certainly it would seem that for there to be any chance of them being successful they must be given repeatedly over a period of time (Roy & Oldham 1976), but even so, several studies, in which this has been done, have given conflicting results.

Hollingworth et al (1983) showed that 73% of a group of patients with tendinitis were successfully treated by injecting a local steroid into the anatomical structure believed to be the source of the pain, but that only 29% of another group were improved when the material was injected into tender points. Weiss (1981) reported considerable success with intra-articular injections of a steroid for tears of the rotator cuff. However, Coomes & Darlington (1976), during the course of comparing the effects of local steroid injections with those of local anaesthetic injections in patients with supraspinatus tears, found that, although a local steroid injection gave pain relief initially, after a month there was little difference between the two groups and concluded that there was no objective evidence to show that local steroids improve the condition.

There would certainly seem to be no evidence that local steroids, or for that matter any other form of treatment presently available, influences the natural history of rotator cuff lesions and it would seem that the best that can be done is to use some type of therapy capable of controlling the pain and thereby improving joint movements during the weeks or months it takes for the underlying lesion to undergo spontaneous resolution.

There are undoubtedly several disadvantages associated with using repeated steroid injections for such a relatively long period of time. A local steroid is not infrequently associated with appreciable post-injection pain. In addition, repeated injections are liable to cause local tissue damage, and when injected into a joint may destroy it (Bentley & Goodfellow 1969). Repeated injections may also have systemic effects; Koehler et al (1974) have shown that the hypothalamic/pituitary/adrenal axis is affected 48 hours after an injection of 80 mg of methyl prednisolone acetate into a knee with plasma cortisol levels being suppressed for 3–6 days. In addition there is always the small but definite risk of infection developing at the site of a steroid injection (Anon 1976).

There is therefore much to be said for using some form of treatment which is equally as effective as a local steroid in alleviating the pain of soft tissue lesions around the shoulder joint but without, at the same time, having its disadvantages. It has for long been known that a local anaesthetic injected into a point of maximum tenderness effectively relieves the pain of such a lesion (Kessel & Watson 1977), and for reasons already discussed (Chs 5 & 8) this can be done even more simply and safely just by stimulating A-delta nerve fibres at such a point with a dry needle. Admittedly the pain relief with either of these two techniques is unlikely to last for long, but at least by repeating acupuncture once a week or as often as is required it is possible to keep the pain under control without any fear of undesirable side-effects occurring as a result of such treatment, and with it therefore being possible to continue with it until such a time as the lesion responsible for the pain spontaneously enters a quiescent phase.

CAPSULITIS (FROZEN SHOULDER)

Frozen shoulder is one of the great enigmas of medicine with there being no general agreement as to its nature, diagnosis or treatment, and with the situation still further confounded by a confusing terminology.

Duplay (1896) first termed the condition periarthrite scapulohumerale, since when it has been known as periarthritis, pericapsulitis, and in 1945 Neviaser coined the term adhesive capsulitis because of appearances he found at operation on

10 cases. These included thickening and contraction of the capsule; also adhesions between opposed synovial surfaces, particularly in the inferior part of the joint. It was not however because adhesions were a striking feature that he described the capsulitis as being adhesive, but rather because he noted that during manipulation of the shoulder after an incision through the anterior capsule that the capsule separated from the head of the humerus in the same manner as adhesive strapping peels from the skin.

There is undoubtedly a widespread acute inflammatory reaction involving the capsule and the rotator cuff with the latter being reported at operation to be extremely friable (Bunker 1985). It is not surprising, therefore, that radioisotope scans show gleaming hot spots in the shoulder region (Binder et al 1984).

Aetiology

The condition is liable to develop whenever movements at the shoulder joint are restricted. It may therefore occur following some injury to the shoulder including repeated episodes of minor trauma (Wright & Haq 1976); or as a complication of a tendinitis; or when the arm remains immobile for some appreciable period of time as may occur with a myocardial infarction or as a result of a hemiplegia.

Clinical diagnosis

Capsulitis is a condition in which there is considerable pain and stiffness around the shoulder with marked restriction of all glenohumeral joint movements, both passive and active. External rotation is more severely affected than abduction or internal rotation. An important characteristic of the pain is that it is particularly pronounced in bed disturbing sleep.

It was because of this marked restriction of all movements that Codman (1934) introduced the term 'frozen shoulder' and although that has since had much popular appeal, as Bunker (1985) recently pointed out, the acute inflammatory nature of the condition makes it somewhat of a misnomer.

The clinical diagnosis may be confirmed by arthrography which shows a marked reduction in the volume of the glenohumeral joint so that it only accommodates a few millilitres of contrast medium instead of the normal 10–15 ml (Bruckner 1982).

Natural history of the condition

It is important when considering the influence of various forms of treatment on this condition including the possible place of acupuncture in its management to have a clear knowledge of the natural history of the disease for as Lloyd-Roberts & French (1959) in writing about this disorder said,

A knowledge of the average time between onset and recovery is of outstanding importance if the effects of treatment are to be assessed in a disease which usually resolves spontaneously.

The pain usually remains severe for about 3 months after which it begins to abate but the restriction of movements continues for much longer. The condition is usually eventually self-limiting, burning itself out within 2 years in the absence of any treatment (Grey 1977). A minority of cases, however, have some permanent disability.

Treatment of capsulitis

A variety of different treatments have been advocated including local steroids, oral steroids, ultrasound, radiotherapy, and sympathetic ganglion block but the reports concerning these have been confusingly inconclusive and conflicting, and as the condition is a naturally resolving one, only those studies that have included controls will be considered.

Lloyd-Roberts & French (1959), in studying a series of patients suffering from what they termed periarthritis or capsulitis of the shoulder, treated one group with an intra-articular injection of hydrocortisone combined with forcible manipulation under anaesthesia followed by active supervised movements; and another group with oral cortisone for 1 month plus active supervised movements. They concluded that the group treated with manipulation and local hydrocortisone did better than the group treated with oral cortisone.

Kessel et al (1981) from a carefully controlled trial concluded that manipulation in combination with systemic steroids is of value. As Bruckner (1982) has pointed out, however, manipulation together with steroids is generally reserved for those patients who have made no improvement 9–12 months from the onset, and therefore after the acute phase of the disease is over. As he says 'it would be very helpful if a simple treatment could be shown to cut short this common and often extremely painful condition'.

The administration of corticosteroids, either locally or systemically, has been popular in the treatment of frozen shoulder ever since they first became available for therapeutic use. Cyriax & Troisier (1953), in treating what they termed 'freezing arthritis', recommended giving an intra-articular injection of hydrocortisone, but the results of this were poor. Subsequently Cyriax (1980) advocated the use of multiple intra-articular injections of hydrocortisone at weekly or biweekly intervals. The dangers inherent in this, however, have already been alluded to when discussing the management of tendinitis.

Lee et al (1974) compared the effects of three forms of treatment (heat plus exercises; intra-articular hydrocortisone plus exercises; hydrocortisone around the biceps tendon plus exercises) with the effect of treatment with analgesics alone. All three groups in which exercise was used obtained a significantly improved range of movements to a similar degree. The analgesic group's response was not as good.

Richardson (1975) showed no difference in relief of pain in one group treated with steroid injections and in another treated with a placebo. And finally, Bulgen et al (1984) have shown that there is no long-term advantage of steroid injection over mobilization, ice, or no treatment in the management of the frozen shoulder.

It is in the light of these conflicting reports that Bruckner (1982) concludes that in the majority of cases, reassuring the patient that it is a self-limiting condition, advising the use of simple 'pendulum' mobilizing exercises, and in the early stages of the condition controlling the pain by some simple means, is as much as can be hoped for.

Acupuncture

It is in the alleviation of the pain during the first few months that acupuncture might seem to have a place.

Camp (1986), one of the few British rheumatologists with experience in the use of acupuncture, has found this form of therapy to be certainly as helpful, if not more so, as corticosteroid injections in the treatment of the frozen shoulder, and states that she advocates 'acupuncture as the treatment of choice in preference to the very painful corticosteroid injections and the largely useless physiotherapy', but makes it clear that, in her opinion, acupuncture, like local steroids, is only of symptomatic benefit and does not alter the natural history of the condition.

There is no doubt, as Bruckner (1982) has said in discussing the shortcomings of numerous reports on the treatment of the 'frozen shoulder', that 'it is essential to design prospective trials which will give definite answers, by carefully defining the condition under study (excluding shoulder pain without passive limitation of movement), treating patients only in the acute stage (first 6 months) and including a proper control group'. It would also seem reasonable, in view of Camp's observations, to include one group treated with acupuncture, but, before doing so, it is necessary to establish which particular acupuncture technique is most suitable for the alleviation of this type of pain. My reason for saying this is because, in my experience, the pain of frozen shoulder can be aggravated by stimulating trigger points too vigorously. Gentle brief stimulation of nerve endings in the tissues overlying these points often seems to give better results and it is interesting to note that Camp (1986) has also found this for she states 'sometimes attempts at needling trigger points simply produces more pain and a violent reaction to acupuncture. Moving the needle away from the trigger points and treating more peripheral points, results almost in complete loss of symptoms in these cases'.

The matter, however, is by no means straightforward. Undoubtedly there are some patients who only respond to strong stimulation and it is for this reason that Mann (1974) has found that on occasions with a persistently painful shoulder, it is necessary to apply a very powerful stimulus by means of 'pecking' the periosteum over the coracoid process.

There is no doubt, as stressed, throughout this book, that, with acupuncture, patients' individual responsiveness to peripheral nerve stimulation varies widely, and it is essential to take account of this, not only in everyday clinical practice, but also when drawing up clinical trial protocols.

Secondary activation of myofascial trigger points in tendinitis and capsulitis

It is common for the persistent pain and restricted movements associated with tendinitis, and in particular with capsulitis, to give rise to the secondary activation of trigger points in muscles in the anterior and posterior axillary folds, the upper arm, the shoulder girdle, and neck.

Those who practise trigger point acupuncture believe that in the treatment of these two conditions it is not sufficient to insert needles into the tissues overlying trigger points locally, without, at the same time, deactivating in a similar manner secondarily activated trigger points in the neighbouring muscles. These latter points have first to be identified by the carrying out of a systematic examination on each individual patient in view of their distribution varying from person to person.

There is, however, no statistical proof that the results of alleviating pain in these conditions by using this somewhat time-consuming procedure are any better than by performing acupuncture with needles inserted into a set number of preselected traditional Chinese acupuncture points; or by injecting a steroid into the tissues around the tendons or capsule. Trials to compare the relative effectiveness and patient acceptability of these three different methods of treatment are therefore indicated.

REFERRAL OF PAIN TO THE SHOULDER JOINT

Pain in the shoulder region may occur in the absence of any lesion in or around the gleno-humeral joint and be due to it being referred there, either because of nerve root entrapment; or because of the primary activation of trigger points in muscles in the neck and shoulder girdle; or because of a lesion around the diaphragm irritating the phrenic nerve.

Referred neurogenic pain

Pain in the shoulder and upper extremity can occur as a result of pressure on a cervical nerve root such as may occur with cervical disc herniation or cervical spondylosis. For reasons given in Chapter 14, there are grounds for believing that these lesions are not responsible for such pain as often as is commonly supposed. Certainly cervical spondylosis cannot be assumed to be the cause just because the characteristic appearances of this degenerative condition are demonstrable radiographically. The only circumstances in which the diagnosis of a nerve root lesion can be made with any confidence is when there are objective neurological signs, and when in particular the electromyogram (EMG) is abnormal. An EMG is, in fact, the only certain means of identifying a radiculopathy (Sola 1984).

On clinical examination, movements of the shoulder are free and do not aggravate the pain, whereas neck movements with, in particular, forced extension and sideways rotation commonly do.

With a C6 nerve root lesion there is usually pain and stiffness in the neck as well as pain in the outer part of the shoulder; pain may also radiate down the arm to the thumb and first finger; there is weakness and wasting of the biceps muscle and depression of the biceps jerk. A C7 nerve root lesion is associated with pain in the upper scapular region and the outer side of the shoulder; it may radiate down the arm to the middle and index fingers; there is weakness and wasting of the triceps muscle and depression of the triceps jerk. A C8 nerve root lesion causes pain to be felt in the outer part of the shoulder and mid-scapular regions.

On careful examination of the muscles in the areas affected by pain, it is often possible to find exquisitely tender trigger points. Although these have become secondarily activated by virtue of the fact that the muscles containing them are in the area affected by neurogenic pain, it is well worth deactivating them by means of inserting dry needles into them as this is often moderately successful in relieving the pain (Sola 1984), and certainly gives far more relief than can be obtained from subjecting the neck to traction or immobilizing it in a collar (see Ch.14).

Referral of pain to the shoulder from primarily activated myofascial trigger points

In addition to pain being referred to the shoulder region from some disorder around the diaphragm irritating the phrenic nerve, pain is commonly referred to this site from myofascial trigger points that have become primarily activated as a result of muscles in the upper part of the chest wall and neck becoming acutely strained or chronically overloaded. For some reason this is still not generally recognized in spite of the fact that attention was first drawn to it by Edeiken & Wolferth as long ago as 1936; Kellgren described cases of it 2 years later; and since then, it has been the subject of several detailed reports.

These include one by Kelly (1942) which he wrote whilst serving in the Australian Army Medical Corps; another by Travell et al (1942) already referred to in Chapter 12; also those of Sola et al (1955), and Sola & Kuitert (1955) based on observations made by them whilst they were serving as medical officers in the United States Air Force.

Unfortunately when these reports were first published, they were, for some reason, largely ignored but in recent years the importance of this particular cause of shoulder pain has once again been stressed (Sola 1984, Simons & Travell 1984) and hopefully it will now begin to receive the recognition it deserves.

The muscles most frequently involved include the supraspinatus, infraspinatus, levator scapulae, trapezius, deltoid, long head of triceps, latissimus dorsi, teres major, biceps, and subscapularis. Trigger points in these muscles can only be found by systematically examining each muscle in turn. The search for these, however, is greatly assisted by every muscle having its own specific pattern of trigger point-pain referral.

Supraspinatus muscle (Fig. 12.14)

Activation of trigger points

Trigger point activity may develop in the supraspinatus muscle when it is subjected to strain, as, for example, by carrying a heavy load such as a suitcase with the arm hanging by the side; or by pulling a heavy object; or by lifting one to, or above, the shoulder level with the arm outstretched. In addition, repeatedly overloading the muscle by such means is liable to convert an acute condition into a chronic one.

Specific pattern of pain referral

Trigger point activity in this muscle causes pain to be referred to the region of the deltoid muscle. Because of its distribution this pain is often erroneously diagnosed as being due to subdeltoid (subacromial) bursitis, which, as explained earlier, is a condition that rarely, if ever, occurs as a primary event. The pain frequently extends down the arm and forearm and, as Travell & Simons (1983a) state, is often felt particularly strongly over the lateral epicondyle (Fig. 13.1).

Movements aggravating the pain

This referred pain is usually a dull ache at rest that is made worse by abducting the arm, and by passively stretching the muscle by adducting the arm behind the back.

Some of the commoner types of movements likely to aggravate the pain include reaching upwards either to brush the hair, or to shave, or to clean the teeth.

Trigger point examination

The patient should sit comfortably, or lie with the affected side uppermost. As the trigger points have to be palpated through the trapezius muscle they are often located more readily if the muscle is put on the stretch by placing the forearm of the patient behind the back at waist level. The trigger points are usually located either at the medial or lateral parts of the muscle, or in both places (Fig. 13.1). In addition, a trigger point may develop in the tendon of the muscle near to its insertion (Fig. 13.2).

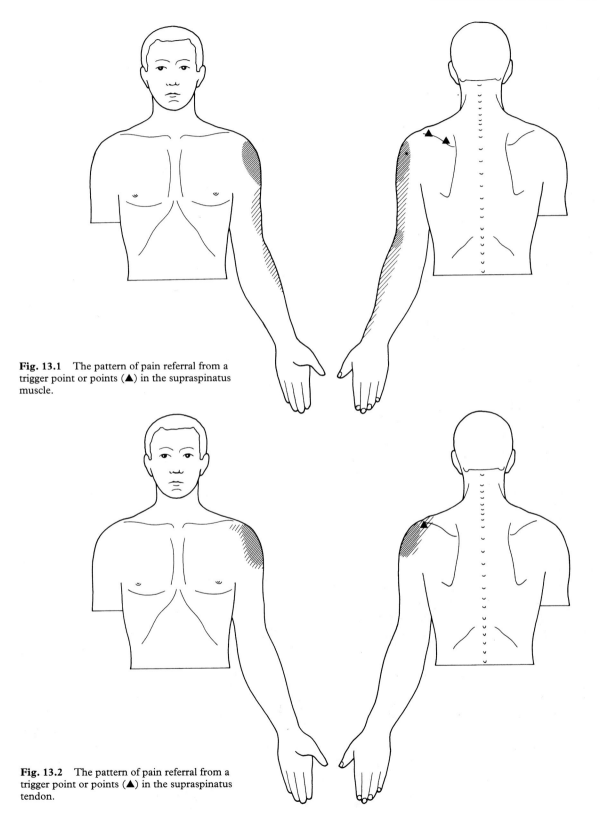

Fig. 13.1   The pattern of pain referral from a trigger point or points (▲) in the supraspinatus muscle.

Fig. 13.2   The pattern of pain referral from a trigger point or points (▲) in the supraspinatus tendon.

Associated trigger points

Trigger point activity may develop in the supraspinatus muscle alone, but more often it develops in the infraspinatus at the same time, and also quite often in the trapezius, levator scapulae and deltoid muscles.

Similarity to neurogenic pain

Referred pain from supraspinatus trigger points is similar in distribution to that from a C5 nerve root lesion (Reynolds 1981). There is, however, an absence of objective neurological signs, and electromyography shows no abnormality.

Deactivation of trigger points

This is most conveniently done with the patient lying on the opposite side. It has to be remembered that the needles must be inserted fairly deeply as this muscle lies behind the trapezius muscle.

Infraspinatus muscle (Fig. 12.14)

Activation of trigger points

This is usually brought about by the muscle being subjected to some sudden strain such as, for instance, when reaching backwards for support when falling; or when it is repeatedly put on the stretch, reaching backwards to pick up objects from, for example, the back of a car when sitting in the front of it.

Specific pattern of pain referral

Referred pain from trigger point activity in the muscle is experienced deep inside the front of the shoulder joint and for this reason is sometimes erroneously thought to be due to an arthritis of the glenohumeral joint which, as stated earlier, is rare. It may also radiate down the anterolateral aspect of the arm and forearm to the radial aspect of the hand, sometimes reaching the thumb and first two fingers (Fig. 13.3) (Travell et al 1942,

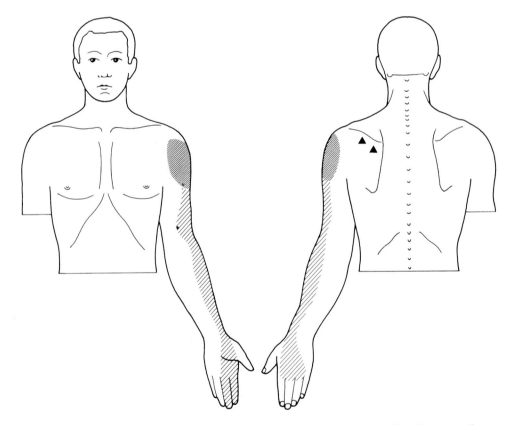

Fig. 13.3   The pattern of pain referral from a trigger point or points (▲) in the infraspinatus muscle.

Travell 1952, Sola & Williams 1956, Pace 1975, Rubin 1981).

This particular type of shoulder pain is particularly disturbing at night because it not only prevents the patient from lying on the affected side but also is troublesome when lying on the unaffected side.

Characteristic disorder of movements

There is an inability to internally rotate and adduct the arm at the shoulder. The hand-to-shoulder blade test in which a normal individual's finger tips can reach the spine of the scapula reveals this typical restriction of movement (Fig. 13.4). It is because of this that a woman has difficulty in doing up buttons or manipulating a zip fastener, and a man has

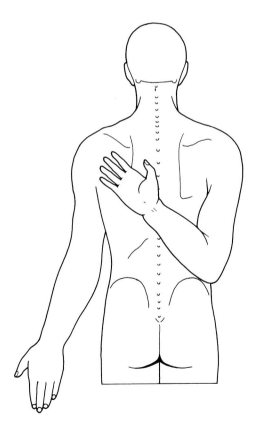

Fig. 13.4 To illustrate how a normal person, on placing an arm behind the back, is able to reach the spine of the contralateral scapula with the finger tips. With trigger point activity in either the supraspinatus or infraspinatus or both, this is not possible.

difficulty in putting his hand into his back trouser pocket.

Trigger point examination

With the patient sitting in a chair, the muscle should be stretched by bringing the hand and arm across the front of the chest to grasp the contralateral arm rest of the chair.

Flat palpation of the infraspinatus fossa should then be carried out systematically. One or more trigger points are usually to be found somewhere along a line immediately beneath the spine of the scapula.

An activated trigger point will be felt as an exquisitely tender taut band which can be rolled under the finger, with sustained pressure on this evoking the specific pattern of referred pain already described. The particular pattern of pain referral called by Long (1956) the scapulo-humeral syndrome has all the features of infraspinatus TP activation but may also include similar activity in the pectoralis and biceps muscles.

Differential diagnosis

Referred pain to the shoulder from trigger point activity in the infraspinatus muscle may closely simulate that arising from glenohumeral joint disease. And as it causes pain to radiate down the arm in a similar distribution to that occurring with irritation of the 5th, 6th and 7th cervical nerve roots, a full neurological examination is essential and, at times, an EMG may be necessary to distinguish between them, confusion being particularly likely to occur in patients who also have neck pain (see Ch. 14).

Deactivation of trigger points

This should be done with the patient lying on the opposite side, with the arm resting on a pillow placed against the chest. The needle is inserted into the tissues overlying a trigger point whilst fixing the latter between two fingers pressed against the scapula. Care must be taken not to push the needle too hard against the scapula as penetration of the infraspinatus fossa with the production of a pneumothorax has been reported (Travell & Simons 1983b).

Teres minor (Fig. 13.4)

This muscle with its attachments immediately adjacent to and just below those of the infraspinatus, and having actions which are almost identical to the latter, has trigger point activation brought about by exactly similar stresses, i.e. stretching and reaching behind the shoulder.

However, unlike the infraspinatus, it is one of the less commonly involved muscles. Sola & Kuitert (1955) found only about 7% of their patients with shoulder pain having TPs in this muscle.

Teres minor is rarely involved without simultaneous involvement of the infraspinatus, and usually notice is drawn to it by the patient continuing to complain of pain in the posterior part of the shoulder, once pain deep in the front of the shoulder has been satisfactorily alleviated

by deactivating TPs in the infraspinatus.

Levator scapulae and trapezius muscles

These muscles are discussed in detail in Chapter 14 as trigger point activity in them is mainly responsible for pain and limitation of movement of the neck. Trigger point activity here is also the cause of pain being referred to the posterior part of the shoulder (Figs 14.1 and 16.6).

Deltoid muscle (Fig. 12.14)

The deltoid muscle, so-called because being triangular in shape it resembles the Greek letter Δ (delta), is made up of three parts — the anterior, middle and posterior.

Activation of trigger points

This occurs mainly in the anterior and posterior parts of the muscle, either as a secondary or a

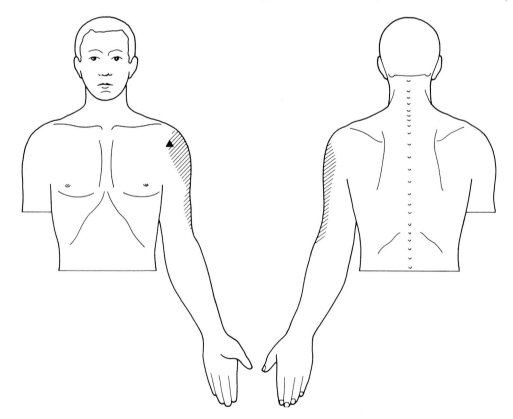

Fig. 13.5   The pattern of pain referral from a trigger point (▲) in the anterior part of the deltoid muscle.

primary event. It often occurs as a secondary phenomenon, both in the anterior and posterior parts simultaneously, when pain is referred to that area from trigger points in the supraspinatus and infraspinatus muscles. The pain from trigger point activity in this muscle remains localized to that area, and is not projected to some distant site.

In the case of primary activity, the clinical picture differs according to whether the anterior or posterior part is involved and so each will be considered separately.

Anterior part

Primary TP activity may be brought about by direct trauma to the upper part of the arm such as may occur with a fall, or when it is damaged by the impact of a ball, or the recoil of a gun. Also when the muscle is subjected to sudden overload such as when grasping a rail to break a fall; or when the muscle is recurrently overloaded such as may occur when some heavy object such as a tool or instrument is repeatedly held at shoulder level.

Symptoms

The patient complains of pain at rest over the anterior part of the deltoid muscle (Fig. 13.5). This is made worse by movement, and in particular there is difficulty in raising the arm to the horizontal so that drinking becomes troublesome.

Signs

Pain is aggravated by asking the patient to abduct the arm with the elbow straight and the palm to the front. The patient also has difficulty in passing the hand across the small of the back. Normally it is possible to rest the hand on the back of the opposite arm. With anterior deltoid TP activity, it may only be possible to reach the midline (Fig. 13.6).

Differential diagnosis

Pain in the deltoid muscle must be distinguished from that arising from a sprain of the acromio-clavicular joint which lies underneath the

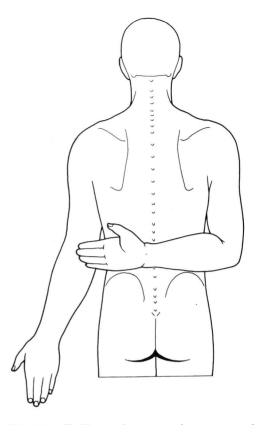

Fig. 13.6 To illustrate how a normal person on putting the arm behind the back can reach across to rest the back of the hand on the opposite arm. With trigger points in either the anterior deltoid or coracobrachialis muscle it is usually not possible to reach past the midline.

proximal attachment of the anterior part of this muscle. This injury, common in rugby players, is characterized by pain and tenderness strictly localized to the shoulder tip and there are of course no TPs to be found in the deltoid muscle itself.

Posterior part

Primary TP activation may occur as a result of injecting some irritant substances such as an antibiotic, vitamin or vaccine into this part of the muscle, or when it is subjected to excessive strain during sporting activities.

Symptoms

The patient complains of pain at the back of the shoulder at rest, and this is made worse by

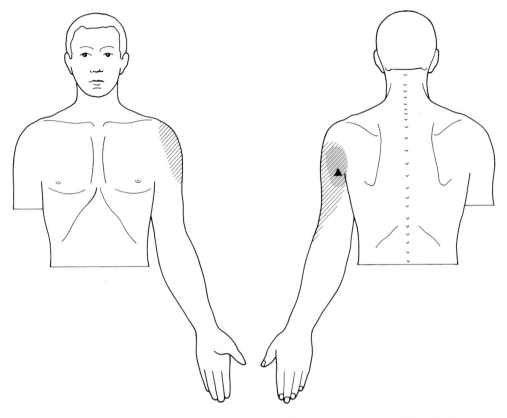

Fig. 13.7   The pattern of pain referral from a trigger point in the posterior part of the deltoid muscle.

movement (Fig. 13.7). External rotation is also limited so that whilst the hand can be brought up to the head it cannot be wrapped around the back of the head.

Signs

Pain is aggravated by asking the patient to abduct the arm with the elbow straight and the palm facing backwards.

Trigger point examination

This is carried out by flat palpation preferably with the muscle under moderate tension by slightly abducting the arm. Trigger points are felt as taut bands and, as the muscle is superficially situated, a local twitch response is readily elicited.

The trigger points in the anterior part of the muscle are usually found high up in the muscle in contrast to those in the posterior part which are

usually found in the lower part of the muscle (Fig. 13.8).

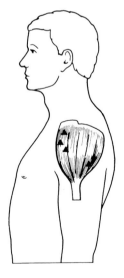

Fig. 13.8   To illustrate the usual location of trigger points in the upper anterior part and lower posterior part of the deltoid muscle.

Trigger point deactivation

This should be done with the patient lying on the opposite side with each trigger point fixed between two fingers. As they are superficially situated, penetration of them with a needle gives a strong twitch response and also evokes referred pain.

Associated trigger points

Trigger point activity is rarely confined to the deltoid alone. In addition to the muscles already mentioned, anterior deltoid TP activity may be associated with similar activity in the biceps brachii, the clavicular section of the pectoralis major, and the coracobrachialis. Posterior deltoid TP activity is often associated with the development of trigger points in the long head of the triceps, and the two muscles forming the posterior axillary fold, namely the latissimus dorsi and the teres major. Each of these will therefore be discussed in turn.

Biceps brachii muscle (Fig. 12.9)

Tendinitis affecting the long head of the biceps has already been discussed. In addition trigger points may become active in the lower part of the muscle just above the elbow (Fig. 13.9), and it is the activation and deactivation of these that will now be considered.

Activation of trigger points

Trigger points in the lower part of the biceps muscle may become activated when the muscle is strained by lifting a heavy object with the arm outstretched, or carrying out some task with the elbow flexed for a long time such as occurs when cutting a hedge; or when supinating against resistance such as when using a screwdriver, or, as with the infraspinatus muscle, when suddenly reaching backwards for support to prevent a fall.

Specific pattern of pain referral

Trigger point activity in the distal part of the muscle near to the elbow causes pain to be referred upwards to the anterior surface of the

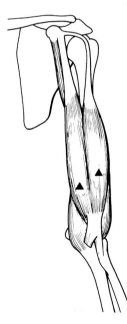

Fig. 13.9   To show the usual location of trigger points in the lower part of the biceps muscle just above the elbow.

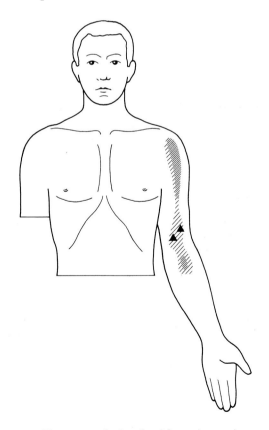

Fig. 13.10   The pattern of pain referral from trigger points (▲) in the lower part of the biceps muscle.

shoulder joint, and sometimes to a lesser extent to the suprascapular region (Fig. 13.10). There is no restriction of movement at the shoulder joint but pain is aggravated by raising the hand above the head.

Trigger point examination

The examination is carried out with the patient seated and with the elbow resting on a table. With the hand supinated, the elbow is slightly flexed to slacken the biceps muscle. Trigger points in the form of elongated tense bands are usually found in the distal part of the muscle (Winter 1944) and may therefore be located by sliding the examining finger across the lower part of both heads.

Deactivation of trigger points

Once a trigger point has been located in this part of the muscle it should be trapped between two fingers whilst a needle is inserted into the tissues overlying it. Care should be taken to avoid penetrating either the median or radial nerves; the one lying along the medial and the other along the lateral border of the lower part of this muscle.

Clavicular section of the pectoralis major muscle

A detailed discussion concerning the activation of trigger points in this muscle is given in Chapter 12, but attention must be drawn here to the fact that trigger points in the clavicular section of this muscle may be responsible for pain in the front of the shoulder, and may also cause abduction of the arm at the shoulder joint to be restricted (Fig. 12.6).

Coracobrachialis (Fig. 12.9)

This muscle, together with the pectoralis minor and the short head of the biceps, is attached at its

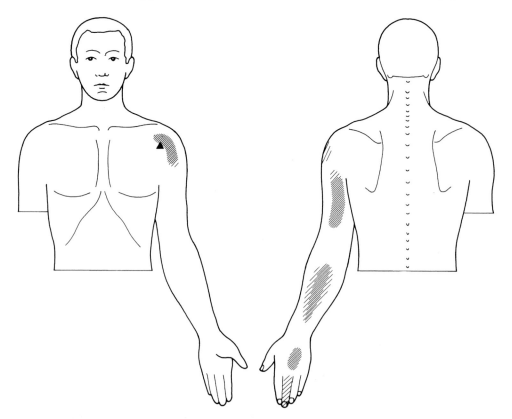

Fig. 13.11 The pattern of pain referral from a trigger point or points (▲) in the coracobrachialis muscle.

upper end to the coracoid process, and at its lower end to the middle of the humerus.

Trigger point activity in this muscle usually does not become evident until trigger points in the other shoulder muscles, particularly the anterior deltoid, have first been successfully deactivated. As Travell & Simons (1983c) state, it should be suspected when in spite of this, the patient continues to complain of pain over the anterior deltoid region, and down the back of the arm to the dorsum of the hand, but sparing for some reason the elbow and wrist (Fig. 13.11). The trigger point usually arises in the upper part of the muscle deep to the anterior deltoid (Fig. 13.11). In order to deactive it, the patient should be placed in the supine position with the arm externally rotated. A needle should then be inserted through the deltoid muscle into the point which is usually to be found just medial to the greater tuberosity of the humerus.

Triceps (long head)

A detailed account of the various parts of the triceps muscle and the effects of trigger point activation in them will be given when discussing pain around the elbow joint in Chapter 15, but reference must be made here to the long head of this muscle (Fig. 13.12) because when TP activity develops in the posterior part of the deltoid it may also arise in the latissimus dorsi, the teres major and this part of the muscle. Trigger points in the long head cause pain to be referred upwards over the back of the arm to the posterior part of the shoulder and sometimes downwards along the back of the forearm (Fig. 13.13). Also a person with this, when instructed to raise both arms above the head with the elbows straight and palms to the front, finds it impossible to hold the affected arm tight against the side of the head (Fig. 13.14).

Trigger point examination

Trigger points are usually found in the mid third of the long head. They are sought by grasping the muscle and rolling its fibres between the thumb and fingers. Pressure exerted in this manner on an active TP should evoke the specific pattern of referred pain already described.

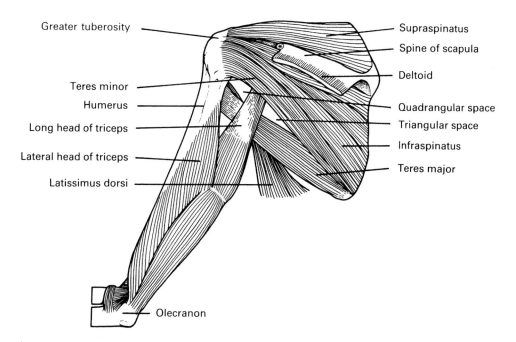

Fig. 13.12 The dorsal scapular muscles and triceps. Left side. The spine of the scapula has been divided near its lateral end and the acromion has been removed together with a large part of the deltoid.

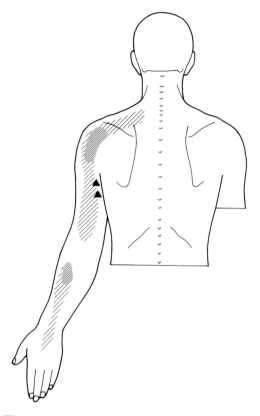

Fig. 13.13 The pattern of pain referral from a trigger point or points (▲) in the long head of the triceps muscle.

Trigger point deactivation

A detailed discussion of this will be given in Chapter 15.

Latissimus dorsi and teres major (Fig. 12.14)

These muscles, which together form the posterior axillary fold, often have trigger point activity in them at the same time.

The latissimus dorsi muscle is considered in detail in Chapter 12 as trigger point activity in this muscle mainly causes pain to be felt in the chest wall around the inferior angle of the scapula. The pain however may also be referred to the back of the shoulder and down the inner side of the arm (Fig. 12.15).

Teres major

This muscle is attached medially to the lower part of the scapula; and laterally converges with

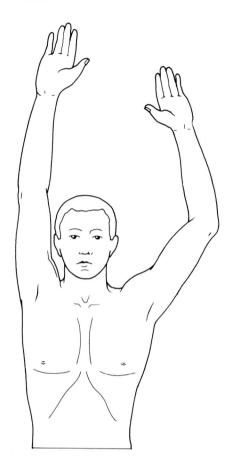

Fig. 13.14 To illustrate the difficulty experienced in bringing the ipsilateral arm up against the ear when there is trigger point activity in either the long head of the triceps or the teres major muscle.

the latissimus dorsi muscle to form the posterior axillary fold before being inserted into the tuberosity close to the latissimus dorsi in the bicipital groove (Fig. 12.14).

Trigger point activity causes pain to be felt in the posterior part of the shoulder when reaching forwards and upwards and occasionally along the back of the forearm (Fig. 13.15). A person with this also has difficulty in pressing the raised outstretched arm tightly against the side of the head in the same way as someone with TP activity in the long head of the triceps (Fig. 13.14).

Trigger point examination

Trigger points may occur at both the inner and outer ends of the muscle (Fig. 13.16). Trigger

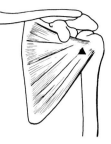

Fig. 13.17   The subscapularis muscle with a trigger point (▲) near to the insertion of this muscle into the humerus.

with the patient lying supine and the arm abducted to 90°.

Deactivation of trigger points

Trigger points in this muscle where it is inserted into the scapula are most readily deactivated with the patient lying on the contralateral side, with each one fixed between two fingers pressed against the back of the scapula. Trigger points in the posterior axillary fold should be deactivated whilst grasping them between finger and thumb, and this is most easily done with the patient lying in the supine position and the arm abducted at a right angle.

Subscapularis muscle

Finally, it is important not to overlook trigger points hidden away in the subscapularis muscle as a cause of persistent pain in the shoulder (Fig. 13.17).

Activation of trigger points

This occurs as a result of repeated movements involving a considerable amount of internal rotation, or with direct trauma to the shoulder, or when the shoulder joint is immobilized for a length of time in the adducted and internally rotated position.

Specific pattern of pain referral

The pain is very severe even at rest and made worse by movement. The pain is predominantly felt over the back of the shoulder but also extends

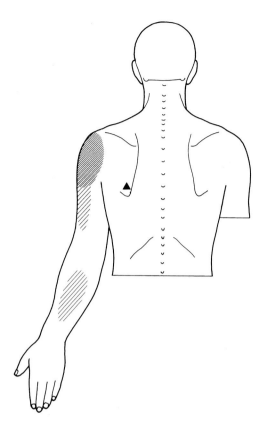

Fig. 13.15   The pattern of pain referral from a trigger point at the inner end of the teres major muscle.

points occurring medially at the insertion of the muscle into the lower lateral border of the scapula may be located by applying pressure against the underlying scapula. Trigger points occurring laterally in the posterior axillary fold may be located by gripping the fold between the thumb and fingers. This may be done with the patient sitting but it is probably easier to do it

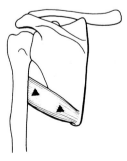

Fig. 13.16   To show sites at which trigger points are liable to become activated in the teres major muscle.

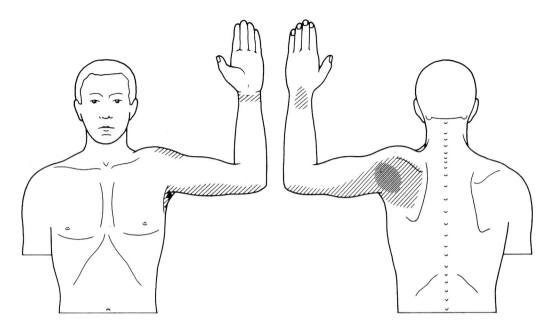

Fig. 13.18 The pattern of pain referral from a trigger point or points (▲) in the axillary part of the subscapularis muscle.

up towards the scapula and down the back of the arm to the elbow. Also there may be some pain around the back of the wrist (Fig. 13.18).

Characteristic disturbance of movements

Progressively painful restriction of abduction and external rotation of the shoulder joint.

Associated trigger points

Once trigger point activation takes place in this muscle it is liable to spread to the pectoralis major, latissimus dorsi, teres major, long head of the triceps, and the anterior and posterior part of the deltoid muscles.

Trigger point examination

Trigger points fortunately are usually to be found along the axillary border of the subscapular fossa

but even here they are difficult to palpate unless the arm is well abducted with at the same time traction on the arm to abduct the scapula. The severe pain and limitation of movement however often makes this difficult, in which case it is better first of all, with the patient lying in the supine position, to apply a vapocoolant spray to the area. Following this the muscle is usually much more readily exposed and firm bands of trigger point activity may then be readily located by means of flat palpation with a finger.

Deactivation of trigger points

The patient should be placed in the supine position with the arm abducted if possible to 90°, with the hand placed behind the head and anchored beneath the pillow. When a trigger point is located, it is fixed between two fingers and a needle inserted parallel to the rib cage into the tissues overlying it.

REFERENCES

Anonymous 1976 Injecting the painful shoulder. Lancet 1: 27
Bentley G, Goodfellow J W 1969 Disorganization of the knees following intra-articular hydrocortisone injections. Journal of Bone and Joint Surgery 51B: 498–502
Berry L, Fernandes L, Bloom B, Clark R J, Hamilton E B D

1980 Clinical study comparing acupuncture, physiotherapy, injection and oral anti-inflammatory therapy in shoulder cuff lesions. Current Medical Research and Opinion 7: 121–126
Binder A I, Bulgen D Y, Hazelman B L, Tudor J, Wraight P

1984 Frozen shoulder: an arthrographic and radionuclear scan assessment. Annals of Rheumatic Diseases 43: 359–369

Bruckner F E 1982 Frozen shoulder (adhesive capsulitis). Journal of the Royal Society of Medicine 75: 688–689

Bulgen D Y, Binder A E, Hazelman B, Dutton J, Roberts S 1984 Frozen shoulder: prospective clinical study with an evaluation of three treatment regimens. Annals of Rheumatic Diseases 43: 353–360

Bunker T D 1985 Time for a new name for 'frozen shoulder'. British Medical Journal 290: 1233–1234

Cailliet R 1981a Shoulder pain, 2nd edn. Davis, Philadelphia, p 48; 1981b: p 53–64

Camp V 1986 Acupuncture for shoulder pain. British Medical Acupuncture Society Journal iii: 28

Codman E A 1934 The shoulder. Todd, Boston

Coomes E N, Darlington L G 1976 Effects of local steroid injection for supraspinatus tears. Annals of Rheumatic Diseases 35: 943

Cyriax J 1980 Textbook of orthopaedic medicine vol. 2 Baillière Tindall, London

Cyriax J, Troisier O 1953 Hydrocortisone and soft tissue lesions. British Medical Journal 11: 966–968

Duplay S 1896 De la periarthrite scapulo-humerale. L'Abeille Medicale 53: 226

Edeiken J, Wolferth C C 1936 Persistent pain in the shoulder region following myocardial infarction. American Journal of Medical Science 191: 201–210

Fernandes L, Berry H, Clark R J, Bloom B, Hamilton E B D 1980 Clinical study comparing acupuncture, physiotherapy, injection, and oral anti-inflammatory therapy in shoulder cuff lesions. Lancet 1: 208–209

Grey R G 1977 The natural history of 'idiopathic' frozen shoulder. Journal of Bone and Joint Surgery 60A: 564

Hollingworth G R, Ellis R M, Hattersley T S 1983 Comparison of injection techniques for shoulder pain: results of a double blind randomised study. British Medical Journal 287: 1339–1341

Kellgren J H 1938 A preliminary account of referred pains arising from muscle. British Medical Journal 1: 325–327

Kelly M 1942 New light on the painful shoulder. Medical Journal of Australia 1: 488–493

Kessel L, Watson M 1977 The painful arc syndrome. Journal of Bone and Joint Surgery 59B: 166–172

Kessel L, Bayley I, Young A 1981 The frozen shoulder. British Journal of Hospital Medicine 25: 334–338

Koehler B E, Urowitz M B, Killinger D W 1974 The systemic effects of intra-articular corticosteroid. Journal of Rheumatology 1: 117–125

Lee P N, Lee M, Haq A M, Longton E B, Wright V 1974 Periarthritis of the shoulder. Annals of Rheumatic Diseases 33: 116–119

Lloyd-Roberts G C, French P R 1959 Periarthritis of a shoulder. British Medical Journal 1: 1569–1571

Long C 1956 Myofascial pain syndromes part II — syndromes of the head, neck and shoulder girdle. Henry Ford Hospital Medical Bulletin 4: 22–28

Mann 1974 The treatment of disease by acupuncture. Heinemann Medical, London, p 196–197

Moore M E, Berk S N 1976 Acupuncture for chronic shoulder pain. Archives of Internal Medicine 84: 381–384

Neviaser J S 1945 Adhesive capsulitis of the shoulder. Journal of Bone and Joint Surgery 27: 211–222

Pace J B 1975 Commonly overlooked pain syndromes responsive to simple therapy. Postgraduate Medicine 58: 107–113

Reynolds M D 1981 Myofascial trigger point syndromes in the practice of rheumatology. Archives of Physical Medicine and Rehabilitation 62: 111–114

Richardson A T 1975 The painful shoulder. Proceedings of the Royal Society of Medicine 68: 731–736

Richardson P G, Vincent C A 1986 Acupuncture for the treatment of pain. A review of evaluative research. Pain 24: 15–40

Roy S, Oldham R 1976 Management of painful shoulder. Lancet 1: 1322–1324

Rubin D 1981 An approach to management of myofascial trigger point syndromes. Archives of Physical Medicine and Rehabilitation 62: 107–110

Simons D G, Travell J G 1984 Myofascial pain syndromes. In: Wall P D, Melzack R (eds) Textbook of pain. Churchill Livingstone, Edinburgh, p 267

Sola A 1984 Upper extremity pain. In: Wall P D, Melzack R (eds) Textbook of pain. Churchill Livingstone, Edinburgh, p 252–257

Sola A E, Kuitert J H 1955 Myofascial trigger point pain in the neck and shoulder girdle. Northwest Medicine 54: 980–984

Sola A E, Rodenberger M L, Gettys B B 1955 Incidence of hypersensitive areas in posterior shoulder muscles. American Journal of Physical Medicine 34: 585–590

Sola A E, Williams R L 1956 Myofascial pain syndromes. Neurology 6: 91–95

Travell J 1952 Pain mechanisms in connective tissue. In: Ragan C (ed) Connective tissues, transactions of the second conference 1951. Josiah Macy Jnr Foundation, New York

Travell J, Rinzler S, Herman M 1942 Pain and disability of the shoulder and arm: treatment by intramuscular infiltration with procaine hydrochloride. Journal of the American Medical Association 120: 417–422

Travell J G, Simons D G 1983a Myofascial pain and dysfunction. The trigger point manual. Williams & Wilkins, Baltimore, p 368; 1983b: p 385; 1983c: p 440

Weiss J J 1981 Intra-articular steroids in the treatment of rotator cuff tear: reappraisal by arthrography. Archives of Physical Medicine and Rehabilitation 62: 555–557

Winter S P 1944 Referred pain in fibrositis. Medical Record 157: 34–37

Wright V, Haq A M M 1976 Periarthritis of the shoulder. I. Aetiological considerations with particular reference to personality factors. Annals of the Rheumatic Diseases 35: 213–219

14. Pain in the neck

INTRODUCTION

Persistent pain in the neck with restriction of its movements and with or without referral of the pain down the arm is a commonly occurring disorder, and before deciding on whether or not to use acupuncture in an attempt to relieve it, it is obviously essential to have first of all established its cause.

Some of the less common causes and ones that require other forms of treatment include primary or secondary malignant disease infiltrating nerve roots or vertebral bodies; a variety of other disorders affecting the vertebrae such as fractures, infective lesions and rheumatoid arthritis; and some disorders of muscle such as polymyalgia rheumatica. The exclusion of these clearly requires the taking of a detailed history, a carefully conducted clinical examination, and some basic investigations including an ESR and cervical radiographs.

It is hardly necessary to cite cases illustrating the importance of making an accurate diagnosis before embarking upon treatment of any type but the following one, although it occurred 25 years ago, is worth quoting as it is firmly imprinted on my mind for reasons that will become obvious.

A man (56) developed persistent pain in the neck with restricted movements. He was treated for several months symptomatically but when, in spite of this, the pain became progressively worse, he was referred to my outpatient clinic for assessment. On examination there were no abnormal neurological signs but whilst he was having X-rays of his neck and chest, he suddenly collapsed due to the development of a quadriplegia! The appearances on the radiographs of the neck at first sight seemed to be normal until it was realized that only six cervical vertebrae were visible,

one having collapsed so completely as a result of metastatic infiltration as to have virtually disappeared. The chest radiograph revealed the site of the primary growth.

This having been said it is now necessary to discuss some of the common causes of persistent neck pain as it is in the treatment of these that acupuncture has much to offer.

During recent years a number of clinicians have presented evidence to show that persistent neck pain with or without referral of this down the arm is often due to the primary activation of trigger points in muscles in the neck and shoulder region (Michele et al 1950, Sola & Kuitert 1955, Long 1956, Sola & Williams 1956, Michele & Eisenberg 1968, Travell & Simons 1983). Neurologists, however, continue to put most emphasis on nerve root entrapment as being the principal cause of this type of pain. With patients under the age of 40, pain is ascribed to acute rupture of an intervertebral disc, and with those older than this, it is considered to be due to cervical spondylosis (Posner 1982, Matthews 1983). These two conditions will therefore be considered first.

ACUTE RUPTURE OF THE ANNULUS FIBROSUS OF AN INTERVERTEBRAL DISC WITH HERNIATION OF THE NUCLEUS PULPOSUS

From early adult life to middle age the intervertebral disc undergoes a degenerative process, and amongst the various biochemical changes taking place in the nucleus pulposus, there is a gradual decrease in its water content and a consequent progressive loss of its fluidity (Urban & Maroudas 1980). At any time during these years the annulus fibrosus is liable to become torn and when this occurs, the nucleus pulposus may protrude through it but only if this should happen in the earlier stages of this degenerative process when the nucleus is still sufficiently fluid to do so. It is, however, in the earlier years of adult life that the annulus fibrosus is least likely to rupture and it is for this reason that herniation of the nucleus pulposus through a tear in this structure is a relatively rare event (Waddell 1982).

Moreover, as at such an early stage of degeneration no abnormality of the disc can be detected on a plain radiograph, and as there are seldom clinical indications for a myelogram and even less for proceeding to surgery, objective proof of a suspected ruptured disc is difficult to obtain. It therefore follows that, although in adults under the age of 40, the sudden onset of severe pain in the neck and arm is often considered to be due to the entrapment of a nerve from a ruptured intervertebral disc, except in the minority of cases with definite physical signs such as weakness of muscles, sensory changes or loss of tendon jerks; or where there is an abnormal EMG, there is never any certainty that this is the cause of the pain and for the reasons given it would seem to be a somewhat rare event.

The commonest cause for acute neck pain would seem to be the primary activation of trigger points in the muscles in that region. In support of this belief are the observations that pain of this type usually develops when these muscles have been subjected to some acute strain and further, that in such circumstances careful examination of the various neck muscles including the levator scapulae, splenius cervicis and trapezius reveals the presence of exquisitely tender trigger points with pressure on these aggravating the spontaneously occurring pain; and that when, at times, acute neck pain is associated with considerable muscle spasm causing the neck to be pulled to one side (acute wry neck) trigger points are also to be found in the sternocleidomastoid muscle. It has to be appreciated, however, that in addition to primary trigger point activation occurring in this manner,

pain may also develop secondary to acute disc prolapse and therefore both of these conditions contribute to what may appropriately be called the acute cervical myofascial trigger point pain syndrome. Acupuncture in the treatment of this syndrome will be considered on page 193.

CERVICAL SPONDYLOSIS

Cervical spondylosis is liable to develop from the age of 40 upwards. It is a very commonly occurring degenerative condition affecting the discs and facet joints of the fifth, sixth and seventh cervical vertebrae. A striking feature of the condition is the development of osteophytes, both anteriorly and posteriorly. It is the posterior osteophytes that are of particular importance because, if sufficiently big, they may cause narrowing of the spinal canal with the gradual onset of a spastic paraplegia; or narrowing of one or other of the intervertebral foramina with the development of nerve root entrapment, giving rise to pain in the neck and arm and the eventual appearance of neurological signs in the arm. In contrast to this, anterior osteophytes and also narrowing of the intervertebral spaces, although often seen on lateral radiographs in this condition, are not a cause of either symptoms or signs. Changes associated with cervical spondylosis are frequently seen in neck X-rays of asymptomatic elderly people (Pallis et al 1954, Friedenberg & Miller 1963, Heller et al 1983).

Pallis et al (1954) carried out a detailed clinical and radiographic study of asymptomatic cervical spondylosis in a random group of 50 inpatients over the age of 50 suffering from a variety of other medical and surgical disorders.

A number of these patients in spite of having no neurological symptoms were found to have pyramidal tract and posterior column signs, together with radiographic evidence of moderate or severe narrowing of their spinal canals from posterior osteophytic, kyphotic, and subluxation changes of cervical spondylosis. However, what was of particular relevance when considering neck pain and the part that cervical spondylosis may play in producing this was that they found that a number of patients, with no pain in the neck or arm, had severe osteophytic narrowing of one or another intervertebral foramen and that approximately one-third of these had neurological signs in an arm of nerve root involvement.

Heller et al (1983) compared the cervical radiographs of two groups of patients. One group included all patients over the age of 60 referred to their department of radiology during the course of one particular year specifically for X-ray examinations of the neck. The other group consisted of all of the patients, also over the age of 60, referred to the department that year for barium studies. They not only found that 85% of those specifically referred for neck X-rays had radiographic evidence of cervical spondylosis but also that there was no significant difference in the prevalence and extent of the radiographic changes in the two groups and, moreover that there was no consistent relationship between symptoms and X-ray appearances.

There are therefore certain enigmas associated with this commonly occurring condition. Foremost amongst these is that whilst the condition causes pain in the neck and arm to develop in some people, others with equally severe radiographic changes remain symptomless. Furthermore, as a corollary to this, the presence of radiographic changes of cervical spondylosis in a person suffering from pain in the neck does not necessarily imply that the pain is due to that condition, such changes often being no more than a fortuitous radiographic finding in someone who, for a variety of different reasons to be discussed later, develops pain that is primarily muscular in origin.

Nerve root entrapment from cervical spondylosis is of course the most likely cause of persistent pain in the neck and arm *when this occurs in association with objective neurological signs*, such as muscle wasting, sensory loss, and depression of one or other of the tendon jerks in an arm (biceps jerk — C5 root; supinator jerk — C6 root; triceps jerk — C7 root) together with, in particular, an abnormal EMG. In such circumstances the presence of posterior osteophytes on the lateral view of a cervical radiograph helps to confirm the diagnosis; nevertheless it has to be remembered that this radiographic abnormality does not necessarily have to be present in order to make such a diagnosis, as nerve entrapment in

cervical spondylosis is sometimes due to the development of fibrosis in a dorsal root sleeve, a tissue reaction that requires a myelogram for its detection (Frykholm 1951).

Although most patients with chronic neck pain over the age of 40 have radiographic evidence of cervical spondylosis the pain, unlike what one might expect, with nerve root entrapment either from well developed posterior osteophytes, or peri-radicular fibrosis, is not persistent but episodic, with each bout lasting from a few weeks to a few months with on average this being about 6 weeks. Although it is reasonable to suppose that pain of this type may at times be due to tissue changes of a reversible nature occurring in cervical spondylosis, similar to those responsible for episodic osteoarthritic pain elsewhere in the body (Ch. 19), what is not sufficiently well recognized is that, in addition, it is often due to the primary activation of trigger points in the muscles of the neck. Jason (1978) in discussing the subject of neck pain states:

It is possible to make a definitive diagnosis of a prolapsed disc or cervical spondylosis in some cases but in many instances the diagnosis is uncertain, and these are best described as non-specific neck pain. There is a wide variety of different forms of neck pain which arise spontaneously or following trivial trauma and associated with little or no radiological changes. Such pain may follow exposure to cold or damp, sleeping in an uncomfortable position, prolonged driving, or any manoeuvre in which the head is held constantly in one position. There may be persistent contraction of the paraspinal muscles, especially in people with chronic anxiety states.

He considers that in some of the cases there may be tears of the paraspinal muscles, ligaments or tendons and then goes on to make the very pertinent observation that sometimes localized tender spots and painful nodules may be palpable.

Many people including myself are prepared to go further than this and to state categorically that everyone with persistent pain in the neck, whether this be due to cervical spondylosis, or whether it is what Jason calls a non-specific type of pain, has exquisitely tender trigger points in the muscles of the neck and shoulder girdle. Also, to state that the aetiological significance of these points with respect to the pain is readily shown by applying pressure to them for this invariably exacerbates any pain felt locally in the neck; and when, in addition, pain is referred down the arm from one of these points, the application of pressure to such a point will often cause pain to shoot down the arm along the same line of referral. The position therefore is that over the age of 40, trigger points in neck muscles are liable to become activated as a secondary event when these muscles happen to be in an area affected by pain from cervical spondylosis. And that, at all ages, trigger points in the neck muscles may become activated as a primary event for one of a variety of reasons to be discussed.

The muscles in which this trigger point activation is likely to take place include the levator scapulae; the splenius cervicis; other posterior cervical muscles; the trapezius; the rhomboids; and the sternocleidomastoid (Ch. 16). The muscles in which trigger points are liable to cause pain to be referred down the arm include the levator scapulae, the scalene muscles (Ch. 12), the supraspinatus and the infraspinatus (Ch. 13).

Each of these muscles, not dealt with elsewhere, will be considered in turn with regard to the sites at which trigger points arise in them, and to their specific patterns of pain referral. This will be followed by a discussion concerning the factors responsible for this trigger point activation and its treatment.

Levator scapulae muscle

When persistent pain in the neck with restriction of its movements is associated with the activation of myofascial trigger points, trigger point activity usually occurs in several muscles at the same time, either on one side but more commonly on both sides of the neck. And, of these muscles, the one most constantly affected is the levator scapulae (Fig. 12.14).

Specific pattern of pain referral

The pain from trigger point activity in this muscle is mainly felt at the base of the neck, but ·it may also extend upwards towards the occiput; outwards to the back of the shoulder and downwards along the inner border of the scapula (Fig. 14.1).

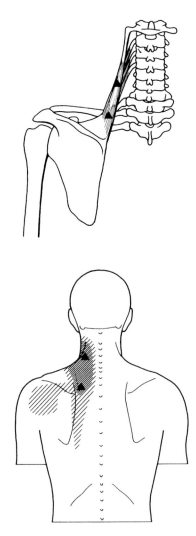

Fig. 14.1   The pattern of pain referral to the neck, shoulder and inner border of the scapula from a trigger point or points (▲) in the levator scapulae muscle. Pain in this distribution occurs as a result of activity in either a trigger point at the angle of the neck or one near to the insertion of this muscle into the superior angle of the scapula, or in both.

The pain may also radiate anteriorly around the chest wall along the course of the fourth and fifth intercostal nerves when it may erroneously be diagnosed as being either anginal or pleural, or even more frequently as being due to intercostal nerve root entrapment. In addition, it quite commonly extends down the arm along the posteromedial aspect of the upper arm and the ulnar border of the forearm and hand to terminate in the ring and little fingers. So this is a pattern of referral that coincides with the

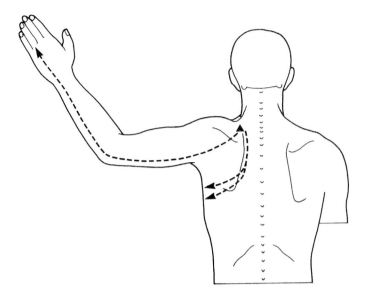

Fig. 14.2 Some other patterns of pain referral from a trigger point (▲) in the levator scapulae near to its insertion into the superior angle of the scapula. These include referral down the inner side of the arm to the ring and little fingers. And referral around the chest wall along the course of the 4th and 5th intercostal nerves.

cutaneous areas of distribution of spinal segments C8, T1 and T2 (Fig. 14.2). ·

Of those patients in whom levator scapulae trigger point pain is referred to these distant parts of the body, some only experience it down the arm; some only feel it around the chest wall; whilst others are aware of it at both sites simultaneously.

Scapulocostal and scapulonumeral syndromes

Michele et al (1950), Russek (1952) and Michele & Eisenberg (1968) in describing the condition in which pain is referred down the arm and around the chest wall from trigger point activity in the levator scapulae muscle, call it the scapulocostal syndrome. Long (1956) more appropriately divides it into the scapulocostal and scapulonumeral syndromes for as he states, trigger point pain around the chest wall and down the arm, although commonly occurring in consort, does not always do so. Moreover, it has to be remembered that pain down the arm from trigger points around the scapula is not only referred from trigger points in the levator scapulae, it may also be referred from either the supraspinatus muscle (Ch. 13) or the infraspinatus muscle with, needless to say, each of

these three muscles having its own specific pattern of pain referral. The use of this particular terminology therefore in my opinion is apt to be confusing, and is better avoided.

Trigger point examination

Trigger points may be found at two separate sites in this muscle. One is at the angle of the neck where the muscle emerges from beneath the anterior border of the trapezius muscle. The other is situated lower down the back at the attachment of the muscle to the superior angle of the scapula (Fig. 14.1).

The point at the angle of the neck is best palpated with the patient sitting comfortably with the elbows supported on arm rests. This helps to relax both the levator scapulae and trapezius and allows the clinician to pull the trapezius out of the way. Once the levator scapulae muscle has been identified, the point of maximum tenderness, i.e. the trigger point, is most readily located by gently turning the head to the opposite side as this puts the muscle on the stretch. The lower trigger point may also be located with the patient in the sitting position. This trigger point is best identified by rolling the fingers across the muscle fibres just above the superior angle of the scapula, when it will be felt as an exquisitely tender taut band.

Splenius cervicis

Specific pattern of pain referral

Trigger point activity may be found in the upper part of the muscle and in the lower part. The trigger point in the upper part refers pain to the head and will therefore be considered in greater detail in Chapter 16.

It is the trigger point in the lower part of the muscle which causes pain to be felt locally around the base of the neck.

Trigger point examination

This trigger point may be located at the angle of the neck where the muscle lies between the trapezius medially and the levator scapulae laterally. It is advisable to rotate the head and neck to the opposite side in order to put the muscle on the stretch when attempting to identify it (Fig. 14.3).

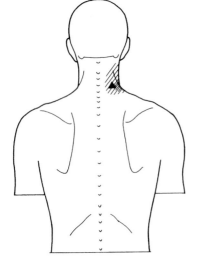

Fig. 14.3 The pattern of pain referral from a trigger point (▲) at the base of the neck in the lower part of the splenius cervicis muscle.

Posterior cervical muscles halfway down the back of the neck

The paravertebrally situated posterior cervical muscles are arranged in four layers. In descending order of depth these layers consist of the upper part of the trapezius; the splenius capitis and cervicis; the semispinalis capitis and cervicis; and the multifidi and rotatores. With a painful stiff neck there is frequently an exquisitely tender trigger point close to the spine in one or other of these posterior cervical muscles at about the level of the 4th or 5th cervical vertebra (Fig. 14.4). The depth at which the trigger point lies and therefore the muscle involved varies from person to person.

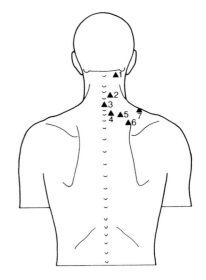

Fig. 14.4   To show the positions of some commonly occurring trigger points at the back of the neck and shoulder girdle.

1. Trigger point in a depression between the upper ends of the trapezius and sternocleidomastoid muscles close to the mastoid process and coinciding in position with the traditional Chinese acupuncture point Gall Bladder 20 (see Ch. 16).

2. Trigger point in a posterior cervical muscle at the level of the 4th cervical vertebra. The particular muscle involved depending on the depth at which the trigger point lies — see text.

3. Trigger point in the ligamentum nuchae.

4. Trigger point in the splenius cervicis muscle at the angle of the neck.

5. and 6. Trigger points in the levator scapulae muscle.

7. Trigger point in the upper free border of the trapezius muscle halfway between the spine and acromion and corresponding in position with the traditional Chinese acupuncture point Gall Bladder 21.

Specific pattern of pain referral

Pain from a trigger point in one of these posterior cervical muscles at this level is referred upwards towards the base of the skull and downwards over the shoulder girdle towards the upper part of the scapula (Fig. 14.5).

Trapezius muscle

Trigger point activity in this muscle is very common. There are several sites where this may develop and therefore reference will first be made to some anatomical features of the muscle. It will be remembered that the two trapezius muscles together take the shape of a diamond. They extend in the midline from the occiput above, to the 12th thoracic vertebra below, and fan out on both sides to be attached to the clavicle in front and the spine of the scapula behind.

For descriptive purposes the muscle may therefore be conveniently divided into an upper part extending from the occiput down to the 5th cervical spine, a middle part extending from the 6th cervical spine to the 3rd dorsal vertebra, and a lower part extending from the 4th to the 12th dorsal vertebra (Fig. 12.14).

Upper part of the muscle

The most frequently occurring trigger point in the trapezius muscle is to be found along the upper border of the shoulder girdle about half way between the spine and the tip of the shoulder. This point therefore coincides in position with the well-known traditional Chinese one known as Gall Bladder 21.

Specific pattern of pain referral

Trigger point activity at this site is the cause of pain being referred up the side of the neck to the base of the skull, and on occasions around the side of the head to reach the temple and back of the eye (TP1 Figs 14.6 and 16.6D).

Trigger point examination

The trigger point is contained in a palpable band that may be located by taking the free edge of the

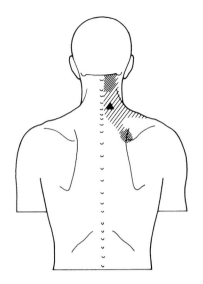

Fig. 14.5 The pattern of pain referral from a trigger point (▲) in a posterior cervical muscle at the level of the 4th cervical vertebra.

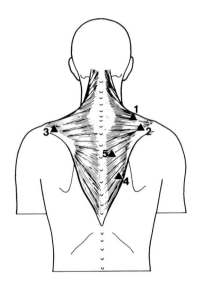

Fig. 14.6 Trigger points (▲) in the trapezius muscle.

muscle in a pincer grasp and rolling the fibres between the fingers and thumb. Sometimes there is also another trigger point in the same part of the muscle situated just below the one already described (TP2 Fig. 14.6). This also causes pain to be referred up the side of the neck.

Middle part of the muscle

A trigger point near to the acromion may be responsible for pain being referred to the posterior part of the shoulder (TP3 Fig. 14.6).

Lower part of the muscle

A trigger point (TP4 Fig. 14.6) may be found in the outer border of the lower part just above the level of the inferior angle of the scapula. Also another one may occur just below the inner end of the scapular spine (TP5 Fig. 14.6). These two trigger points are not often involved but when they are, they may cause pain to be referred to the upper scapular and neck region. They are therefore always worth looking for if neck pain persists after activity in the other trigger points already described has been adequately suppressed.

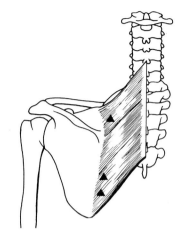

Fig. 14.7 Trigger points (▲) along the medial border of the scapula in the rhomboid muscles.

Rhomboids (major and minor) (Fig. 12.14)

Activation of trigger points

This occurs less frequently than in the other shoulder girdle muscles, but factors which cause it include prolonged working in a round-shouldered position; also strain on the muscles from an upper thoracic scoliosis, such as may occur idiopathically, or following chest surgery.

It may also occur when these muscles, together with the trapezius, become overloaded by having to counteract tension in the pectoralis major and minor brought about by trigger points developing in these latter two muscles.

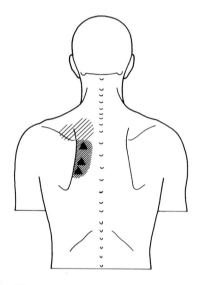

Fig. 14.8 The pattern of pain referral from a trigger point or points in the rhomboid muscles.

Specific pattern of pain referral

Pain from trigger points in these muscles (Fig. 14.7) is confined mainly to an area immediately medial to the inner border of the scapula (Fig. 14.8).

Trigger point examination

With the patient seated and the arms wrapped tightly around the front of the chest in order to bring the scapulae forwards the trigger points are located by means of deep palpation through the trapezius muscle.

Activation of mid-line trigger points in the ligamentum nuchae

Pain on extending or flexing the neck is often associated with the presence of a trigger point or points in the ligamentum nuchae connecting the apices of the cervical vertebral spines (Fig. 14.4). In all such cases therefore it is important to palpate along the length of this ligament from the occiput above to the spine of the 7th cervical vertebra below.

FACTORS RESPONSIBLE FOR THE PRIMARY ACTIVATION OF TRIGGER POINTS IN THE NECK

The factors responsible include acute trauma, acute or recurrent muscle strain, exposure to damp or draughts and anxiety.

This primary activation may take place at any age. And in this connection it is important to remember that in patients over the age of 40 any radiographic evidence of cervical spondylosis *in the absence of physical signs of nerve root entrapment* is usually of little or no significance with the pain most often being due to the primary activation of trigger points.

Acute trauma

Trigger point activation may occur as the result of trauma from any type of accident such as falling from a horse or tripping whilst going downstairs, but one of the commonest nowadays is the whiplash injury liable to affect the occupants of a stationary car when this is hit from behind by another car. Such an accident severely strains the muscles of the neck. The pain from this may spontaneously resolve in a few weeks but often because of the activation of trigger points it persists long after all external evidence of tissue damage such as bruising has disappeared. Failure to recognize this possibility is liable to lead to a totally unwarranted diagnosis of neurosis or even malingering as may be seen from the following case.

A builder (46), as a result of a car accident, was admitted to hospital unconscious and with severe bruising of the right side of the neck, right shoulder and right elbow.

He recovered consciousness within a matter of hours, the bruising disappeared over the next few weeks but he was left with much pain in and restricted movements of the right side of the neck and in spite of physiotherapy, neck traction and the wearing of a collar he still had this pain when seen by an orthopaedic specialist 3 months after the accident. The patient was told at this stage that no further treatment was likely to be helpful but that the pain would disappear spontaneously with time.

When, at follow-up 6 months later, he still had considerable pain and limitation of movements of the neck, and had also by then developed headaches and unsteadiness on sudden movements, the same specialist told him that with patience it would all settle down and that certainly he was unlikely to have trouble once a compensation claim had been settled! The patient felt the implications of such a remark to be totally unjustified particularly as being a self-employed person he was desperately anxious to get back to work. His general practitioner wondered if he might be helped by acupuncture and when seen by me 12 months after the accident he was obviously having much genuine pain in the neck causing him to take large amounts of analgesics.

On examination, there were many exquisitely tender trigger points to be found in several muscles of the neck, and after these had been deactivated by means of dry needle stimulation at weekly intervals on six occasions, his pain was sufficiently well controlled to allow him to return to work, and after two further treatments over the next month it disappeared.

This response to acupuncture was gratifying but of course it would have been possible to have relieved his pain much more quickly if only the development of trigger point activity had been recognized at a much earlier stage.

Postural disorders

Trigger point activity may arise in the neck muscles when some faulty posture is persistently adopted. This not infrequently occurs occupationally as a result of a desk or workbench not being adjusted to an individual's body build. Machine operators and typists are some of those particularly at risk.

A draughtsman (29) had two attacks of severe right-sided neck pain with restricted movements. Each time he was told he must have 'slipped a disc' and was treated by having his neck intermittently stretched and immobilized in a collar.

On each occasion he obtained little or no benefit from these measures, had to take much time off work, and the pain persisted for about 6–8 weeks. In view of this experience, when 1 year later it recurred a third time, he asked his general practitioner about the possibility of acupuncture and was referred to me. I saw him within a week of the pain developing, and found a very sensitive trigger point in the right levator scapulae muscle at the angle of the neck; also one in the free border of the trapezius half-way between the angle of the neck and the tip of the shoulder; and a third half-way down the side of the neck.

When these were deactivated with a dry needle, the pain immediately abated and full movement of the neck was restored. It was only necessary to repeat the procedure once again a week later before lasting improvement was obtained. However, what was of particular importance to him was the fact that he did not have to take any time off work. It is not sufficient to content oneself with effectively alleviating pain, without at the same time seeing whether there is anything that has to be done in order to prevent a recurrence. In this case it was found that each attack had occurred at a time when pressure of work demanded that he sat at his drawing board for a particularly long period, and that because his chair was too low he had to sit during this time with his shoulder girdle in an abnormally elevated position.

Trigger point activity in neck muscles may develop too when the neck has to be turned to one side for long periods such as when a secretary has to read shorthand notes whilst typing, or when the neck is kept fixed in one position for a long time such as when watching a play or driving a car, also when it is repeatedly rotated such as watching a tennis match.

It also may occur during sleep when the neck becomes kinked at an acute angle either due to the pillow being too high or too low.

A girl (14) suffered from severe neck pain that much affected her schooling for 3 years because the significance of too high a pillow was not recognized. During that 3 years she was given several courses of physiotherapy, had had her neck stretched and from time to time had worn a collar. When eventually she was seen by me it only required the deactivation of trigger points on three occasions to bring the pain under control. On investigating the cause of the pain it became apparent that the child for many years had insisted on sleeping with the head resting on three pillows. Since this habit has been changed, she has had no recurrence of pain.

Sagging of the shoulder girdle

The activation of trigger points commonly occurs in those, who because of occupational strains, obesity, or even laziness, have become round shouldered with drooping of the shoulder girdle — the so-called syndrome of the sagging shoulders.

Tilting of the shoulder girdle

This is not an uncommon cause of trigger point activity developing, and occurs either secondary to a pelvic tilt in someone who because of a congenital or acquired defect has one leg longer than the other, or from the habitual use of a walking stick which is too long.

Transmitted strain to the neck

Any painful disorder affecting the lower limb may, by putting a strain on all parts of the spine, cause not only the development of trigger points in the muscles of the lower back but also in the muscles of the neck.

Persistent pressure on the shoulder girdle

Trigger point activity may develop in the neck muscles when they are subjected to persistent strain from the wearing of unsuitable clothing such as an overcoat which is too heavy, or shoulder straps which are too tight.

Environmental factors

These include exposure either to draughts or to damp.

Anxiety

A common cause of trigger points developing in neck muscles is when these are persistently held taut because of nervous tension. When this is the predominant cause, the patient often complains of headaches as well.

PREVENTATIVE MEASURES

It must be stressed that although pain from any of the above causes may readily be alleviated by means of dry needle stimulation of trigger points, such pain will recur unless steps are taken in every case to define the underlying cause so that appropriate measures may be taken either to avoid it or to eliminate it.

TREATMENT

Because of the traditional belief that persistent pain and stiffness of the neck are mainly due to nerve root entrapment, either from an acute prolapse of an intervertebral disc, or from cervical spondylosis, treatment usually includes continuous or more often intermittent traction; the wearing of a specially designed collar; and the use of various forms of physiotherapy.

Pain of this type may persist for many months or years but often it subsides spontaneously after about 6–8 weeks and it is now generally agreed that none of the standard forms of treatment such as neck traction (Steinberg & Mason 1959, British Association of Physical Medicine Trial 1966), the wearing of a collar (Matthews 1983) or different types of physiotherapy including diathermy and ultrasound (Rogers & Williams 1981) significantly influence its course.

There is therefore much need for a new approach to the treatment of persistent neck pain and, now that it is realized that often it is associated with the activation of trigger points in the muscles, we have in trigger point acupuncture one of considerable promise. This first became apparent to me some years ago now, when, as it so happened, one of the first patients to be treated by me with this particular form of therapy had pain of this type.

A housewife (61) was referred to my outpatient clinic with angina but what troubled her even more was that for the past 6 months, since she and her husband had been in a car accident, she had had persistent pain in the neck with marked restriction of its movements. She further informed me that she had not mentioned this to her general practitioner as she could not face having to wear a collar! An X-ray of the cervical spine showed, as might be expected at that age, the characteristic appearances of cervical spondylosis. In addition, however, examination of her neck muscles revealed the presence of trigger points and she was therefore asked to attend my outpatient clinic again for me to attempt to relieve her pain with acupuncture.

It must have been with a certain amount of trepidation that she kept her appointment for this as she brought her husband with her for moral support! Trigger points were found at three similar sites on both sides of her neck. Needles were inserted into these and left in position for 2–3 minutes. Much to her surprise (and to a certain extent mine also!) on withdrawing them she found that her neck was very much more comfortable and that she could move it through a full range of movements. She said that her husband would never believe this and so asked if he could come into the treatment room to witness it!

After expressing pleasure at his wife's response to treatment, he revealed that he too, since the car accident, had had persistent pain in his neck and had experienced severe limitation of its movements. Further, he said that he had had two courses of intensive treatment in the hospital's department of physical medicine for what he had been told was severe arthritis of the neck, and wondered whether as an act of desperation he also might be allowed to try the effects of acupuncture.

The hospital physician concerned agreed to this, and after my examination I found the husband to have several trigger points in both sides of his neck. Once these had been deactivated with dry needles, the immediate results were as gratifying as in the case of his wife.

Ultimately the wife had to have treatment on four occasions and the husband on six in order to obtain lasting relief from their pain. My memory, however, of those two walking down the hospital corridor after their first treatment both joyfully moving their heads from side to side in evident amazement at their new-found freedom of neck movements will forever be indelibly imprinted on my mind, and at the time did much to strengthen my resolve to study acupuncture further!

There can be no doubt that in both these cases the neck pain was due to the activation of trigger points in neck muscles that had become strained as a result of the car accident and that the radiographic changes observed in both of them were chance findings. It is interesting to note that the husband had been told that the reason for his failure to respond to physiotherapy was because the arthritis in his neck was so bad!

Deactivation of trigger points

The two cases just quoted once again serve to illustrate how important it is in all cases of persistent neck pain to examine the muscles of the neck for trigger points. Moreover such an examination has to be carried out in a systematic manner as it is essential to avoid overlooking any of the trigger points that may be contributing to the pain.

The patient should therefore be seated comfortably in a chair, but with the head and arms suitably positioned to put the muscles on the stretch. Each muscle should then be examined in turn in order to ensure that no trigger points are overlooked and that each in turn has a needle inserted into the tissues overlying it. Particular care, however, must be taken when putting needles into muscles around the base of the neck and into the muscles of the chest wall, never to insert them in a vertical direction but always at an angle so as to avoid penetrating the pleura.

As previously stated (see Ch. 8), when treating musculoskeletal pain by inserting needles into the tissues overlying trigger points and stimulating nerve endings at these sites by means of manually manipulating these needles, such stimulation should never be carried out too energetically as otherwise it is liable to cause a temporary exacerbation of the pain. For some reason it would seem that this is especially likely to happen when deactivating trigger points in muscles around the head and neck, and therefore in carrying out acupuncture on this part of the body, it is advisable to be particularly careful not to keep needles in situ for more than a few minutes and to keep any manipulation of them down to a minimum.

This having been said it has to be admitted that somewhat paradoxically some people advocate strong stimulation of acupuncture points by means of passing an electric current through needles inserted into them for up to 40 minutes in the treatment of chronic neck pain (Loy 1983).

It is obvious that statistically-controlled trials will have to be carried out in order to compare the relative efficacy of manual and electro-acupuncture but, in the meantime, my personal preference is for the use of manual acupuncture in the manner described for the routine treatment of persistent neck pain. On occasions, however, in cases where the response is poor it is sometimes helpful to employ transcutaneous electrical nerve stimulation (TENS).

RESULTS OF TRIGGER POINT ACUPUNCTURE

Everyday clinical experience would appear to suggest that the treatment of persistent neck pain with trigger point acupuncture is very rewarding. It would seem that approximately 70% of patients obtain long-term relief from repeating this type of treatment on several occasions but the number of times this has to be carried out is largely dependent on the length of time the pain has been present before treatment is started. A minority of cases only obtain relief for short periods and the treatment therefore has to be repeated on a regular basis at fairly frequent intervals. Such patients however find this a small price to pay for having their pain kept under control. A small group of patients obtain no benefit from this type of treatment. These are usually people with neck pain of many years standing, well-marked neurological signs and radiographic evidence of extensive spondylitis. It must be realized, however, that when considering results it is difficult to generalize, for in the treatment of persistent neck pain, as in the treatment of all types of musculoskeletal pain with acupuncture, the effectiveness of the method seems not only to depend on the underlying pathology, but also on the degree of responsiveness to peripheral nerve stimulation of each individual person's centrally placed pain modulating mechanisms.

Clinical trials

The estimate of results given above based on clinical experience is only very approximate and there is much need for large-scale statistically controlled trials to be conducted in order that the efficacy of trigger point acupuncture in the treatment of persistent neck pain may be evaluated more accurately. Unfortunately up to now such trials that have been carried out have been of somewhat limited value.

Coan et al (1982) carried out a randomized controlled study of traditional Chinese acupuncture in the treatment of chronic neck pain. There were, however, only 15 patients in the treatment group and 15 in the 'no treatment' control group. Admittedly the results seem to have been somewhat impressive because 80% of the treated group showed significant improvement as judged by the amount pain was decreased, medication was reduced and activity was increased; in contrast to only 20% in the control group. However, the subjects were recruited through newspaper advertisements and, therefore, as a group they may have had a greater degree of faith in acupuncture and may have been more responsive to any placebo effect than a group of patients selected at random from those attending a medical clinic.

The trial carried out by Petrie & Langley (1983) on 13 patients with chronic neck pain is notable for the excellence of the type of placebo treatment used in the control group. This consisted of mock transcutaneous nerve stimulation (TENS) presented to the patients who received it as subliminal pulse therapy. Traditional Chinese acupuncture given to another group seemed to be significantly more effective than this type of placebo at the end of 8 twice-weekly treatment sessions but unfortunately there was no follow-up and the small numbers in each group means that the trial can only be regarded as a pilot study.

Matsumoto et al (1974) attempted to compare the relative effectiveness of manual trigger point acupuncture and electroacupuncture in the treatment of chronic neck pain considered by them, from radiographic evidence, to be due to osteo-arthritis of the cervical spine. Unfortunately the smallness of the numbers in the two main groups and various sub-groups made it difficult for them to reach any statistically significant conclusions. Loy (1983), as already mentioned, carried out a study designed to compare the relative effectiveness of electroacupuncture and physiotherapy in the treatment of chronic neck pain, considered by him, also mainly from appearances on X-rays, to be due to cervical spondylosis.

In the light of what has already been discussed in this chapter it would seem unwise to assume that because a group of patients with persistent neck pain show degenerative changes in their cervical radiographs that the pain in all of them is necessarily due to this. There are good reasons for believing that in only a few will this be so and that the others will have pain that is primarily muscular in origin, with in such cases, the X-ray changes being no more than a fortuitous investigatory finding. In view of this difficulty in distinguishing between these two types of pain it would seem better when conducting trials on a group of patients suffering from them to avoid the use of terms such as cervical spondylitis or arthritis and to be content as Coan et al (1982), and Petrie & Langley (1983) were, simply to refer to them collectively as cases of chronic neck pain. Or, alternatively, in view of the fact that the activation of trigger points, either as a primary or secondary event, occurs in all of them and that it is of such considerable significance with respect to treatment, it would perhaps be even more advantageous to refer to them collectively as cases of the chronic cervical myofascial trigger point pain syndrome.

REFERENCES

British Association of Physical Medicine Trial 1966 Pain in the neck and arm. A multicentre trial of the effects of physiotherapy. British Medical Journal 1: 253–258

Coan R M, Wong G, Coan P L 1982 The acupuncture treatment of neck pain: a randomized controlled study. American Journal of Chinese Medicine 9: 326–332

Friedenberg Z B, Miller W T 1963 Degenerative disc disease of the cervical spine. A comparative study of asymptomatic and symptomatic patients. Journal of Bone and Joint Surgery 45A: 1171–1178

Frykholm R 1951 Cervical nerve root compression resulting from disc degeneration and root-sleeve fibrosis. Acta Chirurgica Scandinavica Supplement 160

Heller C A, Stanley P, Lewis-Jones B, Heller R F 1983 Value of X-ray examinations of the cervical spine. British Medical Journal 287: 1276–1278

Jayson M 1978 Back pain, spondylosis and disc disorders. In: Scott J T (ed) Copeman's textbook of the rheumatic disease, 5th edn. Churchill Livingstone, Edinburgh, p 960–985

Long C 1956 Myofascial pain syndromes Part 2 — syndromes of the head, neck and shoulder girdle. Henry Ford Hospital Medical Bulletin 4: 22–28

Loy T T 1983 Treatment of cervical spondylosis. Electroacupuncture versus physiotherapy. Medical Journal of Australia 2: 32–34

Matsumoto T, Levy B, Ambruso V 1974 Clinical evaluation of acupuncture. The American Surgeon 40/7: 400–405

Matthews W B 1983 Lesions of the spinal roots. In: Weatherall D J, Ledingham J G G, Warrell D A (eds) Oxford textbook of medicine. Oxford University Press, Oxford, ch 21, p 43–44

Michele A A, Davies J J, Krueger F J, Lichtor J M 1950 Scapulocostal syndrome (fatigue-postural paradox). New York State Journal of Medicine 50: 1353–1356

Michele A A, Eisenberg J 1968 Scapulocostal syndrome. Archives of Physical Medicine and Rehabilitation 49: 383–387

Pallis C, Jones A M, Spillane J D 1954 Cervical spondylosis. Incidence and implications. Brain 77: 274–289

Petrie J P, Langley G B 1983 Acupuncture in the treatment of chronic cervical pain. A pilot study. Clinical and Experimental Rheumatology 1: 333–335

Posner J 1982 Diseases compressing nerve roots or spinal cord. In: Wyngaarden James B, Smith Lloyd H (eds) Cecil's textbook of medicine, 16th edn. Saunders, Philadelphia, p 2148–2150

Rogers M, Williams N 1981 Rheumatology in general practice. Churchill Livingstone, Edinburgh, p 109

Russek A S 1952 Diagnosis and treatment of scapulocostal syndrome. Journal of the American Medical Association 150: 25–27

Sola A E, Kuitert J H 1955 Myofascial trigger point pain in the neck and shoulder girdle. Northwest Medicine 54: 980–984

Sola A E, Williams R L 1956 Myofascial pain syndromes. Neurology (Minneapolis) 6: 91–95

Steinberg V L, Mason R M 1959 Cervical spondylosis. Pilot therapeutic trial. Annals of Physical Medicine 5: 37

Travell J G, Simons D G 1983 Myofascial pain and dysfunction. The trigger point manual. Williams & Wilkins, Baltimore

Urban J, Maroudas A 1980 In: Graham R (ed) Clinics in rheumatic diseases, vol 6, no 1. Saunders, Philadelphia

Waddell G 1982 An approach to backache. British Journal of Hospital Medicine 28(3) 187–219

15. Pain in the arm

INTRODUCTION

Various causes of pain in the arm will now be considered, some of which are most appropriately treated by acupuncture, but also others which are not. The reason for such a wide ranging discussion is because acupuncture must never be considered to be a panacea for all types of painful disorders, and with arm pain, as with pain in any other part of the body, it is first of all essential to make an accurate diagnosis as to the underlying cause of the pain, and then to decide whether acupuncture or some other form of treatment is most likely to be helpful.

Brachial 'neuritis'

Pain radiating down the arm from the neck was until recently often said to be due to brachial 'neuritis'. However, now that many of the disorders liable to cause pain of this type have become better understood, it is realized that there is no scientific basis for this and that such a diagnosis therefore is no longer acceptable. Nevertheless, whether some of the more precise diagnostic terms, which are now so confidently employed, always accurately reflect the true cause of such pain is certainly very much open to question.

Acute neck and arm pain due either to cervical disc prolapse or to primary myofascial trigger point activation

When pain suddenly develops in the neck and arm of a young adult, it is often assumed to be due to nerve root compression from a lateral disc prolapse. The fallibility of making such a diagnosis in the absence of objective neurological signs, in view of the fact that exactly similar pain may develop as a result of the primary activation of trigger points in the muscles of the neck and shoulder girdle, has already been discussed in Chapter 14. The importance of recognizing myofascial trigger points as a possible source of such pain is, of course, because, when these are present, acupuncture is the most logical and effective form of treatment.

Neuralgic amyotrophy

This is unlikely to be confused with either of the above two conditions because, although it is associated with a sudden onset of severe pain in the shoulder and upper arm, there is also marked weakness and wasting of certain muscles such as the serratus anterior, deltoid, spinati and trapezius. Also, whereas the muscle weakness persists for several months or at times indefinitely, the pain usually subsides spontaneously in the course of a few days. However, the importance of this condition with respect to acupuncture is that when it is associated with long-term wasting of the shoulder girdle muscles, the strain on them is eventually liable to lead to activation of trigger points and a recurrence of pain due to this. Such pain is then best relieved by deactivating these trigger points by means of dry needle stimulation.

Malignant infiltration of the brachial plexus

A more insidious development of pain in the neck with radiation down the arm may on occasions be due to infiltration of the brachial plexus, either by a primary or secondary malignant process. In treating malignant pain anywhere in the body the treatment of first choice is obviously the administration of a powerful narcotic analgesic, but those who develop severe side-effects from a drug of this type or become resistant to it are sometimes helped by acupuncture. Filshie & Redman (1985) using this form of treatment in 36 patients with neurogenic pain in the arm that had failed to respond to conventional drug therapy following surgery, radiotherapy, or chemotherapy for carcinoma of the breast found that 'a significant improvement of power and pain relief occurred in 17 out of the 36'. They noted, too, that for some reason acupuncture was most helpful in those patients whose pain was associated with post-irradiation fibrosis.

Chronic neck and arm pain due either to cervical spondylosis or to primary myofascial trigger point activation

As already stated in Chapter 14, and repeated now, as it cannot be too strongly emphasized, there is no justification for assuming that pain in the neck and down the arm, in the absence of objective evidence of nerve root involvement, is necessarily due to cervical spondylosis, just because changes of the latter happen to be demonstrable radiologically. The reasons for this are that such changes are common in everyone over the age of 40 whether they have symptoms or not, and even more importantly because pain of exactly the same type and distribution may occur as a result of trigger points in the muscles of the neck and shoulder girdle becoming primarily activated for one or other of a variety of reasons.

It has to be admitted that clinically the distinction between the two is sometimes difficult due to the fact that the pain which occurs as a result of nerve root entrapment in cervical spondylosis may itself cause trigger points to become secondarily activated in muscles supplied by the nerve root or roots affected. And at times, therefore, an electromyograph is helpful because, in nerve root entrapment, spontaneous potentials occur in the muscles supplied by the affected nerves, but in primary myofascial disorder there is no such abnormality.

In everyday clinical practice, however, it is usually sufficient to rely on the taking of a detailed history, together with the carrying out of a careful neurological examination and a systematic search for myofascial trigger points. The history is of particular importance as it is only by knowing the exact circumstances prevailing at the time of onset of the pain that an assessment can be made as to whether any factors capable of activating trigger points may have been present.

The following case is a good example of the importance of history taking in deciding both the cause of neck and arm pain and its appropriate treatment.

A physiotherapist (46) on developing pain in both sides of her neck and down the left arm was referred for an X-ray of the cervical spine. As the radiograph showed evidence of cervical spondylosis she was told that the pain in the neck was due to this and that the pain down her arm was also due to it causing a nerve to become trapped. She was then given some intermittent traction and told to wear a collar. When 3 months later there had been no improvement she asked whether she could try the effects of acupuncture, and as a result of this was eventually referred to me.

On taking the history it became apparent that the symptoms started shortly after a serious domestic upset had caused her to become very agitated and distressed.

On examination, she was found to be holding the muscles of her neck and shoulder girdle in a state of persistent tension. There were no abnormal neurological signs but there were trigger points in various muscles of her neck including the levator scapulae and trapezius. Also, on the left side, there was a trigger point in the supraspinatus muscle with pressure on this causing a sensation described as an electric shock to be referred to the shoulder and down the outer part of the upper arm in the same distribution as the spontaneously occurring pain in her arm.

The trigger points were therefore deactivated by means of dry needle stimulation with immediate relief of the pain. However, in spite of repeating this on four occasions at weekly intervals the pain always quickly returned.

It was therefore decided to treat her anxiety state by getting her to talk about her worries and by giving her some hypnotherapy. Once she learnt to come to terms with her problems she lost much of the tension in her muscles. She was then given one further treatment with acupuncture following which she had no further pain.

Characteristics of nocigenic and of neurogenic pain

It is sometimes thought that it is possible to distinguish between referred pain from myofascial trigger points and neurogenic pain because of differences in their character. This however is not so as both may have a deep aching quality. Admittedly, neurogenic pain is more frequently accompanied by various paraesthesiae such as numbness, burning or pins and needles, but as Sola & Kuitert (1955) pointed out, and everyday clinical practice confirms, similar paraesthesiae may at times be present with pain of myofascial origin, and therefore to attempt to differentiate between the two on these grounds alone is impossible.

A publican's wife (56) with a history of intermittent pain in the neck for 12 years, and for which she had frequently worn a collar, once again developed pain in the neck and down the left arm, but what disturbed her most this time was a feeling of 'pins and needles' spreading down both sides of that arm on moving it. She was informed by her doctor that this was because she had a trapped nerve and was given some physiotherapy and told to wear a collar once again, but when after 5 months her symptoms had not improved, she herself asked for some acupuncture.

The most striking feature in this case was that whenever pressure was applied to a trigger point in the supraspinatus muscle, it invariably brought on the sensation of pins and needles in the outer arm, and when pressure was applied to a trigger point in the levator scapulae muscle a similar sensation travelled down the inner side of the arm to the ring and little fingers. There were no abnormal neurological signs. After deactivation of trigger points in these two muscles by means of dry needle stimulation on four occasions, at weekly intervals, she had no further trouble.

REFERRAL OF PAIN DOWN THE ARM FROM TRIGGER POINTS IN THE MUSCLES OF THE NECK AND SHOULDER GIRDLE

As stated in the previous chapter, Michele et al (1950), Russek (1952), Long (1956), and Michele & Eisenberg (1968) were amongst some of the first to draw attention to the importance of myofascial trigger points in causing pain to be referred down the arm from the neck. Then in 1971, Aronson et al published a report on 16 patients seen by them over an 8-month period with pain of this type. They state that they reported these because they felt it was still not sufficiently well recognized that brachial pain of myofascial origin may be readily mistaken for pain of cervical nerve root origin, due to the fact that their patterns of distribution in the arm are similar.

As they pointed out, prior to being seen by them, this particular group of patients, because their pain had a cervical nerve root distribution, had been misdiagnosed by orthopaedic and neurosurgeons as suffering from nerve root entrapment and as a consequence of this had been subjected to prolonged periods of neck traction and the wearing of cervical collars. It was only when these measures failed to help that they were then referred for further investigation, with the majority of them being considered to be possible cases of coronary heart disease.

They stated that what led them to the correct diagnosis was the absence of objective neurological signs, and the discovery that 'on careful palpation of the chest and trunk every patient demonstrated an exquisitely tender trigger area posteriorly above the medial portion of the scapular spine. Palpating this area resulted in pain also along the cervical nerve root distribution. These findings appear to be the pathognomonic hallmark of the syndrome'. They were of course absolutely correct about this because the two essential requirements for the diagnosis of referred myofascial pain anywhere in the body is firstly to be able to find trigger points in the muscles, and secondly to be able to evoke pain in exactly the same distribution as that of the spontaneously occurring pain by applying pressure to such points.

By these criteria it is now evident that pain down the arm from the neck commonly occurs as a result of trigger point activity in the supraspinatus, the infraspinatus, the scaleni, and the levator scapulae.

Trigger point activity in the supraspinatus

As stated in Chapter 13, pain from trigger points in this muscle is referred to the outer side of the shoulder over the area of the deltoid muscle and down the outer side of the upper arm to the lateral epicondyle where it is often felt particularly strongly. Its pattern of referral therefore coincides with the cutaneous area of distribution of the C5 nerve root, and for this reason its clinical presentation is similar to that of pain from entrapment of this nerve (Reynolds 1981).

Trigger point activity in the infraspinatus

As stated in Chapter 13, pain from trigger points in this muscle is referred to the front of the shoulder, the anterolateral border of the arm and forearm and sometimes extends as far as the radial aspect of the hand. Its pattern of referral therefore coincides with the cutaneous area of distribution of the C5, C6 and C7 nerve roots and for this reason its clinical presentation is similar to that of pain from entrapment of these nerve roots (Reynolds 1981).

Trigger point activity in the scalenus anterior

As stated in Chapter 12 pain from trigger points in this muscle is referred down both the anterior and posterior aspects of the upper arm, the radial border of the forearm, and terminates in the thumb and index finger, and therefore may also simulate a C5–C7 nerve root lesion (Reynolds 1981). Such pain is likely to persist for months or years as trigger points in this muscle are particularly liable to be overlooked.

A man (52) was referred to me with a history that for 11 years he had been getting pain down the outer side of the right arm extending from the shoulder to the index finger and thumb. The pain had been intermittent with episodes of it being brought on by bouts of heavy lifting at work. He had had numerous courses of physiotherapy directed to the neck for what he was told was a 'trapped nerve'. Having received no benefit from these he decided to try acupuncture as a last resort!

On examination of the neck there were two exquisitely tender trigger points in the right scalenus anterior muscle with pressure on one of these causing pain to shoot down the arm to the thumb in the same distribution as the spontaneously occurring pain. The deactivation of these by means of dry needle stimulation quickly brought the pain under control.

Trigger point activity in the levator scapulae

As stated in the previous chapter, trigger point activity in the levator scapulae muscle is a common cause of pain being referred down the arm. Michele & Eisenberg (1968) estimated that it is responsible for more than 90% of all cases of cervicobrachial pain. And certainly of all the myofascial trigger point pains which spread down the arm, it is the one most likely to be confused with pain from cervical nerve root entrapment. This is because there is always much pain in the neck itself extending up as far as the occiput, together with much stiffness of the neck and limitation of its movements, in addition to pain which radiates down the inner side of the arm to the ring and little fingers, in a manner similar to that seen with a C8 T1 nerve root lesion.

Electromyography may be required to distinguish a myofascial trigger point pain syndrome from a cervical nerve root lesion but in practice this is rarely necessary because when trigger point activity is responsible for the pain, pressure on the relevant trigger point almost always, in my experience, causes pain to shoot down the arm in the distribution of the spontaneously occurring pain. When this happens, invariably the pain is relieved by deactivating the trigger point by the acupuncture technique of dry needle stimulation. The following case exemplifies this.

A prison officer (54), 2 years before being seen by me, developed pain in his neck as a result of falling off his motor bike. At that time he was told that his neck X-ray showed quite marked arthritic changes, but in spite of this the pain only lasted for 3 weeks. He was then symptom-free until 9 months before being referred to me after a car ran into the back of his stationary car causing a whiplash injury to his neck. At first the neck felt persistently stiff with pain on turning it to the left side. After some weeks, he also began to get pain down the inner side of the left arm with pins and needles in the ring and little fingers.

He was given a variety of different forms of treatment in the physiotherapy department including neck traction, and was told to wear a collar. When after 9 months the pain in the neck and arm had not improved and he had lost much time off work, he informed his doctor he would like to try acupuncture.

On examination there was quite marked limitation of neck movements on the left side; and in addition there were several trigger points to be found in the muscles of the neck and shoulder girdle. In the levator scapulae muscle there were two; one at the angle of the neck, and one at the site where the muscle is inserted into the superior angle of the scapula. These were of particular interest because pressure on each of them in turn caused pain to shoot down the medial side of the arm to the ring and little fingers in exactly the same distribution as that of the spontaneously occurring pain, which obviously closely mimicked the distribution of pain from a C8 T1 nerve root lesion.

The response to dry needle deactivation of these trigger points was dramatic with the patient becoming symptom-free and able to return to work after only two sessions of treatment.

REFERRAL OF PAIN DOWN THE ARM FROM THE HEART AND FROM TRIGGER POINTS IN THE MUSCLES OF THE CHEST WALL

Pain which radiates down the arm does not of course necessarily stem from either a cervical nerve root lesion or from myofascial trigger points in the muscles of the neck or shoulder girdle. It may also, as already stated in Chapter 12, be referred down the arm from trigger points in the muscles of the chest wall and from the heart in coronary artery disease.

Pain down the arm from trigger point activity in muscles of the chest wall is usually readily distinguished from pain emanating from the muscles of the neck, because the pain is almost always felt in the chest as well as in the arm, as may be seen from the diagrams of the trigger point pain patterns of such muscles as the pectoralis major (Fig 12.7), pectoralis minor (Fig. 12.10), serratus anterior (Fig. 12.11), serratus posterior superior (Fig. 12.13) and the latissimus dorsi (Fig. 12.15).

It is important to remember that whilst anginal pain is usually felt across the front of the chest, as well as at other sites such as the neck and arm, at times it may be predominantly felt in the neck and arm, and occasionally it may be confined entirely to the arm. The latter may be somewhat misleading and is not sufficiently well recognized, although well known to William Heberden (1710–1801) nearly 300 years ago as may be seen from reading Chapter 70 *Pectoris Dolor* in his famous *Commentaries on the History and Cure of Diseases* (Heberden 1818).

PAIN IN THE NECK AND ARM FROM MYOFASCIAL TRIGGER POINTS IN THE ARM

The only muscle in the arm in which trigger point activity is likely to give rise to widespread pain affecting both the neck and arm is the triceps. And when this occurs, the trigger points are situated in the long head of this muscle.

Some relevant facts concerning this muscle will therefore now be discussed in detail.

Triceps muscle

Activation of trigger points

Trigger points may become activated in the long, medial or lateral heads of the muscle as a result of subjecting the muscle to strain during sports such as tennis, golf and doing 'press ups' and also, when the muscle is strained by sitting for any length of time with the arm held forwards without the elbow being adequately supported, such as when driving a car for a long distance.

Long head of the triceps

Trigger points in the medial and lateral heads give rise to localized pain around the epicondyles of the humerus and will therefore be referred to later in the chapter when discussing tennis and golfer's elbow.

It is trigger points in the long head of the triceps that cause pain to radiate over a wide area of the neck and arm and therefore only these will be considered at this stage.

Specific pattern of pain referral

Pain from these trigger points is referred upwards over the posterior part of the shoulder, occasionally to the base of the neck and sometimes down the back of the forearm to the wrist (Fig. 13.13). It is because of this pattern that the pain is sometimes confused with that of a C7 radiculopathy.

Trigger point examination

Trigger points in this head are usually to be found deep in the belly of the muscle just below the level of the posterior axillary fold (Fig. 13.13). They are present in taut bands which, when plucked, give local twitch responses. These bands are best found by palpating that part of the muscle between the thumb and fingers.

When trigger points in the long head are the cause of pain it is not possible to press the upraised arm hard against the ear when the elbow is kept straight (Fig. 13.14).

METHODS OF ALLEVIATING WIDESPREAD PAIN IN THE ARM WHEN CAUSED BY ACTIVITY IN MYOFASCIAL TRIGGER POINTS

Non-acupuncture methods

Injection of steroids into trigger points responsible for pain in the neck and down the arm as recommended by Aronson et al (1971), or procaine, as advocated by Michele et al (1950) and by Russek (1952), or a mixture of these two, as suggested by Michele & Eisenberg (1968), are of course unnecessary and have certain disadvantages (see Ch. 8).

Acupuncture

The technique of deactivating such points by means of dry needle stimulation has already been discussed with respect to the levator scapulae muscle Ch. 14, the supraspinatus muscle Ch. 13, the infraspinatus muscle Ch. 13 and the scaleni (Ch. 12).

The triceps

When deactivating trigger points in the triceps muscle, the patient can either lie face upwards with the arm externally rotated and abducted, or lie on the side with the affected arm uppermost.

The choice is determined entirely by which is easier in any particular case, and depending on where in the muscle the trigger points happen to be situated. In either case a palpable band containing a trigger point should be fixed between two fingers in order to facilitate inserting a needle into the tissues overlying it.

BRACHIAL PLEXUS INJURIES

The brachial plexus may be damaged by stab wounds, bullets, or iatrogenically by surgical operations on the neck. The nerves, however, in such cases usually remain in continuity and with present day neurosurgical techniques, repair operations usually result in good functional recovery without any serious residual pain.

When, however, the brachial plexus is damaged during the course of irradiating neoplastic glands in the neck, this may lead many years later to gradual wasting of the muscles of the hand and the development of severe pain. As this type of pain is not readily controlled by drugs, the possibility of treating it with acupuncture may be considered. However, as was explained in Chapter 9, neurogenic pain is not readily controlled by manual acupuncture. There is sometimes a place for electroacupuncture but in general it is probably better relieved by transcutaneous electrical nerve stimulation (TENS).

Avulsion of the cervical nerve roots

By far the commonest type of brachial plexus injury at the present time is the tearing away of nerve roots from the spinal cord during the course of a motor cycle accident. This type of traction lesion unfortunately usually affects an otherwise fit young man leaving him with an irreversibly paralysed and totally anaesthetic arm, and one in which, in almost 90% of cases, there is severe intractable pain.

Wynn Parry (1980, 1984) has made a special study of this type of injury and for further details about its clinical manifestations and management, the reader is referred to excellent accounts of the subject by him. It is only necessary here to say something about the pain, and methods of alleviating it. The pain is usually described as a persistent severe burning as if the arm is on fire (causalgia), superimposed upon which are episodic paroxysms of intense momentary shooting pain through the arm that often take the patient by surprise, and cause him to cry out.

As Wynn Parry (1984) points out, the single most helpful method of gaining some relief from the pain is for the patient to distract his mind from it by concentrating on work or hobbies. By this means it is often possible for him to get through a working day quite comfortably but, as soon as he sits down to relax in the evening, the pain builds up and at times becomes almost unbearable. Drugs are of very little help with this type of neurogenic pain and so anyone who practises acupuncture may be asked to see such a case. However, as has already been said, neurogenic pain in general responds poorly to manual acupuncture. A better response is sometimes obtained with electroacupuncture but the treatment of choice, as has been shown by Wynn Parry, is transcutaneous electrical nerve stimulation (TENS). It has to be remembered, however, that just as acupuncture does not work if the needles, whether they be stimulated manually or electrically, are inserted into a part of the body deprived of feeling, so TENS does not work if the electrodes are applied to skin which is anaesthetic. It is therefore essential in .combating the pain of a nerve root avulsion lesion firstly to map out the area of anaesthesia and then to place the electrodes on skin above the upper level of this.

COMPRESSION OF THE BRACHIAL PLEXUS (THORACIC OUTLET SYNDROME)

Until about 30 years ago, it was widely taught that a common cause of generalized pain spreading down the arm from the neck with pins and needles in the fingers is compression of the lower trunk of the brachial plexus, either by it being stretched, as it passes over a cervical rib, or compressed, as it passes between the scalenus anterior and a normal first rib (the scalenus anterior syndrome).

It is now realized that although a cervical rib is frequently seen on routine X-rays of the neck, only in about 10% of cases does it cause symptoms, and also that entrapment of the brachial plexus by the scalenus anterior muscle with its very similar clinical picture is also uncommon. Nevertheless, when a patient presents with pain in the arm in the distribution of the C8 T1 nerve roots, such causes of what collectively is known as the thoracic outlet syndrome have to be considered.

In this syndrome there is pain down the inner side of the arm, often from the elbow downwards, associated with paraesthesiae such as numbness or pins and needles affecting the ulnar side of the hand; also some sensory loss on the ulnar side of the hand and forearm, and wasting of the small muscles of the hand supplied by the ulnar nerve, such as the interossei and adductor pollicis.

When these neurological symptoms and signs are due to stretching of the brachial plexus over a cervical rib, there may also be evidence of compression of the subclavian artery including a bruit to be heard in the neck on auscultation, and circulatory changes to be found in the fingers; these vascular changes greatly increase the probability of the diagnosis.

The stretching of the brachial plexus over a cervical rib most commonly gives rise to symptoms and signs in middle-aged women when loss of tone in the muscles of the shoulder girdle causes this to droop. Relief from pain may therefore often be obtained by exercises designed to strengthen these muscles. However, when vascular changes predominate, or there is progressive wasting of the muscles of the hand, then the rib should be removed. Before embarking upon this, care should be taken to exclude an ulnar nerve lesion at the elbow as this may cause similar neurological signs in the forearm and hand.

When the underlying cause of the syndrome is a taut shortened scalenus anterior, then the neurological changes may be associated with symptoms from pressure on the subclavian vein, and only rarely with those associated with pressure on the artery.

Scalenotomy for the relief of pain in the scalenus anterior syndrome proved to be disappointing and is no longer performed. If the condition occurs because of myofascial trigger points in the scalenus anterior then these should be deactivated by dry needle stimulation. However, it should be remembered that when trigger points occur in the muscle without it causing pressure on the brachial plexus, then the referral of pain is down the radial side of forearm and hand (Ch. 12).

The position may be summarized by saying that stretching of the lower trunk of the brachial plexus over a cervical rib or pressure on it by the scalenus anterior are now considered to be very uncommon causes of pain down the arm. It cannot be stressed too strongly that in all cases where there is pain down the inner side of the arm from the neck with pins and needles in the ring and little fingers, in the absence of objective neurological signs and of signs of vascular compression, an active search for trigger points in the levator scapulae should always be made, as this is frequently a cause of pain in this distribution (Ch. 14).

LATERAL EPICONDYLITIS (TENNIS ELBOW)

Both of these diagnostic terms in current use for a condition characterized principally by pain in the region of the lateral epicondyle are really misnomers. This is because the disorder is not primarily due to some abnormality of the lateral epicondyle itself, but rather due to pain being referred to this structure from trigger points in muscles adjacent to it. Also this disorder is not only brought on by playing tennis but by any activity which causes excessive strain to be put on the extensors of the wrist at the elbow.

Clinical features

There is usually a persistent dull ache with, at times, bouts of acute pain on the outer side of the elbow. This pain is aggravated by putting the wrist extensors on the stretch, such as when the pronated wrist is passively flexed. It is also made worse by any action that causes these muscles to contract, such as when the wrist is extended against resistance. With this condition it is possible to lift a chair comfortably when it is gripped

with the hand, palm upwards, but there is considerable aggravation of the pain when this is done with the hand palm downwards.

The pain of lateral epicondylitis is also sometimes associated with pain in the region of the wrist. There is usually no mention of this in standard textbook descriptions of lateral epicondylitis and therefore it will be referred to again later in the chapter when discussing wrist pain. The lateral epicondyle is always extremely tender to touch; also the surrounding tissues at times feel warm, and may on occasions appear to be swollen.

There is some weakness of the grip with a tendency to drop objects. Also, any attempt to sustain a grip such as when shaking hands aggravates the pain.

Activation of trigger points in muscles around the outer part of the elbow

It is usually trigger point activity in the supinator muscle which is primarily responsible for the condition (Travell & Simons 1983a) but trigger points may also develop in the brachioradialis, the extensor carpi radialis longus, the extensor digitorum, and in the lateral border of the medial head of the triceps.

Trauma

The main cause for the activation of trigger points in these muscles is trauma. This may occur acutely, such as when there is direct injury to the elbow, or when the muscles and their attachments at or near to the elbow become suddenly wrenched. It may also arise subacutely when the muscles are traumatized as a result of repeated strenuous extensor movements at the wrist. And, on occasions, the activation may occur insidiously without there being any obvious cause.

The supinator, as its name implies, is the principal muscle responsible for supinating the hand and forearm at the radioulnar joint, but the biceps assists with the movement providing the elbow is flexed slightly. It therefore follows that whenever the muscle is liable to be subjected to undue strain, such as when hitting a tennis ball backhanded, both the elbow and wrist should be held in a slightly flexed position. It is when tennis players fail to do this and take backhand shots with the arm straight that the supinator becomes overloaded. This in turn leads to trigger points in the muscle becoming activated and causing pain to be referred to the lateral epicondyle.

It is not, however, only tennis players who are liable to develop the disorder, but anybody who has to hold the arm straight with the forearm in a position of supination for any length of time, or who carries a load with the elbows flexed and the hands held in the pronated position. Heavy objects in fact should always be carried with the hand palm upwards as then much of the strain is taken by the biceps.

Other common activities liable to put an abnormal strain on this muscle include the repeated turning of a stiff door knob, the un-screwing of a tight jar lid, the controlling of a heavy dog straining at the leash, and the raking of leaves.

Similar activities may also sometimes lead to the activation of trigger points in the brachio-radialis and the extensor carpi radialis longus. In addition, trigger points may become activated in the extensor digitorum as a result of force-ful repetitive movements of the fingers by such people as musicians, craftsmen and gardeners.

Inflammation

The trauma responsible for the development of 'tennis elbow' is often the cause of an acute inflammatory reaction developing in the tissues. In some patients these inflammatory changes enter into a chronic phase, and there is no doubt that it is because of this that many such cases fail to respond to medical treatment and have to undergo surgery.

Goldie (1964), during the course of operating on 113 such patients, observed that the aponeur-osis was infiltrated by granulation tissue and that the symptoms were relieved by excising this. Bernhang (1979) reported evidence of chronic synovial inflammation in 11 out of 21 cases subjected to surgery after having proved resistant to medical treatment.

Activation of trigger points in muscles in the neck and shoulder girdle

Pain around the outer part of the elbow is some-times referred to that site from trigger points in the muscles of the neck, particularly the supra-spinatus and the trapezius, and less often the infraspinatus. The activation of trigger points in these muscles may be a primary event but on occasions there are objective neurological signs and EMG changes to show that it is secondary to nerve root entrapment (Gunn & Milbrandt 1976). The referred pain at the elbow is then responsible for the activation of satellite trigger points in muscles situated in the region of the lateral epicondyle.

The important lesson to be learnt from this is that the persistence of 'tennis elbow' pain follow-ing the deactivation of trigger points in muscles around the elbow is on occasions because there are trigger points in the neck muscles that have been overlooked and which also need to be deactivated.

Trigger point examination at the elbow

Trigger points in the supinator are usually to be found at its distal attachment to the anterior surface of the radius just below the insertion of the tendon of the biceps into the radial tuber-osity. When searching for these trigger points, therefore, the hand should be fully *supinated*. Also the brachioradialis should be pushed out of the way in a lateral direction. This is most readily done if the elbow is slightly flexed. Any trigger points present will then be found to lie just under the skin between the biceps tendon medially and the brachioradialis laterally (Fig. 15.1).

The locating of trigger points in the brachio-radialis and extensor carpi radialis longus should be carried out with the elbow slightly flexed and with the forearm resting comfortably on a pillow in the prone position (Fig. 15.2). The trigger points are best found by palpating these muscles between the thumb and fingers about 3 cm or approximately 1 in distal to the lateral epicondyle (Figs 15.9 and 15.10). It has to be remembered that the brachioradialis is a thin muscle lying immediately over the extensor carpi radialis

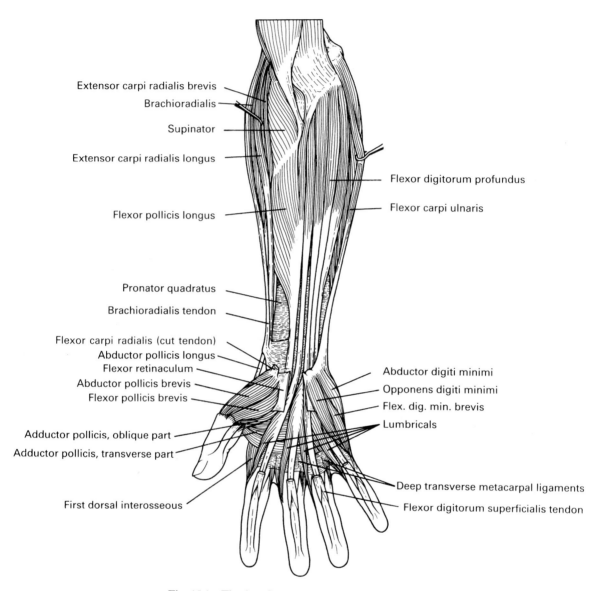

Fig. 15.1   The deep flexor muscles of the right forearm.

longus and that therefore flat palpation should be avoided as with this it is usually difficult to decide which of these two muscles contain trigger points.

The locating of trigger points in the extensor digitorum should be carried out with the arm in the same position as for the brachioradialis and extensor carpi radialis longus. Trigger points in the muscle lie about 6 cm or 2 in below the lateral epicondyle and may be found by flat palpation (Fig. 15.14).

The anatomical arrangement of the triceps

muscle in such that the medial head just above the elbow extends from one side of the arm to the other beneath the muscle's common tendon of attachment to the olecranon process of the ulna. The lower part of the lateral border of the medial head is therefore just above the lateral epicondyle, and the lower part of the medial border of this head is just above the medial epicondyle (Fig. 15.3).

A trigger point in the medial border refers pain to the medial epicondyle and sometimes down

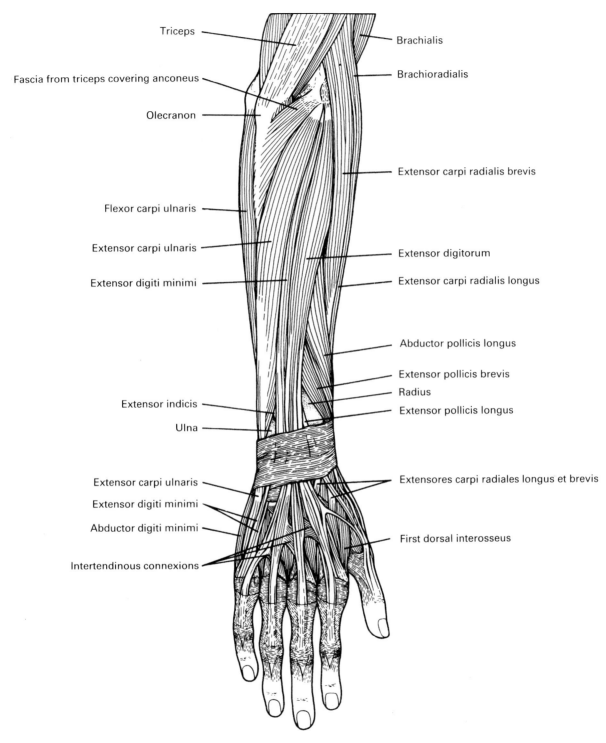

Fig. 15.2   Muscles of the extensor aspect of the right forearm, superficial layer.

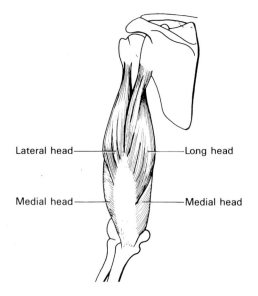

Fig. 15.3   The medial, lateral and long heads of the triceps muscle. It should be noted that the lower part of the medial head just above the elbow extends from one side of the arm to the other beneath the muscle's common tendon of attachment to the olecranon process of the ulna.

the arm to the ring and little fingers and will be discussed again when considering 'golfer's elbow' (p. 212) and when considering the differential diagnosis of ulnar nerve entrapment (p. 219).

It is a trigger point in the lateral border of the medial head just above the elbow which commonly refers pain to the lateral epicondyle in 'tennis elbow'. It is found by flat palpation of the muscle about 4 cm or approximately 1.5 in above the lateral epicondyle near to the attachments of the extensor carpi radialis longus and the brachioradialis (Fig. 15.4A and B).

Motor points, Chinese acupuncture points, and trigger points

When one considers what was said in Chapter 7 about the close spatial correlation between these various points, in spite of the fact that they were discovered by entirely different means, it is not surprising that trigger points and acupuncture points around the elbow are found in close proximity, or as Gunn & Milbrandt (1977) observed, most trigger points around the elbow coincide in position with the muscle's motor points.

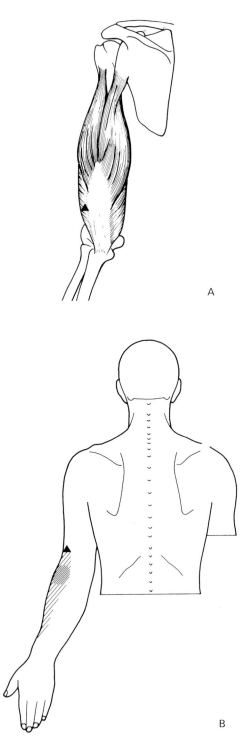

Fig. 15.4 (A) Trigger point in the lateral border of the medial head of the triceps muscle. (B) Pattern of pain referral from this trigger point.

Deactivation of trigger points

In order to deactivate trigger points in the supinator muscle the arm should be placed in the same position as for locating trigger points in the muscle, i.e. it should be placed comfortably on a pillow with the hand fully *supinated*. The elbow should then be slightly flexed as this makes it easier to push the brachioradialis out of the way. A needle should then be inserted into the point of maximum tenderness.

For all the other muscles the arm should also be placed comfortably on a pillow with the elbow slightly flexed, but the hand must be fully pronated. Needles are then inserted into points of maximum tenderness.

Periosteal pecking

In cases which are slow to respond to the deactivation of trigger points in muscles, Mann's method of pecking with a needle the periosteum covering the lateral epicondyle (Mann 1974) is often dramatically effective. Although with this technique there is no post-treatment pain such as there is with a corticosteroid injection, it is nevertheless a somewhat painful procedure at the time of being carried out.

Traditional Chinese approach to acupuncture in the treatment of lateral epicondylitis

The inserting of needles into points of maximum tenderness in the muscles is, as has been emphasized throughout this book, the essential feature of the Western approach to acupuncture but it has to be admitted that up to now there have been no comparative trials to show whether or not, in the alleviation of pain, it is superior to putting needles into pre-determined Chinese acupuncture points.

It is therefore interesting to observe the places into which Brattberg (1983) inserted needles in treating a series of cases of 'tennis elbow' by the traditional Chinese approach to acupuncture, and to compare these with the needle sites often used in Western acupuncture in the treatment of this condition. The traditional Chinese points

used by Brattberg were Large Intestine 10, 11 and 12, Triple Warmer 11 (Fig. 15.5) and Lung 5 (Fig. 15.6), a point situated on the ventral surface of the forearm in the crease of the elbow lateral to the biceps tendon, and therefore close to where Western trigger points are found in the supinator muscles (Fig. 15.8). The Large Intestine points on the dorsum of the forearm are situated in much the same places as trigger points in the brachioradialis (Fig. 15.9), extensor carpi radialis longus (Fig. 15.10) and extensor digitorum (Fig. 15.13). And Triple Warmer 11 (Fig. 15.5) lies posteriorly just above the elbow and therefore not far from where the trigger point in the lateral part of the medial head of the triceps is sometimes found (Fig. 15.4).

Brattberg's patients were divided into two groups. One group, consisting of 34 patients, was treated by traditional acupuncture as just described, whilst a control group of 26 patients was treated with local injections of a corticosteroid.

70% in the acupuncture group had failed to respond to one or more injections of a steroid, and yet in spite of this and the fact that two-thirds of the group had been in pain for more than 6 months, 62% were relieved of pain. In contrast, in the control steroid-treated group, only 31% were relieved of pain, and of the 69% showing no improvement, several of these considered that the treatment had aggravated their condition.

Corticosteroids in the treatment of 'tennis elbow'

The recommended treatment for this condition in all standard textbooks is a local injection of a corticosteroid in combination with a local anaesthetic to counteract the painful effect of this. At the same time there is rarely any indication given as to the exact percentage of those who respond to this particular form of therapy. Any comments concerning the effectiveness of this type of treatment are often couched in very general terms. 'This is a common and disabling lesion which usually responds well to local infiltration with hydrocortisone' is a statement that appears in one well-known textbook of rheumatology (Boyle 1978) and is a typical example.

It is doubtful, however, whether the use of a local injection of a corticosteroid in this condition does give as good results as many of these textbook statements infer, as may be seen from Bernhang's (1979) review of 202 cases treated by this method.

In this series, 88% of cases were given an injection of a corticosteroid and lidocaine (Xylocaine) into one point of maximum tenderness, with this mainly being on the anterior surface of the lateral epicondyle; 27% of cases also received an injection into another point of tenderness in the region of the annular ligament over the radial neck. With this technique, Bernhang obtained partial or complete relief, however, in only 55% of cases.

The practice of injecting a steroid into only one point of tenderness, or at the most two, seems to be fairly widespread with, for example, Boyle (1978) stating 'the most tender point at the external humeral condyle is the site of election for the injection'.

The wisdom of this generally accepted policy must however be challenged in view of the fact that, as indicated earlier in this chapter, the pain in lateral epicondylitis often stems from several trigger points often widely separated in different muscles, and it is because of this that in practising trigger point acupuncture, it is often necessary to insert needles into a number of sites. It is therefore suggested that possibly better results might be obtained with a local steroid if this too was more often injected into several points of tenderness rather than one or two.

There seems, however, to be even more controversy over whether or not, in injecting hydrocortisone into a tennis elbow, the periosteum should be stimulated. Boyle (1978), for example, states that 'the point of the needle should eventually rest on the periosteum of the epicondyle'; Rogers & Williams (1981) believe that 'it is important that the initial half of the injection is into the periosteum of the lateral epicondyle'. Conversely Cailliet (1977) expresses the contradictory view that 'the injection should *not* be into the periosteum of the lateral epicondyle as this sets up a new area of pain without improving the original pathology'.

There can be no doubt that injecting hydro-

cortisone into the periosteum, apart from somewhat paradoxically being a very painful procedure, must have a powerful pain suppressing effect due to its irritant action on the periosteal nerve endings evoking considerable activity in pain-inhibiting mechanisms in the central nervous system, in the same way as the acupuncture technique of periosteal pecking with a dry needle does. And it therefore follows that, in clinical trials designed to compare the relative efficacy of hydrocortisone and acupuncture in the treatment of tennis elbow, it is essential to have uniformity of practice, particularly with regard to any stimulation of the periosteum that may be carried out.

These different methods of using a local corticosteroid in tennis elbow may partially explain the widely varying reported success rates with this type of treatment. For example, Day et al (1978) and Nevelös (1980) achieved improvement in around 90% of cases. Bernhang (1979), however, only obtained complete or partial relief in 55%. And Brattberg (1983), in a well-designed trial comparing the relative effectiveness of acupuncture and a local corticosteroid, found that, whereas acupuncture relieved the pain in 61.8% of one group of cases, a steroid injection only relieved it in 30.8% in another.

It would seem that both these two types of therapies have a place in the treatment of tennis elbow and in considering their relative indications it is first necessary to say something about the mechanisms by which they achieve their effects, and to discuss their individual advantages and disadvantages.

The therapeutic effect of a local steroid, as already stated in Chapter 8, must partly be due to its specific anti-inflammatory action, but also it would seem reasonable to suppose that it is also due to its non-specific painfully irritant effect on the tissues stimulating A-delta nerve fibres with, as a result of this, the evocation of activity in centrally placed pain modulating mechanisms. This is therefore another example of pain driving out pain (see Ch. 10) and explains why Day et al (1978) in comparing the relative efficacy of hydrocortisone, saline and a local anaesthetic in this condition found that 'a painful injection followed by an exacerbation of symptoms for 2–3 days was more likely to be followed by relief than was a painless injection'.

The main advantage of a local corticosteroid is that it has a powerful action and in those cases in which it is successful in relieving symptoms it not infrequently does so after only one or two injections. Its disadvantages are that, as already stated, it is associated with the production of an appreciable amount of post-injection pain for 12–24 hours, this often being severe enough to cause a patient to refuse to have a second injection. Moreover, repeated injections of it are liable to cause tissue damage and this therefore also limits the number of times it can be used.

Acupuncture also achieves its pain-relieving effect by similarly evoking activity in centrally placed pain-modulating mechanisms (Chs 8 and 10), but what is particularly interesting, it too may have a steroid mediated anti-inflammatory action.

Anyone who has used acupuncture extensively for the relief of musculoskeletal pain must have observed how on occasions the inflammatory swelling of tissues subsides following this type of treatment. This, in my experience, has been particularly notable in cases of osteoarthritis and it will therefore be referred to again when discussing the management of this condition in Chapter 19. And, in seeking an explanation for this phenomenon, the recent discovery that there is an elevation of the plasma cortisol level in response to acupuncture would seem to be of considerable relevance. It is necessary therefore briefly to digress in order to consider this subject in general.

Gwei-Djen & Needham (1980) state that as long ago as 1950 research workers at the Chungshan Hospital in Shanghai observed that when experimentally-induced appendicitis in dogs was treated with acupuncture the animals' hydrocortisone blood levels increased by as much as 99%. They also in discussing this matter draw attention to McLeod et al's (1974) report on acupuncture to the Australian Medical Research Council, as this includes personal communications from Chang Hsiang-Thung's group and from Omura Yoshiaki in China stating that the excretion of 17-ketosteroids is significantly increased following acupuncture. Gwei-Djen & Needham also state that Dr Keith Betteridge and

Professor Peter Lisowski in a personal communication to them in 1975 report that Dr Lin Hsü-Kao and his colleagues in Canton have shown that patients who respond well to acupuncture have high adrenocorticoid levels, while those, who do not, have low levels.

This discovery by Chinese research workers that one of the effects of acupuncture is to increase plasma cortisol levels is clearly of considerable importance when assessing the place this type of treatment may have both in allergic disorders such as hay fever and asthma; and in conditions associated with an inflammatory tissue response such as osteoarthritis and lateral epicondylitis (tennis elbow).

The one great disadvantage of using acupuncture in tennis elbow is that long-term relief from pain is rarely obtained with only one treatment. Its outstanding advantages, however, are that, unlike treatment with a local corticosteroid, it is both a well-tolerated procedure and one that does not damage the tissues so that it therefore can be repeated as often as is necessary. Brattberg, for example, found it necessary to give on average 6 treatments at twice-weekly intervals, with the treatment therefore usually lasting for about 3–4 weeks.

It may therefore be seen that acupuncture and local hydrocortisone would seem to achieve their pain-relieving effects by remarkably similar means and that in the treatment of tennis elbow they provide two soundly-based alternatives, each with its own particular advantages and disadvantages. The difficulty that therefore arises in everyday clinical practice is in deciding as to which of the two treatments to use for any particular case. Certainly, if there are only one or two trigger points, it would seem reasonable to inject hydrocortisone into them but often there are several trigger points and in such circumstances acupuncture would seem to be the treatment of choice. It is however somewhat more complex than this because patients' individual responsiveness to these two forms of treatment are somewhat unpredictable with some who fail to respond to acupuncture having their symptoms relieved with a local steroid.

My personal preference, therefore, particularly if there are several trigger points scattered throughout various muscles, is to start treatment with acupuncture as patients find this to be a far more comfortable and therefore more readily acceptable form of treatment. It is necessary however to warn the patient that to obtain long lasting relief with this treatment it may be necessary to repeat it on average 3–4 times at weekly intervals. It is usually possible to deactivate all the trigger points by this method but occasionally one or two continue to remain active in spite of repeated needling and it is then my practice to inject hydrocortisone into these acupuncture-resistant points. Occasionally this disorder fails to respond to either of these two forms of treatment with it then being necessary to release surgically the extensor muscles from the supracondylar ridge.

In general, tennis elbow is a self-limiting disorder with, as previously stated, spontaneous relief from symptoms occurring after 8–12 months. It is of the greatest possible importance to bear this in mind when attempting to evaluate the results of clinical trials in order to avoid automatically assuming that any improvement occurring in a long-standing case is necessarily due to some particular treatment without at the same time considering the possibility as to whether or not it is due to a spontaneous remission.

MEDICAL EPICONDYLITIS (GOLFER'S ELBOW)

This is a similar condition to that which affects the lateral epicondyle, but one which occurs far less commonly. It arises when, as a result of the flexor muscles of the wrist and hand becoming strained, trigger points become activated in these muscles near to their common tendon attachment to the medial epicondyle.

It is characteristic of this disorder that resisted flexion of the wrist, when the elbow is extended, aggravates the pain.

The advantages and disadvantages of a local corticosteroid in this condition are similar to those when using this form of treatment in lateral epicondylitis so they will not be further discussed.

Acupuncture, as in the treatment of lateral epicondylitis, is a worthwhile alternative. There

are two trigger points which usually have to be deactivated. One is to be found in the common flexor tendon near to its attachment to the medial epicondyle, and incidentally not far from the traditional Chinese acupuncture point Heart 3 (Fig. 15.6); the other is to be found along the medial border of the medial head of the triceps immediately above the medial epicondyle (Fig. 15.7), and therefore in the region of the Chinese acupuncture point Small Intestine 8 (Fig. 15.5).

PAIN IN THE WRIST AND HAND

Persistent pain confined to the wrist and hand region may occur as a direct result of some local disorder, or it may arise indirectly as a result of it being referred there from trigger points some distance away in the muscles of the forearm. It is particularly essential to bear the possibility of the latter in mind as otherwise, with there being nothing abnormal to find at the site where the pain is felt, there is always the risk that any patient suffering from it may be considered to be either neurotic or a malingerer.

Although it is now over 40 years since Kelly (1944) first drew attention to the clinical import-

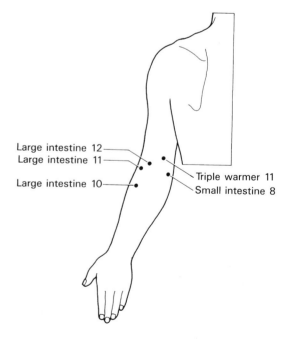

Fig. 15.5   Traditional Chinese acupuncture points at the back of the elbow.

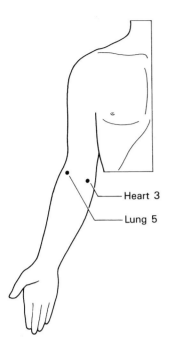

Fig. 15.6 Traditional Chinese acupuncture points on the inner and outer sides of the front of the elbow.

ance of this particular cause of pain in the wrist and hand, too little attention is still being paid to it in current medical teaching, and therefore it will be dealt with at some length.

FOREARM EXTENSOR MUSCLES

The forearm extensor muscles in which trigger point activity is liable to cause pain to be referred to the wrist and hand include the extensor carpi radialis longus, the extensor carpi radialis brevis, the extensor carpi ulnaris, and the extensor digitorum. Trigger point activity in the anatomically closely related brachioradialis and supinator muscles may also be responsible for this (Fig. 15.2).

It will be remembered that in discussing 'tennis elbow' it was stated that trigger points in the supinator, brachioradialis, extensor carpi radialis longus, and the extensor digitorum may also be responsible for pain being felt around the lateral epicondyle.

Activation of trigger points in these muscles

Trigger points in these muscles are liable to become activated as a result of carrying out forceful twisting movements with some tool such as a screwdriver or trowel whilst holding it with a very firm grip.

Specific trigger point pain patterns

Supinator muscle

Trigger points in the supinator muscle refer pain primarily to the lateral epicondyle, but at times they may also cause it to be felt in the region of the first dorsal interosseous muscle (Fig. 15.8).

Brachioradialis muscle

Trigger points in the brachioradialis muscle, in contradistinction to those in the supinator muscle, refer pain primarily to the region of the 1st dorsal interosseous muscle, and only occasionally to the lateral epicondyle (Fig. 15.9).

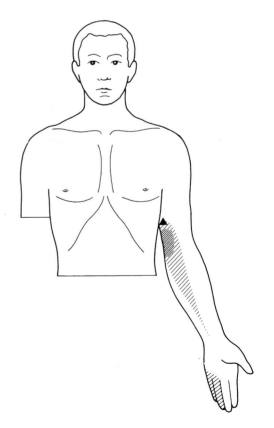

Fig. 15.7 Pattern of pain referral from a trigger point in the medial border of the medial head of the triceps muscle.

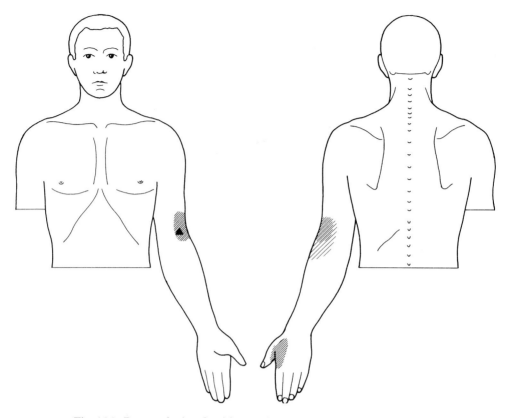

Fig. 15.8   Pattern of pain referral from a trigger point (▲) in the supinator muscle.

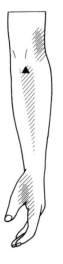

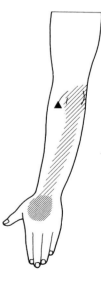

Fig. 15.9   Pattern of pain referral from a trigger point (▲) in the brachioradialis muscle.

Fig. 15.10   Pattern of pain referral from a trigger point (▲) in the extensor carpi radialis longus muscle.

Extensor carpi radialis longus

Trigger points in the extensor carpi radialis longus refer pain to the lateral epicondyle and down the forearm to be felt predominantly on the dorsum of the hand in the region of the anatomical 'snuff box' — the hollow on the outer side of the wrist between the tendons of the extensor carpi radialis longus and brevis (Fig. 15.10).

It has to be remembered that when trigger points in the above muscles refer pain to the region of the 1st dorsal interosseous muscle or the anatomical 'snuff box', satellite trigger points may develop at these sites, and have to be distinguished from primary trigger points which, as will be discussed later, may also develop at these sites as a result of trauma to the wrist.

It is also of interest to note in passing that the Chinese in their traditional system of acupuncture have a well-known point, Large Intestine 4 (Ho-Ku or Hegu), in the first dorsal interosseous muscle (Fig. 15.11), and another point, Large Intestine 5 (Yang Xi in the anatomical 'snuff box', Fig. 15.12).

Extensor digitorum

Trigger points in the extensor digitorum cause pain to be referred down the back of the forearm, back of the hand and into individual fingers depending on which muscle fibres are involved. The middle finger extensor probably is the one most often involved (Fig. 15.13).

Trigger points in the ring and little finger extensors are also liable to cause pain to be referred upwards to the lateral epicondyle (Fig. 15.14).

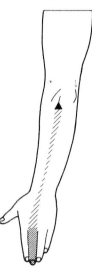

Fig. 15.13 The pattern of pain referral from a trigger point (▲) in the extensor digitorum muscle (middle finger extensor).

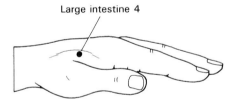

Fig. 15.11 The traditional Chinese acupuncture point Large Intenstine 4 (Hoku or Hegu) in the 1st dorsal interosseous muscle.

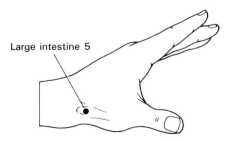

Fig. 15.12 The traditional Chinese acupuncture point Large Intenstine 5 (Yang Xi) in the anatomical snuff box — the hollow on the outer side of the wrist between the tendons of the extensor carpi radialis longus and brevis muscles.

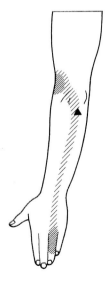

Fig. 15.14 The pattern of pain referral from a trigger point (▲) in the extensor digitorum muscle (ring finger extensor).

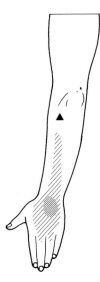

Fig. 15.15 The pattern of pain referral from a trigger point (▲) in the extensor carpi radialis brevis muscle.

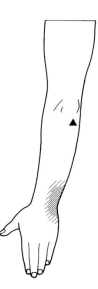

Fig. 15.16   The pattern of pain referral from a trigger point (▲) in the extensor carpi ulnaris muscle.

Extensor carpi radialis brevis

Trigger points in the extensor carpi radialis brevis are found below the level of those occurring in the extensor carpi radialis longus at about 6 cm (or approximately 2 in) below the elbow crease. Pain from these trigger points is referred to the back of the hand and wrist (Fig. 15.15).

Extensor carpi ulnaris

Trigger points in this muscle occur at about the same level in the forearm as those in the extensor carpi radialis brevis, and refer pain to a localized area around the ulnar side of the back of the wrist. Gutstein (1938) was one of the first to draw attention to this but it would seem to be rare and so far no patient with this particular pain pattern has come under my care (Fig. 15.16).

The following case illustrates how trigger points in several extensor forearm muscles may be responsible for the development of a composite pain pattern.

A housewife (60), who was also a keen gardener and who frequently gripped the handle of a trowel tightly whilst weeding, presented with a 9-month history of pain at the back of the wrist, at the base of the thumb, and in the fingers, together with some discomfort in the outer part of the elbow.

She complained that the fingers felt bloated and as if they were going to burst. She also complained that the grip of her hand was becoming increasingly weak, and that this, together with the pain and swelling of her fingers and consequent difficulty with bending them, had led her to become concerned that she might be developing arthritis.

The patient was examined sitting comfortably on a chair with the forearm resting on a pillow, and the elbow slightly bent.

The weak grip was confirmed by getting the patient to squeeze two of my fingers. This action also increased the pain both at the elbow and in the hand.

Flat palpation of the extensor muscles just below the lateral epicondyle revealed trigger points in the extensor carpi radialis longus, and these must have been partly responsible for the lateral epicondyle pain, and pain at the base of the thumb. There were also trigger points in the extensor carpi radialis brevis, which must have been responsible for the pain at the back of the wrist and trigger points in the extensor digitorum that must have been partly responsible for the pain at the elbow, and also in the fingers.

Deactivation of these trigger points by means of the acupuncture technique of dry needle stimulation on four occasions at weekly intervals relieved her of the pain, but on going back to gardening she again developed pain in the hand from the reactivation of trigger points in the forearm and eventually she decided it was better to employ someone to do the weeding!

FOREARM FLEXOR MUSCLES

The forearm flexor muscles in which trigger point activity is liable to cause pain to be referred to the front of the wrist and hand include the flexor carpi radialis, the flexor carpi ulnaris, and the flexor digitorum (superficialis and profundus), all of which are attached proximally to the medial epicondyle by means of a common tendon. Also the flexor pollicis longus which is attached proximally to the radius.

Anatomical relationships of the muscles

In order to be able to identify in which of these various muscles a particular trigger point is located, it is helpful to remember that they are arranged in three layers with the superficial layer consisting of the flexor carpi radialis, and the flexor carpi ulnaris, separated by the palmaris longus; the intermediate layer consists of the flexor digitorum superficialis (Fig. 15.17); and the deep layer consists of the flexor digitorum profundus, and the flexor pollicis longus (Fig. 15.1).

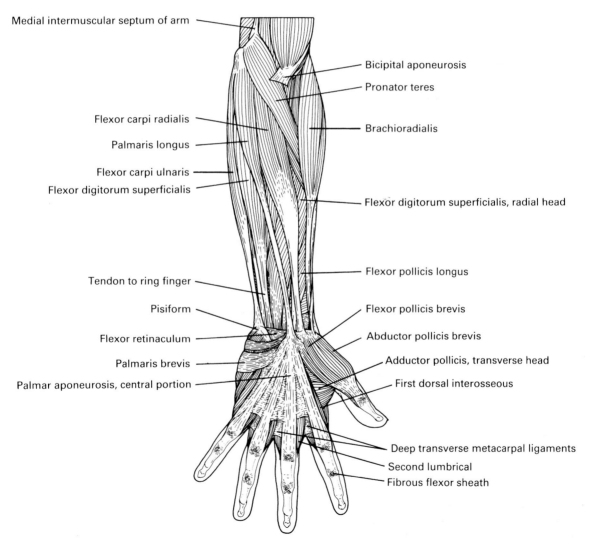

Fig. 15.17 The superficial flexor muscles of the left forearm, the palmar aponeurosis and the digital fibrous flexor sheaths.

Activation of trigger points

Trigger points situated in the hand and finger flexor muscles in the forearm are liable to be activated by prolonged gripping. It commonly occurs, for example, when the steering wheel of a car is gripped tightly during a long journey, particularly when the hands are placed on the top of the steering wheel in the flexed position.

Trigger points in the flexor pollicis longus become activated as a result of gripping tightly with the thumb whilst carrying out any twisting pulling movement such as may occur when weeding.

Specific pain patterns and trigger point locations

Flexor carpi radialis and flexor carpi ulnaris

Trigger points in these two muscles cause pain to be referred either to the radial aspect or the ulnar aspect of the palmar surface of the wrist according to which one is involved (Fig. 15.18). The trigger points in either of these muscles are to be found high up the forearm just below where each muscle is attached to the medial epicondyle (Fig. 15.18). As both muscles are in the superficial layer, the trigger points in each of them are easily recognized by their exquisite tenderness to light touch and by the fact that pressure on them causes a readily visible local twitch response, and the evoking of the specific pain pattern of the particular muscle involved.

Flexor digitorum superficialis and profundus

Trigger points in various parts of these two muscles refer pain to individual fingers. Such trigger points are to be found at almost the same level in the forearm as those in the flexor carpi radialis and ulnaris (Fig. 15.19). However, as the digital flexors lie deep to the hand flexors, any trigger points in them are more difficult to locate, and require firm pressure to elicit the deep seated tenderness associated with their presence, and even with this, neither a local twitch response nor any of the various specific pain patterns can be evoked.

Flexor pollicis longus

Trigger points in this muscle cause pain to be felt in the thumb. As this muscle also lies in the deep layer, firm pressure is required to elicit any trigger point in it. Such a point is usually found on the radial side of the forearm about one-quarter way up from the wrist crease (Fig. 15.20).

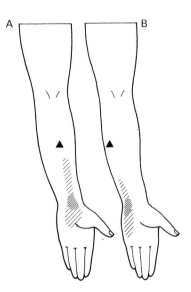

Fig. 15.18 The patterns of pain referral from trigger points (▲) in (A) the flexor carpi radialis muscle and (B) the flexor carpi ulnaris muscle.

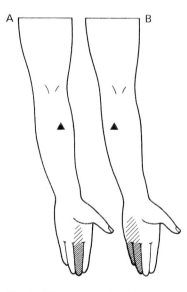

Fig. 15.19 The patterns of pain referral from trigger points (▲) in the flexor digitorum superficialis (A) radial head (B) humeral head.

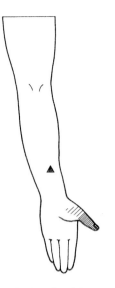

Fig. 15.20 The pattern of pain referral from a trigger point (▲) in the flexor pollicis longus muscle.

Ulnar nerve entrapment at the elbow — the cubital tunnel syndrome

Whilst discussing the part played by trigger points below the medial epicondyle in the flexor muscles of the hand and fingers, it is necessary to say something about ulnar nerve entrapment at the elbow – the cubital tunnel syndrome. It will be remembered that the ulnar nerve at the elbow is held in a groove behind the medial epicondyle by a fibrous expansion of the common flexor tendon. It then enters the forearm beneath an arch formed by the humeral and ulnar heads of the flexor carpi ulnaris muscle to occupy a space bounded by the flexor carpi ulnaris superficially and medially; the flexor digitorum superficialis superficially and laterally, and the flexor digitorum profundus behind it.

The ulnar nerve is at risk of being damaged either by external pressure being applied to it where it lies behind the medial epicondyle; or by it becoming constricted in the cubital tunnel by arthritic or other structural changes affecting the elbow joint. Not infrequently, however, this entrapment may occur in the absence of structural pathological changes. In some of these cases there is evidence of trigger point activity in the forearm flexor muscles, but exactly how this leads to pressure being exerted on the nerve is far from clear (Travell & Simons 1983b).

The symptoms of ulnar nerve entrapment are gradual in onset with numbness and tingling affecting the fifth finger and the ulnar half of the ring finger, followed at a later stage by weakness and wasting of the small muscles of the hand. If the ulnar nerve becomes damaged where it lies behind the medial epicondyle, then pressure on the nerve at that site will reproduce the symptoms. The only effective treatment when the nerve is bound down by fibrous tissue is a surgical operation to release it from the groove and transpose it to the front of the elbow. If, on the other hand, there is evidence of trigger points just below the medial epicondyle in the flexor muscles, then deactivating these trigger points may in some cases, presumably by reducing tension in the muscles, be sufficient to relieve the pressure on the nerve.

It should be noted that pain is not an outstanding feature with ulnar nerve entrapment and therefore in all cases when pain affects the medial side of the forearm and hand, an alternative diagnosis should be sought. The differential diagnosis including cervical nerve root entrapment (C8 T1 nerve roots), trigger point activity in the levator scapulae muscle (Ch. 14) and trigger point activity in the medial border of the medial head of the triceps.

Trigger point in the medial distal border of the medial head of the triceps

This point is found in the medial border of the medial head of triceps just above the medial malleolus.

Specific pattern of pain referral

This trigger point refers pain to the medial epicondyle (p. 212) and down the inner side of the anterior forearm to terminate in the ring and little fingers (Fig. 15.7).

Trigger point location

The trigger point is best located and then deactivated with a dry needle, with the patient lying down in the supine position, the arm externally rotated; the forearm supinated; the elbow slightly flexed; and the whole of the arm supported comfortably on a pillow.

The following case illustrates how failure to recognize trigger point activity in muscles around the medial epicondyle could have resulted in an unnecessary operation.

A ward sister (36) complained that for 1 year she had had pain around the left elbow radiating down the inner side of the arm with some discomfort in the little and ring fingers. An orthopaedic surgeon thought it was due to ulnar nerve root entrapment and recommended that the nerve should be transposed from behind the medial epicondyle to the front of the joint. The patient, not liking the thought of having an operation, asked to be referred to me to see whether acupuncture had anything to offer.

On examination there were two exquisitely tender trigger points, one in the medial border of the medial head of the triceps just above the medial epicondyle and another just below it. After deactivating these by means of dry needle stimulation on three occasions, she was relieved of her symptoms.

Palmaris longus and pronator teres muscles

Trigger point activity in these two forearm muscles may also cause pain to be referred to the hand.

Palmaris longus

This vestigial muscle is not always present but when it is, it also is attached proximally to the medial epicondyle and distally to the palmar fascia and has as its main action the cupping of the hand. It also assists flexion of the hand at the wrist.

It lies, as previously stated, in the superficial layer of the flexor forearm muscles, between the flexor carpi ulnaris and the flexor carpi radialis (Fig. 15.17).

Location of trigger points

Trigger points in this muscle are found high up in the forearm just below the medial epicondyle (Fig. 15.21).

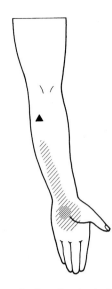

Fig. 15.21 The pattern of pain referral pain from a trigger point (▲) in the palmaris longus muscle.

Activation of trigger points

These trigger points may become activated as a result of repeatedly gripping some object such as a tennis racquet or tool excessively tightly. They may also become activated as a secondary event whenever pain is referred to the upper part of the forearm from trigger points just above the medial epicondyle in the medial head of the triceps muscle. In addition, Travell & Simons (1983c) have observed that patients with Dupuytren's contracture invariably have one or more active trigger point(s) in this forearm muscle.

Specific pattern of pain referral

There is a persistent unpleasant tingling sensation in the palm of the hand; and the patient complains of discomfort on applying pressure to any object held in the palm. This therefore makes the handling of tools difficult.

Deactivation of trigger points

Deactivation of these trigger points just below the elbow is carried out with the forearm extended and well supported.

Pronator teres

This forearm muscle, whilst not a flexor of the hand or fingers, is conveniently dealt with here in view of its anatomical relationship in the flexor forearm muscles. This muscle is attached above by two heads, the humeral head being attached to the medial epicondyle, and the ulnar head to the coronoid process of the ulna. The median nerve enters the forearm between these two heads. The muscle distally is attached to the lateral surface of the radius (Fig. 15.17).

Location of the trigger point

A trigger point in this muscle may be found just below the crease of the elbow, in the proximal part of the muscle, to the medial side of the biceps tendon (Fig. 15.22).

Activation of this trigger point

This sometimes occurs as a result of a fracture at either the elbow or wrist.

Specific pattern of pain referral

Pain from a trigger point in this muscle may be referred down the anterior surface on the radial side to be felt in particular around the radial side of the wrist, in much the same area as pain from trigger point activity in the flexor carpi radialis (Fig. 15.22).

A patient with an active trigger point in this muscle finds it difficult to turn the hand into the fully supinated position and usually is not able to turn it beyond the mid position.

PAIN IN THE WRIST AND HAND FROM LOCAL TRIGGER POINTS

It is not difficult to understand that any activity which puts a strain on the muscles in the region of the wrist or hand, including the thumb and fingers, may lead to the development of persistent pain at one or more of these sites. And, further, it can readily be appreciated that such pain, as the following account will show, may emanate from local trigger points in these

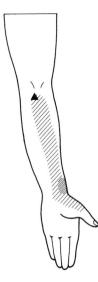

Fig. 15.22 The pattern of pain referral from a trigger point (▲) in the pronator teres muscle.

muscles. However, what is not so obvious is that pain in exactly the same distribution, and due to exactly the same types of strain on the muscles locally in the hand, may also occur because of trigger points becoming activated some distance away in the muscles of the forearm. It therefore follows that in every case of pain in the hand, occurring as a result of trigger point activity, it is essential to ascertain whether such activity is occurring locally in the hand, or high up in the forearm, or both, before any decision can be made as to where acupuncture needles should be inserted.

It is because this is of such fundamental importance that a somewhat lengthy account of myofascial trigger points in the forearm has just been given, and it is hoped that this will help to clarify any confusion concerning the subject prior to turning to the more straightforward concept of wrist and hand pain occurring as a result of local trigger point activity.

However, before doing this, consideration must be given to pain at the wrist occurring as a result of median nerve compression in the carpal tunnel, and also as a result of tenosynovitis around the wrist joint.

CARPAL TUNNEL SYNDROME

Although this syndrome became recognized as a clinical entity soon after the Second World War (Brain et al 1947), and there are now good descriptions of it in standard textbooks, a brief account of it must be given here as the pain at the wrist, which often radiates up the arm, sometimes as far as the shoulder, has to be distinguished from other causes of pain in the arm, and particularly from pain ascending up the arm as a result of myofascial trigger point activity.

It occurs principally in middle-aged women, but may occur in younger women and is occasionally seen in men. The cause of compression of the median nerve in the carpal tunnel is usually not known but it is sometimes due to a tenosynovitis in rheumatoid arthritis, fluid retention during pregnancy, and soft tissue swelling in either myxoedema or acromegaly.

The essential symptoms are pain in the arm and paraesthesiae in the fingers. The pain is characteristically nocturnal, awaking the patient in the early hours of the morning. It is felt at the wrist, but often ascends up the arm, at times as high as the shoulder. The paraesthesiae usually affect the index, middle and radial side of the ring finger, but surprisingly on occasions may involve the little finger.

These nocturnal symptoms are often relieved by hanging the arm over the side of the bed. On waking in the morning, the hand often feels stiff and swollen.

During the day, the arm is not troublesome but the paraesthesiae persist and are made worse by any activity such as knitting or holding a book.

The condition, as might be expected, most often affects the dominant side but eventually it may become bilateral. The nocturnal pain and the nocturnal and diurnal paraesthesiae may persist for many months without any objective neurological signs developing, but eventually weakness and wasting of two of the thenar muscles (abductor pollicis brevis and opponens pollicis) cause flattening of the outer half of the thenar eminence.

On examination, the pain and tingling can often be provoked by applying pressure to a point of exquisite tenderness over the anterior carpal ligament. If any doubt as to the diagnosis remains, an electrical conduction test may be carried out but it has to be remembered that this test may be misleadingly normal in cases with a short history.

Treatment

When symptoms are of long standing and particularly when there is evidence of muscle wasting, decompression of the median nerve by division of the flexor retinaculum is essential.

When the history is short, conservative measures are justifiable. The avoidance of activities which aggravate the symptoms is advisable, and the wearing of a splint at night is beneficial. In addition, the local injection of a corticosteroid is often extremely helpful. One has to guard against injecting the material into the median nerve, or into the tendon of palmaris longus. So before embarking upon this, it is worth trying the effect of simply inserting an acupuncture needle into the transverse carpal ligament at the point of maximum tenderness, because, due to the ability of acupuncture to reduce tissue oedema (Ch. 19), this sometimes proves to be equally as effective although it is a procedure that may have to be repeated on several occasions at weekly intervals before there is any lasting relief of symptoms.

TENOSYNOVITIS OF THE WRIST

This is a common cause of pain in the region of the wrist. Inflammation of the synovial sheaths surrounding the tendons around the wrist joint is liable to occur whenever the forearm muscles are used excessively or the fingers are worked both hard and rapidly. The condition may therefore occur as a result of recreational pursuits or occupational tasks.

Pain, which can be quite severe, is felt along the line of one or more tendons at the wrist. It is usually associated with swelling, and characteristically crepitus will be detected on moving the tendon. The tenosynovitis affecting the conjoined tendons of the extensor pollicis brevis and abductor pollicis longus as they pass over the styloid process of the radius (de Quervain's disease) is liable to occur as a result of any activity associated with strenuous repetitive movement of the thumb. In this condition there is pain and tenderness over the styloid process and, in particular, crepitus may be elicited on extending the thumb.

Treatment

For this disorder, rest of the affected part on a splint or in plaster is helpful. Cases which do not respond to this should have an injection of a corticosteroid into the tendon sheath. Extreme care, however, has to be taken not to inject the material into the tendon itself as this may cause it to rupture.

TRIGGER POINT ACTIVITY OCCURRING LOCALLY IN THE MUSCLES OF THE WRIST AND HAND

Pain due to trigger point activity in muscles around the wrist and hand will now be considered but, as this may readily be confused with pain in exactly the same distribution from trigger point activity higher up in the elbow, the opportunity will be taken to summarize what has already been said concerning the latter.

PAIN IN THE THUMB

Pain in the thumb may occur as a result of it being referred there from trigger points in the muscles of the forearm or from trigger points locally in the muscles around the thumb. The muscles around the thumb liable to contain these include the adductor pollicis, and a muscle mass consisting of the opponens pollicis covered by the abductor and flexor pollicis brevis. In practice, it is difficult to differentiate between these three muscles when attempting to locate trigger points but as probably it is the opponens pollicis in which they most commonly occur, this muscle will be referred to in particular.

When trigger points become activated in these muscles they will frequently also be found in the 1st dorsal interosseous muscle and in addition there is often a point of exquisite tenderness in the anatomical snuff box.

The relative anatomical relationship of the adductor and opponens pollicis, the approximate position of their trigger points, and their specific patterns of pain referral are shown in Figures 15.23, 15.24 and 15.25. The action of the adductor pollicis is to bring the thumb adjacent to and parallel with the index finger. The action of the oppones pollicis is to bring the thumb across the palm to touch the pads of the ring and little fingers. Trigger point activity is liable to arise in these muscles whenever the thumb is strained by some form of sustained gripping action. Writing or sewing therefore may do this when continued for long periods, but perhaps the commonest activity to cause it is weeding when the ground is dry.

Gardening is therefore a good example of an activity liable to give rise to pain in the thumb developing either from trigger points in muscles in the forearm or locally in the muscles around the thumb. It will be remembered that trigger points some distance above the wrist in the flexor pollicis longus may also be activated by twisting and pulling movements associated with pulling out weeds, and that trigger points just below the lateral epicondyle, in either the extensor carpi radialis longus or the brachioradialis, are likely to be activated by tightly gripping the handle of a trowel whilst shifting heavy soil.

Post-traumatic pain in the thumb

When pain following trauma to the thumb persists long after any tissue damage has resolved, it is usually due to activation of trigger points in muscles in that region. Such pain, if not treated appropriately, may persist for a long time; or it may recur intermittently, spontaneously disappearing when the trigger points pass into a latent phase, but returning again when they become reactivated in response to some further often quite minor trauma. The following case is a good example of this.

A housewife (50) fractured her left wrist. Soon after the plaster was removed she noticed pain at the base of the left thumb which persisted for about 2 months. It then recurred intermittently, 2–3 times a year, for about 3–4 weeks at a time. After this had gone on for about 4 years, she was referred to me for assessment.

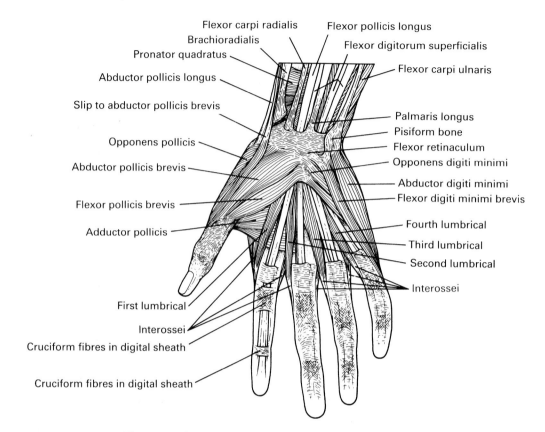

Fig. 15.23   Superficial dissection of muscles of the palm of the right hand.

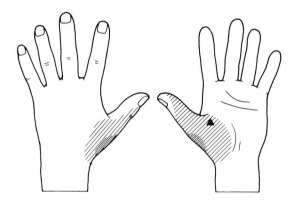

Fig. 15.24   The pattern of pain referral from a trigger point (▲) in the adductor pollicis muscle.

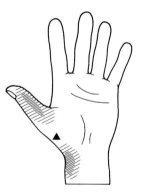

Fig. 15.25   The pattern of pain referral from a trigger point (▲) in the opponens pollicis muscle.

On getting her to analyse in detail any particular circumstances associated with the onset of the pain, it soon became apparent that this always started when she cooked for more than two people, and used especially large and heavy saucepans, which for some inexplicable reason, considering she was right-

handed, she was always in the habit of lifting off the stove with the left hand.

On examination, the appearances of the thumb were normal but there were exquisitely tender trigger points in the adductor pollicis, the opponens pollicis, and the 1st dorsal interosseous muscle. Deactivation of these trigger points by means of dry needle stimulation on two occasions relieved the pain, and as she has also made a determined effort to lift the saucepans with her right hand, she has had no further trouble.

When post-traumatic pain in a peripheral structure such as the thumb has persisted continuously for some time, it may eventually start to spread up the limb. Undoubtedly, Leriche (1939) was referring to this when he described 'post-traumatic spreading neuralgia' and also Taylor (1938) when referring to 'ascending neuritis'.

As this type of antidromic referral of pain is not well recognized, other than with median nerve entrapment, two examples of it occurring following trauma will be described.

A 16-year-old schoolgirl tripped and, in falling, wrenched her right thumb backwards by catching it on the edge of a desk.

There was much immediate pain with, according to her, considerable swelling and bruising of the tissues at the base of the thumb. When, after 6 weeks, the latter disappeared but the pain persisted, she was referred to an orthopaedic specialist. An X-ray of the hand showed no abnormality and in particular no evidence of a fractured scaphoid. However, in view of the persistent pain, he immobilized the thumb and wrist in a plaster, but on removing this 6 weeks later, the pain was as bad as ever, and in addition the thumb felt stiff and weak. Physiotherapy was therefore given and a month later she was discharged from his care. The pain persisted making gripping a pen difficult and interfering with her school work. As the appearances of the thumb and wrist were normal, her doctor began to wonder whether anxiety about forthcoming exams was a factor in the prolongation of her symptoms, but he became concerned when the pain started to spread up the outer side of her arm, at first as far as the elbow, but eventually up to the shoulder.

Eight months after the accident she was referred to me for assessment as to whether acupuncture might be helpful. On examination there was nothing abnormal to be seen but there was some generalized tenderness of the thumb with restriction of its movements, and also there were points of exquisite tenderness (trigger points) on the outer, inner and dorsal aspects of the base of the thumb and in the anatomical 'snuff box'. Three needles were therefore inserted around the base of the thumb and one into

the anatomical 'snuff box'. When a needle was put into the latter site, pain immediately shot up the outer side of the arm towards the elbow along the line of distribution of the spontaneously occurring pain.

When seen 1 week later, she reported she had experienced relief from pain but only for 3 days. On re-examining her, it became obvious that satellite trigger points in the extensor muscles just below the lateral epicondyle, in the deltoid, and in the supraspinatus had been overlooked on the first occasion. Needles were therefore inserted into the tissues overlying these points as well as the ones around the base of the thumb. Treatment at regular intervals had to be given for another 2 months before lasting relief from the pain was obtained.

The second case is that of a 40-year-old woman whose mentally defective son attacked her and caught hold of her right thumb, wrenching it backwards. Bruising and swelling around the joint fairly quickly subsided, but it left her with persistent pain, which was not only felt around the thumb but after a time gradually spread up the outer side of the arm.

When seen by me 1 year after the injury, the pain in her thumb at rest and, in particular, on using it, was seriously affecting her life. Trigger points were found around the base of the thumb, and satellite ones at the elbow and in the shoulder girdle. These had to be deactivated nine times over the course of the next 3 months before permanent control of the pain was finally obtained.

PAIN IN THE PALM OF THE HAND

It will be remembered from what was said earlier that a persistent prickling type of discomfort in the palm of the hand may develop when trigger points become activated just below the elbow in the palmaris longus muscle. This sometimes occurs in patients with contracture of and tender nodules in the palm from the development of Dupuytren's contracture. In addition, localized pain in the palm, also in association with the presence of a tender nodule, may occur in the disorder known as trigger finger.

Trigger finger

Repeated trauma to the hand may lead to the development of a reaction in the sheath of one of the digital flexor tendons in the palm and when this occurs the finger when flexed becomes locked.

In this condition, usually referred to as a trigger finger, there is an exquisitely tender point at the site of a nodule in the palm just proximal to the head of the metacarpal bone.

Traditionally it is taught that a corticosteroid should be injected locally into the synovial sheath but this is not necessary and, of course, if by a mistake it should happen to be put into the tendon, it can cause this to rupture. However, there is no need to use this form of treatment as the condition can be relieved equally well simply by inserting a needle into the point of maximum tenderness, and stimulating the nerve endings at that site by rotating the needle a few times.

There are three aspects concerning this which never cease to surprise me. Firstly that the needle only has to be inserted a short distance into the skin. Secondly that the response to needle stimulation in this condition is good with it usually only being necessary to carry it out on one or two occasions even when the disorder has been present for some considerable time. Thirdly that with this technique not only is the pain readily controlled but the finger movement is also quickly restored to normal. The following case is quoted as a typical example.

A 62-year-old company director had had a trigger finger (ring finger on the right hand) for 6 months. It was not so much the locking of the finger on flexion that worried him as the discomfort in the palm when trying to grip a golf club! His doctor somewhat surprisingly did not inject hydrocortisone into the tendon sheath but contented himself with telling the patient that the condition was not bad enough to warrant an operation! Eventually the patient persuaded the doctor to let him try the effects of acupuncture and so he was referred to me.

On examination, there was the usual exquisitely tender point in the palm. A needle was inserted into the skin overlying this and then subjected to a rotary movement until the immediate pain induced by the needle penetrating the skin had been replaced by a feeling of numbness. This occurred after about 20 rotary movements of the needle. On withdrawing the needle, there was no residual tenderness at the site, and not only could he move the finger freely but more important from this particular patient's point of view,

he could grip a golf club comfortably! Since having treatment on two occasions he has had no further trouble.

PAIN IN THE FINGERS

As has already been said, pain and swelling of the fingers may occur as result of the activation of trigger points high up in the forearm in either the flexor digitorum (p. 218) or the extensor digitorum (p. 215).

Pain in the fingers with stiffness of their movements may also occur because of the activation of trigger points in the interosseous muscles of the hand. Trigger points in these may be activated as a primary event when even a small object has to be held firmly for a long time, such as a needle by a seamstress, or a paint brush by an artist.

Heberden's nodes

A Heberden's node is a small nodule which develops on the dorsolateral or dorsomedial aspect of a terminal phalanx at its joint. At first it may be painful and tender but eventually it is symptomless.

The significance of Heberden's nodes is still no more certain than when Heberden (1818b) asked 'What are these little hard knobs, about the size of a small pea, which are frequently seen upon the finger, particularly a little below the top, near the joint?'

In more recent years it has become customary to associate these with the development of osteoarthritis of the finger joints but Travell & Simons (1983d) state that in addition they are frequently associated with the primary activation of trigger points in the interossei.

Trigger points around arthritic small joints of the hand

Exquisitely tender trigger points are often to be found in palpating the tissues around osteoarthritic and rheumatoid arthritic small joints of the hands. There are no absolute rules as to their distribution and one has to palpate carefully around a painful joint in order to find them. Deactivation of such trigger points in the tissues around an osteoarthritic joint often has a markedly pain-relieving effect. It is also sometimes a worthwhile procedure in the later stages of rheumatoid arthritis. The activation of trigger points in these two conditions, however, will be discussed at greater length in Chapter 19.

REFERENCES

Aronson P R, Murray D G, Fitzsimmons R M 1971 Myofascitis: a frequently overlooked cause of pain in cervical root distribution. North Carolina Medical Journal 32: 463–465

Bernhang A M 1979 The many causes of tennis elbow. New York State Journal of Medicine 79: 1363–1366

Boyle A C 1978 Injection techniques. In: Scott J T (ed) Copeman's textbook of rheumatic diseases, 5th edn. Churchill Livingstone, Edinburgh, p 1034–1035

Brain W R, Wright A D, Wilkinson M 1947 Spontaneous compression of both median nerves in the carpal tunnel. Lancet 1: 277–282

Brattberg G 1983 Acupuncture therapy for tennis elbow. Pain 16: 285–288

Cailliet R 1977 Soft tissue pain and disability. Davis, Philadelphia, p 176

Day B H, Govindasamy N, Patnaik R 1978 Corticosteroid injections in the treatment of tennis elbow. Practitioner 220: 459–462

Filshie J, Redman D 1985 Acupuncture and malignant pain problems. European Journal of Surgical Oncology 11: 389–394

Goldie I 1964 Epicondylitis lateralis humeri — a pathogenetical study. Acta Chiurgica Scandinavica supplement 339

Gunn C C, Milbrandt W E 1976 Tennis elbow and the cervical spine. Canadian Medical Association Journal 114: 803–809

Gunn C C, Milbrandt W E 1977 Tennis elbow and acupuncture. American Journal of Acupuncture 5: 61–66

Gutstein N 1938 Diagnosis and treatment of muscular rheumatism. British Journal of Physical Medicine 1: 302–321

Heberden W 1818 Pectoris dolor. In: Commentaries on the history and cure of diseases. Wells & Lilly, Boston, ch 70; 1818b 'Digitorum nodi', ch 28

Kelly M 1944 Pain in the forearm and hand due to muscular lesions. Medical Journal of Australia 2: 185–188

Leriche R 1939 The surgery of pain. Translated and edited by A. Young Archibald. Bailliére Tindall & Cox, London

Long C 1956 Myofascial pain syndromes — Part II. Syndromes of the head, neck and shoulder girdle. Henry Ford Hospital Medical Bulletin 4: 22–28

Lu Gwei-Djen, Needham J 1980 Celestial lancets. A history and rationale of acupuncture and moxa. Cambridge University Press, Cambridge, p 213–214

McLeod J G, Sainsbury M J S, Joseph D 1974 Acupuncture: A report to the National Health and Medical Research Council. Australian Government Publications Service, Canberra

Mann F 1974 Periosteal acupuncture. In: The treatment of disease by acupuncture, 3rd edn. Heinemann Medical, London, p 197

Michele A A, Davies J J, Krueger F J, Lichtor J M 1950 Scapulocostal syndrome (fatigue — postural paradox). New York State Journal of Medicine 50: 1353–1356

Michele A A, Eisenberg J 1968 Scapulocostal syndrome. Archives of Physical Medicine and Rehabilitation 49: 383–387

Nevelös A B 1980 The treatment of tennis elbow with triamcinolone acetonide. Current Medical Research and Opinion 6: 507–509

Reynolds M D 1981 Myofascial trigger point syndromes in the practice of rheumatology. Archives of Physical Medicine and Rehabilitation 62: 111–114

Rogers M, Williams N 1981 Rheumatology in general practice. Churchill Livingstone, Edinburgh, p 130

Russek A C 1952 Diagnosis and treatment of scapulocostal syndrome. Journal of the American Medical Association 150: 25–27

Sola A E, Kuitert J H 1955 Myofascial trigger point pain in the neck and shoulder girdle. Northwest Medicine 54: 980–984

Taylor J 1938 Surgical treatment of pain. Lancet II: 1151–1154

Travell J G, Simons D G 1983a Myofascial pain and dysfunction. The trigger point manual. Williams & Wilkins, Baltimore, p 510; 1983b: p 541; 1983c: p 526; 1983d: p 565

Wynn Parry C B 1980 Pain in avulsion lesions of the brachial plexus. Pain 9: 45–53

Wynn Parry C B 1984 Brachial plexus injuries. British Journal of Hospital Medicine 32(3): 130–139

16. Pain in the head and face

HEADACHE

It has been estimated by Blau (1983) that a busy general practitioner may see 500–1000 patients with headache every year. Occasionally it is a symptom of glaucoma, cranial arteritis, or a space occupying lesion, and occurs in conjunction with other symptoms and signs of these conditions. Most often, however, it is due to one of the primary cephalalgias of which there are four main types — muscle contraction headaches, tension headaches, migraine and cluster headaches. It is in the treatment of the first three of these that acupuncture has proved to be of benefit, and these will therefore be considered in some detail.

Muscle contraction headache

Tension and muscle contraction headaches are often considered to be synonymous but as Blau (1982) points out there are advantages in separating them because of certain differences in their aetiology and management. Muscle contraction headache develops when trigger points become activated in the muscles of the neck as a result of some locally occurring disorder. As discussed in Chapter 14, it may occur in association with a painful stiff neck when, for example, the muscles in the neck are sprained by a whiplash injury, or when pain and stiffness of the neck develop as a result of cervical spondylosis. This type of headache may also occur, as will be discussed later in this chapter, in the absence of a painful stiff neck when there is activation of trigger points in the sternomastoid muscle.

Firstly, however, attention will be directed to the use of acupuncture in the treatment of two conditions that commonly occur together in the same patient, namely tension headaches and migraine. In order to be able to understand how this technique can be applied in a rational manner as part of the general management of these disorders, it is necessary to consider their clinical manifestations, and in the case of migraine, its aetiology and pathophysiology.

Tension headache

This is by far the commonest of the primary type headaches (Caviness & O'Brien 1980). It usually takes the form of a persistent ache or tightness affecting any part of, or the whole of the head. It is often described as a constricting tight band around, or heavy pressure on, the head. The discomfort tends to recur every day and to last for many hours whilst at the same time rarely interfering with normal activities. Vomiting is not a feature (Hunter & Phillips 1981).

In this condition, anxiety or depression causes the muscles of the neck and scalp to be held in a state of persistent tension and, as a result of this, trigger points in certain muscles of the neck become activated. The condition may occur alone or in association with migraine, or, as discussed in Chapter 14, as part of the painful stiff neck syndrome.

Migraine

Migraine may conveniently be divided into the classical and common types.

Classical migraine usually takes the form of self-limiting episodes of severe throbbing pain affecting one side of the head, often in association with nausea, vomiting, photophobia, and facial pallor. An attack is generally preceded by one or another prodromal symptom including, most commonly, a disturbance of vision but at times tingling and numbness down one side of the body, and occasionally a disturbance of speech.

Common migraine, as its name implies, occurs far more often. It is less likely to be unilateral, and although it may be associated with nausea and vomiting, there are no prodromal symptoms.

Aetiology

A striking feature of migraine and one that is of considerable relevance when considering its aetiology is that it is three times commoner in women than men. This female preponderance would seem to be associated with vascular changes that occur as a result of fluctuations in oestrogen and progesterone levels, and there is a tendency for the disorder to occur in association with menstruation, early pregnancy, the menopause, and the taking of the contraceptive pill.

Attacks may also be brought on in some people by the intake of certain foodstuffs such as chocolate, citrus fruits, tyramine-containing cheeses, and alcohol, especially red wine. Alcohol is a non-specific vasodilator, whereas tyramine leads to the release of noradrenaline in migrainous patients that causes a cerebral vasoconstriction followed by a rebound vasodilation.

Attacks may also be associated with a fall in the level of blood sugar, either from fasting or as a reactive hypoglycaemia following the ingestion of an excessive amount of carbohydrate. As will be discussed later, when attempting to prevent the recurrence of migraine it is essential to exclude, as far as possible, these various causative factors before turning to the use of acupuncture.

Pathophysiology

In attempting to place the use of acupuncture in migraine on a scientific basis it is necessary to know as much as possible about the pathophysiology of the disorder, but unfortunately, as Sovak et al (1980) state, the lack of an animal model and the impossibility of obtaining samples of affected tissue ensures that this remains unclear.

Although the ingenious blood flow studies in migraine with the radioisotope xenon, carried out by Oleson & Lauritzen (1982), have shown that the circulatory changes in this condition are not as straightforward as previously thought, it is still generally agreed that in classical migraine the prodromal phase is associated with cerebral vasoconstriction, and that in both common and classical migraine the painful stage is characterized by a significant dilation of extracranial and intracranial blood vessels.

There is therefore no argument about migraine being a vasomotor disorder but, as Dalessio (1984) points out, such a disorder by itself is not necessarily painful unless it occurs in association either with ischaemia or inflammation, and that there are reasons for believing that the throbbing headache in this condition occurs as a result of both a vasodilation and a self-limiting sterile local inflammatory reaction in the vessels. Moreover, this reaction is associated with the production of various pain-producing inflammatory mediators including serotonin (5-hydroxy tryptamine), histamine, plasma kinins, and prostaglandins, and the liberation of these substances into the surrounding tissues coincides with an increased vascular permeability (Dalessio 1976).

It would therefore seem reasonable to postulate that, as extracranial vessels as well as intracranial vessels are involved in this inflammatory reaction, the focal areas of tenderness so commonly found in the muscles of the neck and scalp, both during and in between attacks of migraine, occur as a result of superficially placed nerve endings such as at the motor points of these muscles being rendered supersensitive by these various pain-producing inflammatory substances.

Tfelt-Hansen et al (1981) systematically examined the muscles of the neck and scalp in 50 patients during typical common migraine attacks and found tender points in all cases. Moreover, by infiltrating these tender points during an attack, either with a local anaesthetic, or with saline, both proving to be equally effective, they rendered 24 out of 48 of these patients symptom-free within 70 minutes; this is a much shorter time than the average natural duration of an attack. And furthermore, as their results with saline were as good as those obtained with a local anaesthetic, it is reasonable to conclude that the effectiveness of the latter when injected into tender points in migraine is not as Hay (1976) suggests, because it blocks the flow of nerve impulses from these points, but because, like saline, it has a non-specific stimulating effect on peripheral nerve endings, with this in turn evoking activity in the central nervous system's pain-modulating mechanisms. This is an effect that can be obtained even more simply by employing the acupuncture technique of dry needle stimulation.

When Loh et al (1984) compared the effects of acupuncture and drug therapy in patients with migraine and muscle tension headaches, they found tender points in the neck and scalp muscles in 34 out of 41 cases examined in between attacks, and not surprisingly, considering what has just been said, found acupuncture to be a worthwhile prophylactic when these points were present, but not when they were absent. As the stimulation of peripheral nerve endings at tender points in the muscles of the neck and scalp in migraine, either by injecting a chemical into them, or by inserting a dry needle into them, during the time that a headache is present, is sometimes capable of foreshortening the time for which it lasts, and as when this is carried out during the interval between headaches it often prevents them from recurring, it seems reasonable to conclude that these tender points must be important sources of pain in this condition, and that they are in fact trigger points. In favour of this also is the clinical observation that the over-zealous stimulation of these points with dry needles in a migrainous subject is liable to bring on an attack of migraine.

These trigger points in the muscles of the neck and scalp will be referred to again when discussing the treatment of migraine with acupuncture, but before turning to this, it is necessary to draw attention to some of the changes observed in the plasma and CSF levels of endogenous opioid substances in simple and migrainous headaches, as these may have some relevance when considering the rationale for using this form of therapy.

Sicuteri et al (1978) found low concentrations of a morphine-like substance in the cerebrospinal fluid of chronic headache patients. Anselmi et al (1980) in a study of idiopathic headache sufferers found similarly low levels both in the CSF and

plasma. And Baldi et al (1982) showed that during a migraine attack the plasma beta-endorphin levels are significantly lower than in between attacks. It would seem possible therefore that the periodicity of migraine may in part be related to fluctuations in the levels of these naturally occurring pain suppressors. The discovery by Facchinetti et al (1981) that a group of patients with chronic headache, who reacted poorly to acupuncture, had low levels of plasma beta-endorphin may also be of much significance when one considers the manner in which acupuncture is thought to achieve its analgesic effect (Ch. 10).

USE OF ACUPUNCTURE IN THE TREATMENT OF MIGRAINE

As already indicated, acupuncture is capable of aborting an attack of migraine but its main use is in the prevention of attacks. It is of course remarkable that it is possible to prevent migraine developing by stimulating nerve endings in between headaches. The only other painful disorder that comes to mind in which acupuncture is used prophylactically in this manner is dysmenorrhoea, when according to traditional Chinese teaching it is helpful, premenstrually, to stimulate the so-called Spleen 6 point situated in the lower part of the leg about a hand's breadth above the medial malleolus (Fig. 16.1).

When considering the place of acupuncture relative to other forms of therapy in the prophylaxis of migraine, it has to be remembered that it is a time-consuming procedure. Each treatment session lasts for about 20–30 minutes, and, in those cases in which the technique proves to be helpful, treatment has to be repeated on a number of occasions at frequent intervals. There is moreover no way of predicting which patients will benefit from it, and for this reason, every patient has to be given a preliminary trial of three treatments at weekly intervals before a decision can be made as to whether or not to continue with it.

My policy, therefore, when presented with a patient whose attacks of migraine are sufficiently frequent as to require prophylactic treatment, is firstly to ascertain whether or not food substances, alcohol, the contraceptive pill or psychogenic factors are contributing to the situation. It has to

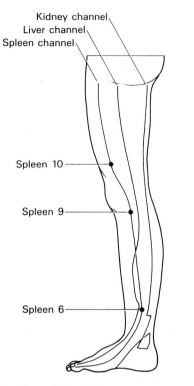

Fig. 16.1 The traditional Chinese acupuncture points Spleen 6, 9 & 10.

be admitted that the exercise of excluding a suspect food substance or a particular type of alcoholic drink does not usually seem to be particularly rewarding. The reduction of nervous tension, however, by means of hypnotherapy, and teaching the patient to practise autohypnosis on a daily basis, is, in my experience, often very helpful. Most cases also require prophylactic drug therapy. Some patients find the beta-adrenoceptor blocking drug propranolol effective, others obtain greater benefit from the anti-serotonin agent pizotifen, whilst others prefer the alpha-2 receptor agonist drug clonidine. Plum (1982), however, finds the most effective and the safest agent in migraine prophylaxis to be amitriptyline, thus confirming Lance & Curran's (1964) carefully conducted cross-over trial which showed this drug to be the best of a number of drugs in the treatment of chronic tension headache. That trial was particularly noteworthy as it showed that the response to amitriptyline could not be correlated with the presence or absence of depressive symptoms. Since

then, others have shown that this drug may be an even more effective migraine prophylactic in non-depressed patients than in those overtly depressed (Couch et al 1976, Couch & Hassanein 1976).

It is now recognized that the tricyclic group of drugs have both an antidepressant effect and an entirely separate analgesic effect with the latter not only coming on more rapidly than any mood change but also being obtained with a relatively low dosage (average 75 mg each evening). This is mentioned not only because of its importance so far as the treatment of migraine and other types of chronic pain are concerned, but in particular because it is now known that both the analgesic and the antidepressant effects of tricyclic drugs are brought about by their action on the central serotoninergic system, and because of this, they help to potentiate the effectiveness of acupuncture, a technique which it will be remembered (Ch. 10) depends largely for its action on evoking activity in the serotonin-mediated descending inhibitory system in the central nervous system.

The implications of all this, so far as migraine is concerned, are that this disorder is sometimes responsive to amitriptyline, sometimes to acupuncture, and that there are good grounds for believing that a combination of the two might be even more effective but statistically controlled trials to confirm this have yet to be carried out.

The situation may therefore be summarized by saying that the place for acupuncture is when for one reason or another the various drugs already mentioned are contraindicated, or when side-effects from them leads to them being discontinued, or when they fail to reduce the frequency and severity of the headaches.

Location of points to be stimulated

Acupuncture is usually only of value in the treatment of migraine when there are tender points in the muscles of the neck and scalp. For reasons previously given, there are good grounds for referring to these as trigger points, and some people, including myself, believe that the most logical means of carrying out acupuncture in this condition is to insert needles into the tissues overlying them. The identification of these points therefore necessitates a systematic search of the muscles down the back of the neck, across the top of the shoulders, and over the scalp, each time a person is treated. However, as will be seen from some of the clinical trials to be discussed later, many physicians, with considerable experience in the use of needle stimulation therapy, prefer to use the same set of predetermined traditional Chinese acupuncture points in every case. Classical Chinese acupuncture points include one just medial to the mastoid process (Gall Bladder 20), one over the middle of the upper border of the trapezius (Gall Bladder 21) and points in the temporal region also on the Gall Bladder meridian (Fig. 16.2) together with a point in the first dorsal interosseous muscle

of the hand (Large Intestine 4) (Fig. 15.11) and one in the first dorsal interosseous muscle of the foot (Liver 3) (Fig. 16.3).

The muscles in which activated trigger points are to be found in migraine and tension headaches include the paravertebrally situated posterior cervical muscles, the trapezius muscle at the highest point of the shoulder girdle, the sternocleidomastoid muscle and the temporalis muscle. These latter two muscles will be further discussed later in the chapter when all the various causes for trigger point activity in them will be considered together (p. 242 and p. 245 respectively).

Posterior cervical muscles

Sites at which trigger points may become activated in the four layers of the posterior cervical muscles (in descending order of depth — the trapezius, the splenii, the semispinalis muscles, and multifidi together with the rotatores) are shown in Figure 16.4. The referral of pain from these trigger points varies somewhat according to the particular point or points involved and the muscle or muscles in which they are situated, but in general it is to the occiput, and from there along the side of the head to the temporal region, and in some cases, to the eye (Fig. 16.5).

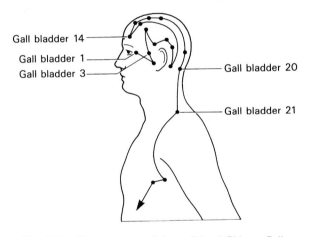

Gall bladder 14
Gall bladder 1
Gall bladder 3
Gall bladder 20
Gall bladder 21

Fig. 16.2 The upper part of the traditional Chinese Gall Bladder meridian. The lower part, not shown, extends down the outside of the trunk, leg and foot to terminate at the base of the 4th toe.

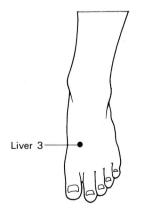

Liver 3

Fig. 16.3 The traditional Chinese acupuncture point Liver 3.

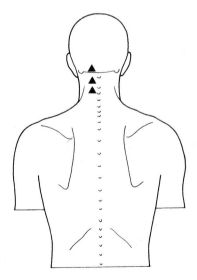

Fig. 16.4 Trigger points (s) in the posterior cervical muscles at the upper part of the back of the neck.

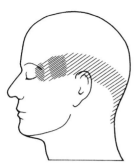

Fig. 16.5 A commonly occurring pattern of pain referral from the posterior cervical muscle trigger points shown in Figure 14.4

When palpating a trigger point in the posterior cervical group of muscles, it is not usually possible to be certain in which particular muscle it lies but this does not matter as the deactivation of any of these points, as with trigger points in general, is best carried out by means of light manual stimulation of a needle inserted superficially to a depth of approximately 5 mm. This is particularly important when treating migraine as any form of vigorous stimulation may cause an attack of pain to develop.

Trapezius muscle

There is almost invariably an exquisitely tender trigger point in the upper free border of the trapezius muscle about midway between the spine and the acromium, corresponding in position with the traditional Chinese acupuncture point Gall Bladder 21. The referral of pain from this trigger point is up the side of the neck, and when particularly severe, it is also referred along the side of the head to the temple and eye (Fig. 16.6D). The deactivation of this point should be carried out in a similar manner.

There is such a close spatial correlation between Western style trigger points and traditional Chinese acupuncture points around the head and neck involved in the treatment of migraine that it probably makes little difference to the outcome as to which are used. But what does require to be carefully investigated is whether in the treatment of this disorder, there is anything to be gained by following the traditional Chinese practice of

inserting needles into points some distance away in the hand and foot.

Distant points

It will be remembered from Chapter 1 that according to the traditional Chinese approach to acupuncture various parts of the body are said to be linked by channels known as acu-tracts or meridians so that pain in one part of the body can be treated either by inserting needles locally at that site, or by inserting them into points some distance away from the area of pain, providing that both the latter and the distant points lie along the same meridian. As discussed in Chapter 2, ever since the Western world first heard about acupuncture 300 years ago, it has always been very sceptical about acu-tracts or meridians, knowing that contrary to the teaching of the ancient Chinese, they are anatomically not demonstrable. It is therefore extremely interesting that in recent years neuroanatomical research has shown that certain parts of the body are linked in a manner hitherto not thought possible. For example, studies by Rossi & Brodal (1956) and those by Torvik (1956) show that there are direct projections from the spinal cord to the trigeminal nucleus. The micro-electrode studies recently carried out in cats by Sessle et al (1981) also demonstrate that the responsiveness evoked in individual neurones in the trigeminal subnucleus caudalis as a result of stimulating the tooth pulp is considerably inhibited by stimulation of the forepaws.

Such observations have considerable relevance to the practice of acupuncture. For example, Mann et al (1973), in discussing some cases of chronic pain treated with acupuncture, stated 'In the case of pain in the distribution of the trigeminal nerve, acupuncture was applied to the ipsilateral extremities.' And they went on to explain that this was done because 'there is a projection from the spinal cord to the spinal trigeminal nucleus of both sides, and stimulation of limb nerves can bring about primary afferent depolarisation in the spinal trigeminal nucleus'.

Neuroanatomical studies carried out in the Western world during recent years therefore give credence to the ancient belief of the Chinese that by stimulating a point called by them Hoku (The

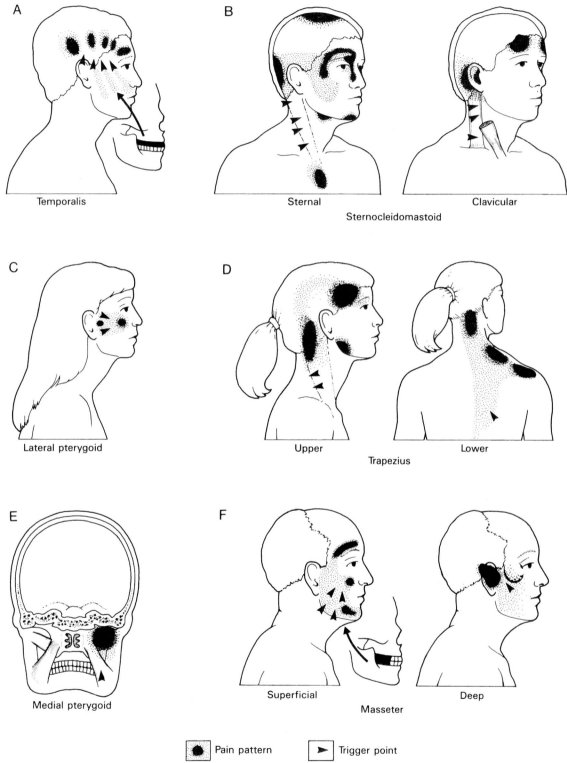

A Temporalis

B Sternal — Clavicular

Sternocleidomastoid

C Lateral pterygoid

D Upper — Lower

Trapezius

E Medial pterygoid

F Superficial — Deep

Masseter

Pain pattern   Trigger point

Fig. 16.6 Patterns of pain referral from trigger points in masticatory muscles and two neck muscles. (Reproduced with permission of D. G. Simons and J. G. Travell from Wall P. D. and Melzack R. (eds) 1984 *Textbook of Pain*.)

Joining of the Valleys) or Large Intestine 4, in the first dorsal interosseous muscle of the hand (Fig. 15.11), it is possible to control pain occurring in the face and scalp.

It will be remembered, however, from Chapter 10, that several investigators, including Andersson & Holmgren (1975), Jeans (1979), and also Chapman et al (1980) who have compared the relative effectiveness of near and distant points, have concluded that stimulating points near to the site of pain is more effective than stimulating distant ones.

Certainly when attempting to alleviate musculoskeletal pain by Western-style stimulation-produced analgesia, it is only considered necessary to stimulate the trigger points that are considered to be the source of pain. It is therefore interesting to note that when it comes to alleviating the pain of migraine, or to preventing it from recurring, many physicians in the Western world with considerable experience in the use of acupuncture employ both proximal and distal points. Loh et al (1984), for example, in their statistically controlled trial of acupuncture versus drug therapy, in cases of migraine and muscle tension headaches of such severity as to warrant referral to the National Hospital for Nervous Diseases in London, used local traditional acupuncture points around the neck and scalp (Gall Bladder 20 and 21 in the neck; Gall Bladder 3 in the temple and 14 in the forehead (Fig. 16.2)) together with two distant points — one in the first dorsal interosseous muscle in the hand (Large Intestine 4 — Fig. 15.11), and the other in the first dorsal interosseous muscle in the foot (Liver 3 — Fig. 16.3). And by using this combination of points, they were able to conclude 'that acupuncture is a beneficial treatment for headache and migraine for some patients, and that its more widespread use is justified'.

Vincent (1989) also stimulated local and distant traditional Chinese acupuncture points in a well-designed, carefully conducted, randomized, controlled trial in which he was able to show that 'true acupuncture was significantly more effective than the control procedure (see Ch. 11) in reducing the pain of migraine'.

It has to be said, however, that the situation is far from straightforward for Jensen et al (1979) in their placebo versus acupuncture trial in university students in Denmark suffering from repeated headaches used only the distal point, Liver 3 in the foot, but, nevertheless, in spite of employing this point alone concluded 'that acupuncture is a relevant therapy for headache with a definite symptomatic effect'.

In view of these diverse but seemingly successful methods of using acupuncture in the prevention of primary headaches, there is, in my opinion, a pressing need for controlled trials to be set up in order to compare the relative efficacy in migraine of stimulating:

1. local and distant points
2. local points only
3. distant points only.

Unfortunately one of the difficulties in assessing the value of any type of treatment in migraine is that it is a type of disorder that is liable to be readily responsive to a placebo. Matthews (1983) in discussing this matter states,

the placebo effect in migraine is so marked that virtually any form of treatment administered with sufficient aplomb, as for example, acupuncture, will produce a remission in a high proportion of patients.

The results of Dowson et al's trial (1985), in which the effect of traditional Chinese acupuncture and that of a placebo in the treatment of simple and migrainous headache were compared, tend to confirm this view. This was an extremely well conducted, single blind randomized study with certain particularly commendable features including the use of pain diaries in which patients conscientiously recorded their treatment responses for 4 weeks prior to treatment, during 6 weeks of treatment and for 24 weeks follow-up; and, the employment of an extremely well-thought-out type of placebo treatment that involved the placing of two electrodes on the skin over the mastoid process connected to a TENS stimulator, the circuitry of which was so adjusted as to allow the red light on the machine to flash whilst preventing any current from reaching the patient. The authors admit that,

the numbers entered into the study are small and we have analysed those suffering from simple headache and migrainous headaches together. It is possible that a larger study with a separate analysis for specific types of headache might reveal that acupuncture is successful in some instances, but not in others.

And they conclude:

it appears that the complaint of headache is very sensitive to placebo therapy, but it is possible that acupuncture has a real therapeutic effect of approximately 20% over placebo. We would, therefore, recommend that future studies should be planned with more patients and on the basis of this assumption.

Cluster headaches (migrainous neuralgia)

This is a relatively rare disorder but one that has to be distinguished from migraine, particularly as both may occur in the same patient, also because the management is different and because, so far as my limited experience is concerned in attempting to treat it with acupuncture, it is not relieved by this form of treatment. It is a condition that predominantly affects men in the 40–60 age group. It is characterized by an excruciating pain around the eye, spreading to the face and temple with profuse watering and redness of the eye and stuffiness of the nose. Each attack lasts from about 20–120 minutes once or several times every day in a 'cluster' lasting 3–8 weeks. The symptom-free intervals between the clusters are widely variable.

The patient usually knows what time of day or night to expect an attack and a prophylactic ergotamine suppository inserted some hours before will often abort it.

PAIN IN AND AROUND THE TEMPEROMANDIBULAR JOINT

It must be emphasized at the outset that pain in and around this joint is rarely due to arthritis. Admittedly, patients with rheumatoid arthritis sometimes have radiographic evidence of this in the joint but pain from it is uncommon (Chalmers & Blair 1973). Similarly, osteoarthritic changes shown on an X-ray of this joint are usually no more than a fortuitous radiological finding (Cawson 1984). In the later years of adolescence, pain in the region of this joint is very commonly due to caries in a partially erupted wisdom tooth, but, at all ages, pain in this vicinity may also be

due to what Schwartz (1956) called the temperomandibular joint pain-dysfunction but what is more commonly referred to now as the myofascial pain-dysfunction syndrome (Laskin 1969, Mikhail & Rosen 1980). It is as well to avoid the eponymous term Costen's syndrome because Costen's (1934) original description was somewhat confusing.

The myofascial pain-dysfunction syndrome

This disorder, which mainly affects females, may develop at any age. The patient experiences a dull, continuous, poorly localized ache mostly around the ear, the angle of the mandible and the temporal area but also often in the jaws, teeth and side of the face. The continuous ache is punctuated by momentary jabs of sharp pain (Bell 1977). The patient may also complain of various clicking or popping noises in the joint on opening the mouth, and also of limited mouth opening and dizziness (Sharav et al 1978).

On examination, the limited mouth opening and the abnormal sounds in the joint that sometimes are produced on attempting this may be confirmed. The muscles around the joint are tender and systematic palpation of these reveals the presence of focal points of exquisite tenderness, or trigger points, particularly in the lateral pterygoid, the masseter, and the medial pterygoid muscles (Travell & Simons 1983a). The exact location of these trigger points will be described later but first it is necessary to say something about the aetiology of the syndrome and its management in general, for it is certainly no good directing treatment at these points alone without at the same time correcting other disorders.

Aetiology of the syndrome and its management

There would seem to be a triad of factors responsible for the condition including occlusal disturbances, psychological disorders, and perhaps because of one or other or both of these, the activation of trigger points in the masticatory muscles.

Occlusal disturbances

There is much controversy concerning the part played by occlusal disturbances in the aetiology of this syndrome. Some authorities such as Clarke (1982) believe there is no significant difference between those occurring in patients with this syndrome and those found in asymptomatic controls. Others such as Sharav (1984) consider that such disturbances are a prerequisite for the development of dysfunction and pain. And it should be noted in relationship to this that the American Dental Association (Ayer 1983) has recently lent its support to the view that the use of dental appliances designed to temporarily modify the occlusion are helpful in the treatment of this condition.

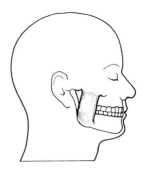

Fig. 16.7   The masseter muscle.

Psychological disorders

Since Schwartz (1956) first drew attention to the importance of psychological disorders in the aetiology of this condition, it is generally agreed that anxiety, depression, frustration, and resentment may singly or collectively contribute to this syndrome with bruxism — a purposeless grinding or gnashing of the teeth — being an outward manifestation of such disorders of mood.

Treatment must therefore include the prescribing of an antidepressant or tranquillizer according to whichever is most appropriate, or the use of various relaxation techniques such as biofeedback (Stem et al 1979) or hypnotherapy. My preference is for the latter and to teach the patient to practise autohypnosis on a regular basis each day.

Myofascial trigger points

The masticatory muscles in which activated trigger points are likely to be found include the lateral pterygoid, the masseter, the medial pterygoid, and the temporalis muscles. Greene et al (1969) in a study of 277 patients with TMJ pain dysfunction found that, of those in pain, 84% had tenderness of the lateral pterygoid and 70% had tenderness of the masseter muscle.

Sharav et al (1978) observed much the same in a series of 42 patients, with active trigger points occurring in the lateral pterygoid in 83% and in the masseter in 69%.

As in practice, it is better to deactivate trigger points in the masseter muscle before dealing with

those in the more deeply lying lateral pterygoid muscle, the masseter muscle will be considered first.

Masseter muscle

The masseter muscle consists of a superficial and deep part. The superficial part which is the larger of the two arises from the zygomatic process of the maxilla, and the zygomatic arch. Its fibres pass downwards and backwards to be inserted into the angle and lower half of the ramus of the mandible. The deep part, much of which is concealed by the superficial part arises from the zygomatic arch, and its fibres pass vertically downwards to be inserted into the lateral surface of the coronoid process and upper half of the ramus of the mandible (Fig. 16.7).

Activation of trigger points

Trigger points in this muscle may become activated as part of the myofascial pain syndrome, but additionally when there is prolonged over-stretching of the muscle as sometimes occurs during a dental operation or as a result of the direct trauma of an accident, and secondarily, when pain is referred to the region of this muscle from trigger point activity in the sternocleidomastoid muscle. The trigger point activity is the cause of referred pain, restriction of jaw opening, and somewhat surprisingly tinnitus (Travell 1960).

Specific pattern of pain referral

Trigger points in the superficial layer of the muscle are responsible for pain being referred along both the maxilla and mandible, around the molar teeth, and in and around the temperomandibular joint (Fig. 16.6F).

Those in the deep layer refer to the region of the temperomandibular joint and ear (Fig. 16.6F). They may also be responsible for the development of tinnitus. Deafness or giddiness, however, never occur.

Trigger point examination

In locating trigger points, it is necessary to put the muscle on the stretch by propping open the mouth. A cylindrical cardboard air-tube used for respiratory function measurements is very useful for this purpose.

Trigger points in the superficial part of the muscle usually occur near to either the upper or lower attachments, where they are best located by flat palpation. On occasions they may be found in its belly and are then best located by gripping the muscle between a finger inserted into the mouth and the thumb pressed against the cheek. Trigger points in the deep part are located by palpating it where it overlies the posterior part of the ramus of the mandible, just in front of the external auditory meatus.

Deactivation of trigger points

When deactivating a trigger point with a dry needle, the point should be either fixed between two fingers placed side by side extra-orally, or it should be held in a pincer grip, between a finger inside the mouth, and the thumb on the outside pressing against the cheek.

Lateral (external) pterygoid muscle

The lateral pterygoid muscle lies deep to, and mainly behind, the coronoid process and zygomatic arch. It is made up of two divisions — the superior and inferior.

Attachments

The superior division is attached in front to the sphenoid bone and behind to the capsule of the temporomandibular joint. The inferior division is attached in front to the lateral pterygoid plate and behind to the neck of the mandible (Fig. 16.8).

Activation of trigger points

This occurs with malocclusion of the teeth or with overuse of the muscle as a result of anxiety-induced bruxism, or both.

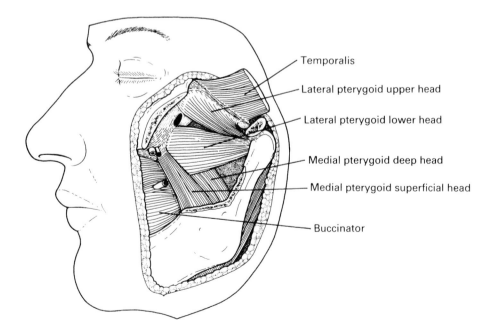

Temporalis

Lateral pterygoid upper head

Lateral pterygoid lower head

Medial pterygoid deep head

Medial pterygoid superficial head

Buccinator

Fig. 16.8   The left ptyerygoid muscles. The zygomatic arch and part of the ramus of the mandible have been removed.

Specific pattern of pain referral

Trigger points in this muscle are responsible for pain being referred to the temperomandibular joint and around the region of the maxillary sinus (Fig. 16.6C).

Trigger point examination

The locating of trigger points at the anterior attachment of the inferior division is best carried out by intraoral palpation. With the mouth open and the lower jaw drawn towards the side to be examined, a finger is squeezed between the maxilla and the coronoid process of the mandible, along the roots of the upper molar teeth. If the space is too narrow to admit a finger, some instrument such as the handle of a dental mirror should be employed. The finger is slid as far along the length of the coronoid process as possible, a manoeuvre facilitated by having the mouth partially closed. Pressure is then applied in an inwards direction towards the lateral pterygoid plate to test for the exquisite tenderness of trigger point activation. Similar tenderness from a trigger point in the temporalis muscle at its attachment to the coronoid process may be elicited by pressing with the finger, at exactly the same site but in an outwards direction.

Trigger points in other parts of the muscle are best located by extraoral examination. It must be remembered, however, that it is impossible to palpate the muscle from the outside with the mouth closed because the superior division is then behind the zygomatic arch, and the inferior division behind the ramus of the mandible. The examination therefore must always be carried out with the mouth open. It is then possible to palpate the mid parts of both the superior and inferior division through the bony aperture, bounded above by the zygomatic arch, and below by the coronoid process anteriorly and the condyloid process posteriorly (the mandibular notch). In order to palpate the mid part of the superior division, pressure should be exerted in an upwards and forwards direction, and for the inferior division it should be applied in a downwards and forwards direction. It is only possible to elicit tenderness at these sites, however, if trigger points in the overlying masseter muscle have previously been deactivated.

Deactivation of trigger points

Intraoral approach

It is possible to deactivate trigger points in the anterior part of the inferior division by inserting a needle intraorally, but this should only be attempted by someone skilled in manipulating needles within the mouth. Otherwise it is better to use an external approach.

Extraoral approach

In order to deactivate trigger points in the lateral pterygoid muscle extraorally, the patient should be placed in the supine position and the mouth propped open.

For trigger points in the anterior part of the inferior division, the needle is inserted through the masseter muscle, and then through the mandibular notch in the direction of the upper molar teeth.

For trigger points in the anterior part of the superior division, the needle is passed under the zygomatic arch just anterior to the temperomandibular joint in an upwards and forwards direction towards the orbit.

For trigger points further back, in either division of the muscle, the needle is inserted through the mandibular notch perpendicular to the surface and slightly posteriorly. To reach the superior division, the needle is directed upwards beneath the zygomatic arch, and to reach the inferior division the needle is directed downwards towards the angle of the mandible.

Medial pterygoid muscle

If, after deactivating trigger points in the masseter and lateral pterygoid muscles, opening the mouth is still painful and restricted, with in addition some difficulty in swallowing, then it is possible that there are active trigger points in the medial pterygoid muscle.

Attachments

The medial pterygoid muscle is attached below to the angle of the jaw and above to the lateral pterygoid plate (Fig. 16.8).

Trigger point examination

The patient should be placed in the supine position, with the mouth propped open. The muscle is first palpated from the outside by pressing a finger against the inner surface of the mandible at its angle. At this site the lower end of the muscle is just within reach of the finger. An intraoral examination is then carried out in order to reach parts of the muscle higher up. With the pad of the finger facing outwards, it is inserted into the mouth and slid behind the lower molar teeth until it encounters the bony edge of the ramus of the mandible, and just behind this, it comes up against the muscle running in a vertical direction (Fig. 16.6E).

Deactivation of trigger points

Deactivation of trigger points in this muscle is technically difficult but fortunately as Travell & Simons (1983b) point out it is usually possible to control the pain by stretching the muscle, and then applying a vapocoolant spray to it. The patient is placed in the supine position and encouraged to stretch the muscle by placing two fingers behind the lower incisor teeth, and the thumb under the chin, and then pulling the mandible forwards and downwards to open the jaws fully. Whilst this is being done, the vapo-coolant spray is swept from the neck below upwards towards the temperomandibular joint. It is important to ensure that the spray does not go into the eye by placing a pad over it.

Temporalis muscle

The temporalis muscle is the third most commonly involved of the masticatory muscles after the masseter and lateral pterygoid in the myofascial pain dysfunction syndrome (Greene et al 1969) but as the activation of trigger points in this muscle may also occur for many other reasons, all of the various causes will be considered together later in the chapter.

TRIGEMINAL NEURALGIA

Trigeminal neuralgia clearly has to be included in the differential diagnosis of pain in and around the face, but as this book is primarily concerned with musculoskeletal pain, only brief reference will be made to its clinical features in order that it may be distinguished from other causes of facial pain. This condition of unknown aetiology may develop at any age but it is most commonly seen from the age of 50 onwards. In young people, it occasionally heralds the onset of multiple sclerosis.

The pain usually involves the 2nd or 3rd divisions of the nerve. It commonly takes the form of uni-lateral, brief, very severe electric-shock like stabs repeated at frequent intervals in short-lasting bouts with intervals of freedom from pain varying in duration from minutes to hours. After several weeks, the pain spontaneously remits but recurs some time later. Unfortunately, there is a tendency over the course of time for the remission periods to get shorter whilst the bouts of pain in an attack get progressively more severe, and the attacks last longer.

Each bout of pain is usually precipitated by some non-noxious stimulus such as shaving, washing, or even just touching or moving the face. Also, in some people, eating, drinking or brushing the teeth may bring on an attack.

It is important to note that with idiopathic trigeminal neuralgia there are no abnormal physical signs including no sensory loss.

Treatment

Carbamazepine is the drug of choice in the treatment of this condition but unfortunately in about 25% of patients it is ineffective and in about 25% of patients it cannot be tolerated. Therefore only about 50% can be successfully treated with it (Loeser 1984).

Those not helped by carbamazepine should be given diphenylhydantoin but again only a pro-portion of people are helped by it. The usually recommended alternative is destruction of the trigeminal nerve but, before embarking upon this, it is always worth trying the effect of some form of hyperstimulation analgesia such as electroacu-puncture (Hester 1984) or transcutaneous electrical nerve stimulation (Eriksson et al 1979).

ATYPICAL FACIAL PAIN

Pain in the face, which from its character is clearly

not due to trigeminal neuralgia, and which, following careful investigation, is not found to be due to disease of the teeth, bones, or sinuses, is often diagnosed as atypical facial pain. The very term signifies how ill-defined the condition is, and regrettably all too often the possibility of the pain being referred from trigger points in muscles in this region is not considered. It must be admitted, however, that there is a group of patients who have pain in the face, which, unlike that of trigeminal neuralgia, is persistent in character, is often associated with an area of sensory loss, and not infrequently is bilateral. Also, on examination, in addition to there being no evidence of disease of any of the structures of the face, there is also no evidence of trigger point activity in the neighbouring muscles, and therefore by a process of exclusion the only diagnosis possible is one of atypical facial pain (Weddington & Blazer 1979).

As patients with atypical facial pain often show some evidence of emotional instability, treatment usually consists of giving an antidepressant, sometimes in combination with a phenothiazine. Such drugs however are only occasionally helpful in this condition. The anticonvulsants, carbamazepine and diphenylhydantoin, are also sometimes recommended but there seems to be no scientific basis for this and only a small number of patients are likely to be helped. Side-effects from any of these drugs are common and such treatment should never be embarked upon until by careful examination the possibility that the pain may be coming from myofascial trigger point activation has carefully been excluded. The muscles, in which trigger point activity most commonly causes pain in the face and head, are the sternocleidomastoid and the temporalis, and each will now be considered in turn.

Sternocleidomastoid muscle

Many errors in diagnosis, and consequently much inappropriate treatment, are due to a lack of awareness that the activation of trigger points in the sternocleidomastoid muscle is an important cause of persistent pain in the head and face, and also in certain cases is the cause of a distressing type of postural dizziness.

Activation of trigger points

Trigger points frequently become activated in the upper part of this muscle on one side of the neck in patients with tension headaches, in those with migraine, and in those with both. They may also become activated in any part of this muscle when the neck is kept turned to one side for any length of time, such as, for example, when typing a long report from shorthand notes.

They may become activated in the muscles on both sides of the neck as a result of the head being tilted backwards for some time such as, for example, when painting a ceiling or sitting at the front of the theatre watching a play being performed on a high stage. However, one of the commonest causes of bilateral activation of trigger points in this muscle is when the muscles on both sides of the neck become strained as a result of a whiplash injury occurring as a result of one car running into the back of another. When this happens, trigger points in the levator scapulae, posterior cervical, and the trapezius muscles also become activated with the development of a painful stiff neck (Ch. 14); whilst trigger points in the sternocleidomastoid muscle are liable to give rise to a variety of symptoms including pain in the head and face, and postural dizziness.

Symptoms from trigger point activation in the sternocleidomastoid muscle

Trigger points at the upper part of the sternal division of the muscle near to its insertion into the mastoid process are responsible for pain being referred to the occipital region and to the top of the head, often with marked tenderness of the area of the scalp affected (Fig. 16.6B). Those in the mid-part of this division refer pain along the supraorbital ridge, around the eye, and into the cheek (Fig. 16.6B). The activation of trigger points in this part of the muscle sometimes occurs in association with trigger point activity in other muscles such as the temporalis, the masseter, the external pterygoid, the orbicularis oculi and the zygomaticus, and unless the presence of trigger points in these muscles is recognized, the composite pain pattern is liable to be misdiagnosed as that of atypical facial neuralgia.

Travell (1981) reported a very interesting case of trigger point activity in muscles such as those just mentioned that had been the cause of intractable pain in the face for 13 years before the true cause of the pain was finally established. It is perhaps unfortunate that she referred to this as a case of atypical facial neuralgia for, in my view, such a diagnosis should be reserved for that group of cases in which myofascial trigger point activity is not present, and that cases in which pain is due to this are better referred to as examples of the chronic facial myofascial trigger point pain syndrome.

Trigger points at the lower end of this division near to its attachment to the sternum refer pain in a downwards direction over the upper part of the sternum. The pattern of this is such that it is liable to be mistaken for pain that is myocardial in origin (Fig. 16.6B).

Trigger points in the deeper clavicular part of the muscle are likely to refer pain either into the ear and postauriclar region, or across the front of the forehead (Fig. 16.6B).

Trigger point activity in the sternal division also affects the autonomic nervous system and may be the cause of conjunctival redness and watering of the eye and nose similar to that seen with migrainous neuralgia (Travell 1960, 1981). This is liable to be very confusing when this trigger point activity is responsible for pain developing around the eye, except of course that in migrainous neuralgia an attack of pain, although very intense, usually only lasts for less than an hour. Trigger point activity in this muscle may also cause disturbed proprioception with the development of postural dizziness.

Disturbances of proprioception brought about by trigger point activity in the sternocleidomastoid muscle

Cohen's investigations (1959, 1961) into body orientation carried out in monkeys have shown that whilst it is the function of the labyrinths to give information concerning the position of the head in space, information concerning the position of the head in relationship to the body comes from proprioceptive mechanisms in the neck. In man, the main muscle concerned with this would seem to be the sternocleidomastoid and it is because of this that unilateral trigger point activation in it is often the cause of postural dizziness developing.

In my experience, it never takes the form of giddiness or vertigo if, by these terms, one means a sudden disturbance of balance associated with a sensation of rotation either of the person concerned or of their surroundings, but rather it is a sensation of unsteadiness and loss of balance with a tendency to veer to one side when attempting to walk in a certain direction. This disorientation and loss of co-ordination is mainly postural and occurs when movements of the body or head involve a change in tension in the affected sternocleidomastoid muscle. Such symptoms may be associated with nausea but never with vomiting, tinnitus, or nystagmus. In the differential diagnosis, an anxiety state, and also in the elderly, vertebrobasilar ischaemia have to be considered. Postural dizziness due to sternocleidomastoid trigger point activity may occur at any age, with Weeks & Travell (1955) reporting a case of it occurring in an 11-year-old girl.

Travell, who was one of the first to recognize this condition, and who in 1955 published a report of 31 adults suffering from it, maintains that the trigger points responsible for this phenomenon are always situated in the clavicular part of this muscle, and that therefore it is associated with frontal headache with either the one or the other dominating the clinical picture (Travell 1967).

Most of the cases of this type of postural imbalance that have come under my care have been in patients who, in addition to having trigger point activity in this muscle, also have had painful stiff necks due to similar activity occurring in other muscles of the neck as a result of whiplash injuries. It is always interesting to observe how often in the referral letter this unsteadiness is assumed to be due to 'nerves' brought on by the shock of the accident. It is also remarkable how often the disorder disappears once the appropriate trigger points have been deactivated by inserting dry needles into them.

In considering the mechanism by which postural dizziness occurs as a result of trigger point activity in the sternocleidomastoid muscle, it has to be remembered that the sensory innervation of this muscle comes from the anterior primary rami of the 2nd and 3rd cervical nerves, and that Cohen (1961) in experiments on monkeys and baboons produced an exactly similar type of unsteadiness and loss of balance in these animals by artificially cutting off the sensory input from these two nerves.

Furthermore, the clinical implications of this are that when pain in the head, superficial tenderness of the scalp, postural dizziness and nausea occur as a result of some injury in which there has been marked hyperextension of the neck the two possibilities that have to be considered are that the symptoms may be due either to trigger point activation in the sternocleidomastoid muscle, or to direct injury to an upper cervical spinal nerve.

Behrmann (1983) reviewed 17 cases in which these symptoms were due to a traumatic neuropathy of the 2nd cervical spinal nerve, and in 12 of them the injury to the nerve was caused by exactly the same type of acceleration-deceleration road traffic accident, with a wrenching movement of the head, as that which is liable to cause trigger point activation in the sternocleidomastoid muscle. The main distinguishing feature would seem to be that with the trigger point syndrome there is no sensory loss, but with trauma to the second cervical spinal nerve, there is diminished sensation to pin prick over one side of the head or localized to the periorbital, temporal, or suboccipital areas.

POST-TRAUMATIC HEADACHE

The post-concussional syndrome of headaches, persistent tenderness of the scalp, postural dizziness, irritability, and failure of concentration is a well-recognized entity but one about which there is considerable diversity of opinion concerning its aetiology. Many experienced clinicians such as Matthews & Miller (1972) incline to the belief that it is psychogenic in origin. In support of this view Matthews & Miller point out that the condition is commoner after minor head injuries than it is after major ones, and that it rarely occurs in head injuries sustained in the house or during sport. Indeed it arises most often from trauma incurred during a traffic accident, and even more frequently from trauma associated with an industrial accident, and particularly in those circumstances when

there is a claim for compensation — and to quote these authors '"treatment" is fruitless'. From the few cases of post-traumatic headache either with or without a history of concussion that have come under my care, it is my belief that trigger point activation in the muscles of the neck, such as the splenii, trapezius and sternocleidomastoid muscles, is an important cause, not only of persistent headache but also of persistent scalp tenderness, and postural dizziness, and that in all such cases a systematic search for trigger points is mandatory, for when present, deactivation by means of dry needle stimulation is likely to prove helpful. This is a view also supported by the observations of Rubin (1981). There is therefore a pressing need for a large-scale survey of cases of post-traumatic headache and dizziness in order to establish the true incidence of myofascial trigger point activity in this condition.

Certainly the post-traumatic headache syndrome does not only occur as a result of head injuries but may develop whenever the muscles of the neck are subjected to the trauma of being held persistently in a state of hyperextension, as for example in the following case, when this occurred as a result of a meningitis.

A female business executive (41) developed severe retraction of her neck during the course of what was said to be a viral meningitis. The illness was sufficiently bad for her to be kept in hospital for 6 weeks. Shortly after getting over the acute stage of the illness, she began to develop severe bilateral temporal headaches, a painful stiff neck, and a feeling of unsteadiness on walking. Eighteen months later, because of these symptoms persisting, she was admitted to a neurological unit for investigations including a brain scan. No abnormality was found but she continued to have these symptoms and by the time she was referred to me 3 years later she was frequently off work because of the severity of the headaches and was taking 8 Ponstans a day. On examination, there were exquisitely tender trigger points in the posterior cervical muscles, the levator scapulae, the trapezius, and the sternocleidomastoid muscles. Deactivation of these with a dry needle gradually caused her symptoms to abate but the procedure had to be repeated at regular intervals over the course of the next 3 months before the headaches and postural dizziness were finally brought under control.

TORTICOLLIS

Torticollis (Latin, *tortus* — twisted, *collum* — neck) is of two distinct types. The one is a spasmodic contraction of the neck muscles due to a lesion in the basal ganglia and the other, a constant pulling over of the neck muscles due to the activation of trigger points in them.

The clinical picture of spasmodic torticollis is one in which there is paroxysmal contraction of the neck muscles causing the head to be frequently and involuntarily turned forcibly to one side. This is a very distressing condition and one in which eventually the head may become permanently turned to one side. On examination, there is an obvious severe and painful contraction of the sternocleidomastoid muscle but, on closer inspection, it becomes obvious that all of the muscles of the neck are involved. This is not, however, a local disorder but one that is due to some unknown disturbance of the basal ganglia. Treatment is far from satisfactory although stereotaxic surgery is sometimes helpful.

The other type of wry neck, and one that it is essential to distinguish from the spasmodic type as it is so far more readily treatable, is the one in which there is persistent contraction of the neck muscles causing the neck to be constantly pulled over to that side, and occurring as a result of the activation of trigger points in various muscles of the neck, including the posterior cervical muscles, the levator scapulae, the trapezius and the sternocleidomastoid muscle.

A man (30) had in his early teens, been accidentally shot in the head causing him to have a depressed fracture of the skull and a hemiplegia. Since that time he had had much pain in the neck with restriction of neck movements and recurrent headaches. He was referred to me, both because of these persistent symptoms and also because during the previous 18 months he had developed a constant and painful spasm of his neck muscles causing the neck to become increasingly pulled over to the affected side. On examination, there were numerous, obviously very active, trigger points in the muscles of the neck just mentioned. These were deactivated by dry needle stimulation once a week.

After 4 weeks, the pain in the neck became appreciably less, but treatment had to be continued for another 4 weeks before he could begin to keep his neck upright without discomfort. Eventually, however, with further treatment spread over several months, his long-standing headaches and pain in the neck disappeared. Also, he entirely lost any evidence of a torticollis and regained full movements of the neck. Another interesting aspect of the case that is worth noting is that on the initial examination there was exquisite tenderness of the scalp around the craniotomy scar and, on closer examination, it became apparent that there was one focal point of maximum tenderness in the scar itself. It was considered therefore that this must be a trigger point, and although needling it was difficult due to the scar being tough, and also because it was a very painful procedure, the treatment nevertheless very quickly brought about a dramatic lessening of the generalized tenderness around the scar; and as a result of repeating it a few further times, the tenderness disappeared altogether.

Temporalis muscle (Fig. 16.9)

This muscle, which is attached to the temporal bone above and the coronoid process of the mandible below, quite commonly develops activated trigger points in it. This may occur in people

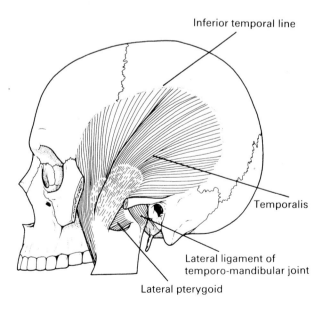

Fig. 16.9 Left temporalis. The zygomatic arch and masseter have been removed.

who are tense, in migrainous subjects, and in those who because of bruxism develop the myofascial pain-dysfunction syndrome. It is also liable to occur when the muscle is suddenly cooled by being exposed to a draught, or when it is subjected to direct trauma such as may occur with a fall on the head or being hit by a golf ball. In addition it may develop as a secondary event when pain is referred to the temporal region from trigger points in the sternocleidomastoid or upper trapezius muscles.

Location of trigger points and their specific pain patterns

The sites at which trigger points are likely to be found include:

1. the anterior part of the temple at the lateral end of the supraorbital ridge
2. midway between this point and the ear along the line of the zygomatic arch
3. on the same line just in front of the ear
4. just above the ear.

The referral of pain from a trigger point at site 1 is along the supraorbital ridge and on occasions towards the upper incisors; that from a trigger point at sites 2 and 3 is locally in the region of the temple and sometimes downwards into the teeth of the upper jaw; that from a trigger point at site 4 is in a backwards and upwards direction from it (Fig. 16.6A).

Locating trigger points

When examining the temporalis muscle for trigger points, they are more readily found if the muscle is put slightly on the stretch by having the mouth propped partially open.

Trigger point deactivation

It is relatively easy to deactivate trigger points in this muscle with a dry needle provided that they are first trapped between two fingers. Care, however, must be taken to avoid puncturing the temporal artery.

Differential diagnosis

It has to be said that although persistent pain in the temporal region is commonly due to trigger point activation, when it occurs in the middle-aged and elderly, the possibility that it may be due to giant cell arteritis must always be considered. In this disorder the pain may be in any part of the head but is commonest in the temporal region and when this is so, it is often made worse by mastication — a state of affairs sometimes somewhat ineptly referred to as jaw claudication considering that the jaw is incapable of limping! On examination, the temporal artery is characteristically thickened and pulseless, there is much surrounding tenderness, and, in some cases, the overlying skin is reddened. The physical signs, however, are often by no means obvious and in any case of doubt it is essential to have the ESR measured as with this condition it is invariably appreciably elevated.

This disorder has been discussed at some length because unless the possibility of it occurring is taken into consideration, the pain and tenderness associated with it may all too readily be assumed to be due to trigger point activation. This is a mistake that could have far reaching consequences because whilst time is being wasted treating the condition with acupuncture rather than with a corticosteroid, there is always the risk of blindness developing.

Finally, it is necessary to say something about trigger point activity in three skin muscles — the orbicularis oculi, the zygomaticus, and the occipitofrontalis (Fig. 16.10).

The orbicularis oculi

Trigger points may become activated in this muscle as a primary event in someone who persistently frowns, or as a secondary event when pain is referred to the orbit from trigger points in the sternomastoid muscle.

The trigger point lies above the eyelid just beneath the eyebrow against the bone of the orbit. The referral of pain from this is down the side of the nose (Fig. 16.11).

In deactivating this point with a dry needle, superficial needling is particularly necessary because

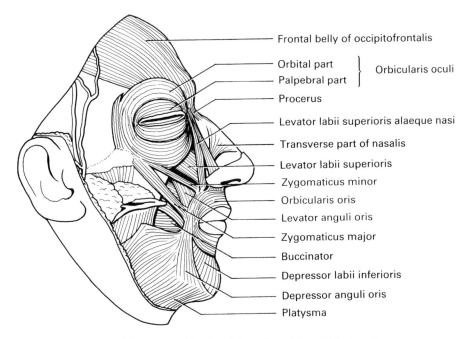

Frontal belly of occipitofrontalis

Orbital part ⎫
Palpebral part ⎭ Orbicularis oculi

Procerus

Levator labii superioris alaeque nasi

Transverse part of nasalis

Levator labii superioris

Zygomaticus minor

Orbicularis oris

Levator anguli oris

Zygomaticus major

Buccinator

Depressor labii inferioris

Depressor anguli oris

Platysma

Fig. 16.10   Muscles of the scalp and face. Right lateral aspect.

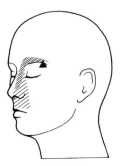

Fig. 16.11   The pattern of pain referral from a trigger point in the orbicularis oculi muscle.

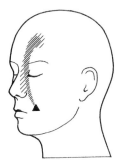

Fig. 16.12   The pattern of pain referral from a trigger point in the zygomaticus muscle.

due to the laxity of the tissues at this site there is a risk of a haematoma developing.

Zygomaticus major

This muscle, which assists in controlling facial expression by drawing the angle of the mouth upwards and backwards, attaches above to the zygomatic bone, and below to the angle of the mouth.

A trigger point in it may become activated either as a result of direct trauma to the face or secondary to trigger point activation in the masticatory muscles. This point is usually situated just

above the corner of the mouth and is best located with the mouth propped wide open and the muscle held in a pincer grip with one digit intraorally and the other extraorally. Pain from it is referred upwards along the side of the nose to the forehead (Fig. 16.12). The trigger point is generally to be found in a palpable band of muscle and to deactivate it, a needle is inserted into the point of maximum tenderness.

Occipitofrontalis muscle

This cutaneous muscle of the scalp is in two parts — the frontalis situated anteriorly, and the

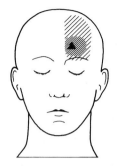

Fig. 16.13   The pattern of pain referral from a trigger point in the frontalis belly of the occipitofrontalis muscle.

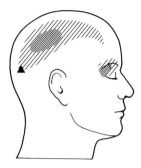

Fig. 16.14   The pattern of pain referral from a trigger point in the occipitalis belly of the occipitofrontalis muscle.

occipitalis situated posteriorly. The action of both of them acting together is to wrinkle the forehead.

A trigger point in the frontalis is liable to become activated in someone who persistently frowns, and also, when trigger points in the sternomastoid muscle refer pain to the frontal region of the head.

The trigger point is usually situated above the inner end of the eyebrow. Pain from this is referred locally around the trigger point site. In order to deactivate it, a needle should be inserted superficially and obliquely into the skin (Fig. 16.13). A trigger point in the occipitalis part of the muscle often becomes activated as a result of trigger points in the posterior cervical muscles referring pain to the occipital region. It refer pain over the side of the head from the occiput to the orbit (Fig. 16.14). It is readily identified by palpating gently over the back of the head and this point also should be deactivated by inserting a needle superficially and obliquely into the skin.

REFERENCES

Andersson A, Holmgren E 1975 On acupuncture analgesia and the mechanism of pain. American Journal of Chinese Medicine 3: 311–334

Anselmi B, Baldi E, Casacci F, Salmon S 1980 Endogenous opioids in cerebrospinal fluid and blood in idiopathic headache sufferers. Headache 20: 294–299

Ayer W 1983 Report of the president's conference on the examination, diagnosis and management of temperomandibular disorders. Journal of American Dental Association 106: 75–77

Baldi E et al 1982 Intermittent hypoendorphinaemia in migraine attacks. Cephalgia 2: 78–81

Behrmann S 1983 Traumatic neuropathy of second cervical spinal nerves. British Medical Journal 286: 1312–1313

Bell W E 1977 Management of masticatory pain. In: Alling C C, Mayhan P E (eds) Facial pain, 2nd edn. Lea & Febiger, Philadelphia, ch 12

Blau J N 1983 Chronic headaches in general practice. British Medical Journal 286: 1375–1376

Blau J N 1982 A plain man's guide to the management of migraine. British Medical Journal 284: 1095–1097

Caviness V S, O'Brien P 1980 Headache. New England Journal of Medicine 302: 446–450

Cawson R A 1984 Pain in the temperomandibular joint. British Medical Journal 288: 1857–1858

Chalmers I M, Blair G S 1973 Rheumatoid arthritis of the temperomandibular joint. Quarterly Journal of Medicine 42: 369–386

Chapman C R, Colpitts Y M, Benedetti C, Kitaeff R, Gehrig J D 1980 Evoked potential assessment of acupuncture analgesia, attempted reversal with naloxone. Pain 9: 183–197

Clarke N G 1982 Occlusion and myofascial pain dysfunction; is there a relationship? Journal of American Dental Association 85: 892

Cohen L A 1959 Body orientation and motor coordination in animals with impaired neck sensation. Federation Proceedings 18: 28

Cohen L A 1961 Role of eye and neck proprioceptive mechanisms in body orientation and motor co-ordination. Journal of Neurophysiology 24: 1–11

Costen T B 1934 A syndrome of ear and sinus symptoms dependent upon disturbed function of the temperomandibular joint. Annals of Otology Rhinology and Laryngology 43: 1–15

Couch J R, Hassanein R S 1976 Amitriptyline in migraine prophylaxis. Archives of Neurology (Chicago) 36: 695–699

Couch J R, Ziegler D K, Hassanein R S 1976 Amitriptyline in the prophylaxis of migraine. Effectiveness and relationship of antimigraine and antidepressant effect. Neurology (Minneapolis) 26: 121–127

Dalessio D J 1976 The relationship of vasoactive substances to vascular permeability and their role in migraine. Research and clinical studies in headache. S. Karger, Basle, vol IV, p 76–84

Dalessio D J 1984 Headache. In: Wall P D, Melzack R (eds) Textbook of pain. Churchill Livingstone, Edinburgh, p 277–292

Dowson D I, Lewith G T, Machin D 1985 The effects of acupuncture versus placebo in the treatment of headache. Pain 21: 35–42

Eriksson M B E, Sjölund B H, Nielzen S 1979 Long term results of peripheral conditioning stimulation as an analgesic measure in chronic pain. Pain 6: 335–347

Facchinetti F, Nappi G, Savoldi F, Genazzi A R 1981 Primary headaches: reduced circulating beta-lipoprotein and beta-endorphin levels with impaired reactivity to acupuncture. Cephalgia 1: 95–203

Greene C S, Lerman M D, Sutcher H D, Leskin D M 1969 The TMJ pain-dysfunction syndrome: heterogeneity of the patient population. Journal of American Dental Association 79: 1168–1172

Hay K M 1976 The treatment of pain in trigger areas in migraine. The Journal of the Royal College of General Practitioners 26: 372–376

Hester J 1984 Aspects of facial pain. British Medical Acupuncture Society Journal (May) 9

Hunter M, Phillips C 1981 The experience of headache — an assessment of the qualities of tension headache pain. Pain 10: 209–219

Jeans M E 1979 Relief of chronic pain by brief, intense transcutaneous electrical stimulation — a double blind study. In: Bonica J J, Liebeskind J C, Albe-Fessard D G (eds) Advances in pain research and therapy 3. Raven Press, New York, p 601–606

Jensen L B, Melsen B, Jensen S B 1979 Effect of acupuncture on headache measured by reduction in number of attacks and use of drugs. Scandinavian Journal of Dental Research 87: 373–380

Lance J W, Curran D A 1964 Treatment of chronic tension headache. Lancet 1: 1236–1239

Laskin D M 1969 Etiology of the pain dysfunction syndrome. Journal of American Dental Association 79: 147–153

Loeser J D 1984 Tic douloureux and atypical facial pain. In: Wall P, Melzack R (eds) Textbook of pain. Churchill Livingstone, Edinburgh, p 430

Loh L, Nathan P W, Schott G D, Siekha K J 1984 Acupuncture versus medical treatment for migraine and muscle tension headaches. Journal of Neurology, Neurosurgery and Psychiatry 47: 333–337

Mann F, Bowsher D, Mumford J, Lipton S, Miles J 1973 Treatment of intractable pain by acupuncture. Lancet II: 57–60

Matthews W B, 1983 Headache. In: Weatherall D A, Ledingham J G G, Warrell D A (eds) Oxford textbook of medicine. Oxford University Press, Oxford, p 145–149

Matthews W B, Miller H 1972 Diseases of the nervous system. Blackwell Scientific Publications, Oxford p 122–123

Mikhail M, Rosen H 1980 History and etiology of myofascial pain-dysfunction syndrome. Journal of Prosthetic Dentistry 44: 438–444

Oleson J, Lauritzen M 1982 Spreading cerebral oligaemia in classical and normal cerebral blood flow in migraine. Headache 22: 242–248

Plum F 1982 Headache. In: Wyngaarden J B, Smith L (Jnr) (eds) Cecil's textbook of medicine, 16th edn. Saunders, Philadelphia, p 1948–1951

Rossi G F, Brodal A 1956 Spinal afferents to the trigeminal sensory nuclei and to the nucleus of the solitary tract. Confinia Neurologica 16: 321–322

Rubin D 1981 Myofascial trigger point syndromes. An approach to management. Archives of Physical Medicine and Rehabilitation 62: 107–110

Schwartz L L 1956 A temperomandibular joint pain-dysfunction syndrome. Journal of Chronic Diseases 3: 284–293

Sessle B J, Hu J W, Dubner R, Lucier G E 1981 Functional properties of neurons in cat trigeminal subnucleus caudalis (medullary dorsal horn) II. Modulation of responses to noxious and non-noxious stimuli by periaqueductal grey, nucleus raphe magnus, cerebral cortex, and afferent influences, and effect of naloxone. Journal of Neurophysiology 45: 211–255

Sharav Y 1984 Orofacial pain. In: Wall P D, Melzack R (eds) Textbook of pain. Churchill Livingstone, Edinburgh, p 338–349

Sharav Y, Tzukert A, Refaeli B 1978 Muscle pain index in relation to pain dysfunction and dizziness associated with the myofascial pain-dysfunction syndrome. Oral Surgery 46: 742–747

Sicuteri F, Anselmi B, Curradi C, Michelacci S, Sassi A 1978 Morphine-like factors in CSF of headache patients. In: Costa E, Trabucci M (eds) Advances in biochemical psychopharmacology 18. Raven Press, New York, p 363–370

Sovak M, Dalessio D J, Kunzel M, Sternbach R 1980 Current investigations in headache. In: Bonica J J (ed) Pain. Raven Press, New York, p 261–282

Stem P G, Mothersill K J, Brooke R I 1979 Biofeedback and a cognitive behavioral approach to treatment of myofascial pain-dysfunction syndrome. Behavior Therapy 10: 29–34

Tfelt-Hansen P, Lous I, Oleson J 1981 Prevalence and significance of muscle tenderness during common migraine attacks. Headache 21: 49–54

Torvik A 1956 Afferent connections to the sensory trigeminal nuclei, the nucleus of the solitary tract and adjacent structures. Journal of Comparative Neurology 106: 51–132

Travell J 1955 Referred pain from skeletal muscle. I. Pectoralis major syndrome of breast pain and soreness II. Sternomastoid syndrome of headache and dizziness. New York State Journal of Medicine 55: 331–339

Travell J 1960 Temporomandibular joint pain referred from muscles of the head and neck. Journal of Prosthetic Dentistry 10: 745–763

Travell J 1967 Mechanical headache. Headache 7: 23–29

Travell J 1981 Identification of myofascial trigger point syndromes: a case of atypical facial neuralgia. Archives of Physical Medicine and Rehabilitation 62: 100–106

Travell J G, Simons D G 1983a Myofascial pain and dysfunction — The trigger point manual. Williams & Wilkins, Baltimore, p 168–182, 1983b: p. 254

Vincent C A 1989 A controlled trial of the treatment of migraine by acupuncture. The Clinical Journal of Pain 5 (4): 305–312

Weddington W N, Blazer D 1979 Atypical facial pain and trigeminal neuralgia: a comparison study. Psychosomatics 20: 348–356

Weeks V D, Travell J 1955 Postural vertigo due to trigger areas in the sternocleidomastoid muscle. Journal of Pediatrics 47: 315–327

17. Low-back pain

INTRODUCTION

The main indication for acupuncture in the alleviation of low-back pain is when such pain is mechanical in its relationship to activity, and due to some structural dysfunction at that site. It therefore follows that before contemplating the use of such treatment it is necessary to exclude other causes of low-back pain of a non-mechanical nature including inflammatory, metabolic, and neoplastic disorders of the spine; also referred pain from abdominal or pelvic organs; and the pain of peripheral vascular disease.

It is only possible to do this by taking a careful history, by carrying out a detailed physical examination including in particular a systematic search of the musculature of the lower back for trigger points, and by carrying out certain investigations. With respect to the latter, it is essential in all cases to measure the erythrocyte sedimentation rate (ESR) and to have radiographs (PA, oblique and lateral views) of the spine. In certain circumstances it may also be necessary to carry out more highly specialized radiographic investigations and, on occasions, certain specific biochemical blood tests.

DIFFERENTIAL DIAGNOSIS BETWEEN MECHANICAL AND NON-MECHANICAL LOW-BACK PAIN

Although it would clearly be inappropriate in a book of this type to enter into a detailed discussion of all the various diagnostic features which help to separate mechanical from non-mechanical low-back pain, it nevertheless may help to ensure that acupuncture is not used inappropriately if brief reference is made to a few of the more important ones.

Mechanical low-back pain

The history given by a patient with low-back pain of mechanical type is quite different from that when the pain is due to some non-mechanical cause, and therefore simply by listening to the patient carefully one can often obtain considerable help in distinguishing between these two fundamentally different types of pain.

The commonest form of low-back pain is that which occurs as a result of some structural dysfunction and, because of the direct relationship it has with activity, it may be said to be of the mechanical type. It tends to be more noticeable in carrying out movements after sitting or lying down for some time. Also, twisting, lifting, bending, and coughing often make it worse. It is relieved by resting and therefore, as might be expected, there is often a history of it being most troublesome during the course of day-time activities. It may nevertheless come on in bed at night as a result of turning or lying awkwardly, but when this occurs it is quickly eased once a comfortable position is found.

There is sometimes a complaint that the pain becomes worse on sitting down. This may, at first sight, seem surprising but the reason for it will be explained later when discussing the location of trigger points.

It has to be remembered that a history of pain in the buttocks and thighs, brought on by walking and relieved by resting, may be vascular in origin, and develop as a result of aorto-iliac occlusion (Leriche's syndrome). In addition, it is possible for sciatica to occur as a result of atheromatous obstruction in the internal iliac artery causing ischaemia of the sciatic nerve (Lamerton et al 1983). This is why history-taking must be supplemented by a careful physical examination including palpation of the femoral pulses.

Further, when a patient with low-back pain complains that the legs become painful, weak, and affected by paraesthesiae on walking, and that this is relieved by resting, and in particular by adopting a squatting position, the possibility of stenosis of the spinal canal, either congenital or acquired, has to be considered (Porter 1987), and investigated accordingly by tomography, or by ultrasonic measurements (Porter et al 1978) or preferably by computerized axial tomography (Schumaker et al 1978).

Non-mechanical low-back pain

Non-mechanical low-back pain occurs far less commonly than that of the mechanical type. It occurs as a result of neoplastic, infective, inflammatory, or metabolic disease of the spine, and for several reasons, including the fact that its intensity bears no relationship to physical activity, the history tends to be different.

The onset is usually insidious, with the pain gradually increasing in intensity, and being as severe when resting at night as it is during the day. It may in fact seem to be worse at night because there is nothing to distract the mind from it, and unlike mechanical type pain it cannot be eased by a change of position.

Ankylosing spondylitis, the principal inflammatory disease affecting the lower back, will be singled out for special mention because of certain distinctive features in the history (Calin et al 1977), and because it is the one non-mechanical disorder in which acupuncture may be of much help in relieving pain. The disease, which affects men five times more commonly than women, declares itself in early adult life by the insidious onset of pain affecting both sides of the lower back and spreading to the buttocks. This pain characteristically causes early morning waking, and on rising there is considerable stiffness, but this is relieved by activity. In addition there may be a history of iritis, and a family history of the

disease. Careful attention to the history is essential because although, once the disease has become established, the ESR is elevated, and there are diagnostic radiographic changes in the sacroiliac joints and lumbar spine, in the early stages both the ESR and the X-ray appearances may be normal. In such circumstances it may sometimes be necessary to carry out technetium scanning of the sacroiliac joints in order to demonstrate the presence of sacroiliitis. When the clinical picture is not straightforward, the HLA-B27 test may also be helpful, as a positive test is strongly suggestive of this disease being the cause of the pain. At the same time, it has to be remembered that it may only be a reflection of a carrier state, with the pain being due to some other cause.

Pain referred to the back from abdominal and pelvic organs

When pain in the lower part of the back occurs as a result of it being referred to that site from some abdominal or pelvic disorder, it is usually accompanied by other symptoms which direct attention to the organ involved. This, however, is not invariable, particularly in the initial stages, and one has to be particularly wary when there is a history of recent trauma to the back as this may be diagnostically misleading.

A woman (54) developed persistent pain across the lower back shortly after being involved in a car accident. The pain was unremitting and in spite of it being present day and night, and not relieved by rest, the trauma was assumed to be responsible, and in view of this she spent several months having physiotherapy. By the time she was referred to me for an opinion as to whether acupuncture might be helpful, the character of the pain together with the fact that she was losing weight, and feeling generally unwell, led to further investigations which ultimately revealed the presence of a carcinoma of the body of the pancreas.

Dual pathology

When taking the history it has to be remembered that in spite of the philosophical maxim of the 14th-century Franciscan, William of Occam, that

'Entities are not to be multiplied without necessity' (Occam's razor), symptoms indicative of abdominal or pelvic disease, and low-back pain may not necessarily be due to the same cause.

Several cases have been referred to me by a gastroenterological colleague for acupuncture because, although there have been symptoms of an abdominal disorder, such as the irritable bowel syndrome, or diverticulitis, there has in addition been low-back pain which from its relationship to posture and movement has clearly been of a mechanical type, and therefore eminently suitable for this form of treatment.

CLINICAL EXAMINATION

As a detailed account of the proper manner in which to examine the back is to be found in any standard textbook, only some of the more salient features will be mentioned here with special reference to those of particular importance in coming to a decision as to whether or not acupuncture might be helpful in the symptomatic relief of lumbosacral pain.

The examination really begins as soon as the patient enters the room, and particularly whilst taking the history, as observations at that stage concerning the patient's appearance, expression, and manner of describing symptoms often give a good indication as to whether or not there is likely to be an underlying debilitating disease; also as to the degree to which the pain is affecting the patient; and above all these observations are of help in determining the psychological make-up of the individual. As will be explained later, there is often a complex interrelationship between psyche and soma in the pathogenesis of mechanical type low-back pain which often influences the response to any form of treatment including acupuncture, and which often makes it necessary to treat both the mind and the body.

The first part of the formal examination of the back should be carried out with the patient standing and with sufficient clothes removed to give an uninterrupted view of the whole length of the spine and legs.

On inspection, the trained eye will readily note the café-au-lait patch possibly indicative of a neurofibroma; the midline dimple or tufts of hair over a spina bifida occulta; the patch of erythema ab igne from prolonged usage of a hot water bottle; and the lower lumbar hump characteristics of spondylolisthesis; but from an everyday practical point of view, and particularly when acupunture is likely to be used, the most important observations at this stage are those concerning whether or not there is inequality of the length of the two legs.

Short-leg syndrome

A short leg, either when this is of congenital origin, or when it is acquired, usually as a result of a fracture, puts a considerable strain on the muscles of the lower back, so that when trigger points in these muscles become activated for one reason or another, the effect of this strain is to nullify any attempt to deactivate these points. It is therefore a waste of time employing any technique such as acupuncture for this purpose without at the same time correcting the deformity.

The physical findings associated with relative shortness of one leg include the pelvis being seen to be tilted in association with a compensatory scoliosis; also, on the side of the short leg, the shoulder is held lower, the hip is less prominent, there is a loss of the hollow of the flank, and the gluteal fold is lower than the one on the opposite side (Nichols 1960).

Travell & Simons (1983a) consider that a discrepancy in leg length of 1.3 cm ($\frac{1}{2}$") may cause no symptoms throughout a lifetime if myofascial triggers do not become activated, but if, for one reason or another, this occurs, then it only needs a discrepancy of 0.5 cm ($\frac{3}{16}$") to perpetuate this trigger point activity.

Travell (1976) believes that the quadratus lumborum is the one muscle in particular in which trigger point activity is most likely to persist in the presence of a short leg.

It is important to realize that an uncorrected short leg has far-ranging consequences because it may not only cause low-back pain to become chronic, but it may also, by putting a strain on the ipsilateral muscles of the neck, cause trigger points to become activated in those mucles with the consequent development of persistent neck pain and headaches.

Two commonly used techniques for assessing differences in leg length, carried out with the patient lying down, are unreliable because the paitent is non-weight bearing. These include one where a tape measurement is made from the anterior superior iliac spine to the tip of the medial malleolus; and the other where, with the knees straight, the distance is measured between comparable points on the medial malleoli. A better method is to have the undressed patient in the standing position with the feet together. An approximate estimate of the comparative length of two legs can then be made by palpating the iliac crests, or posterior superior iliac spines. Pages of a journal should then be placed under the foot of the short leg, and the number of these gradually increased until the pelvis and shoulder are level. This gives a measure as to how much the shoe on the affected side should be raised, a task which incidentally in my experience is best done by a cobbler with a special interest in and experience of this type of work.

Curves of the lumbar spine

On inspection of the back with the patient standing, the curves of the lumbar spine should also be observed. Loss of its normal lordosis may occur with certain inflammatory conditions but it may also result from pregnancy and obesity. Any scoliosis also should be noted. This may develop in painful conditions as a result of muscle spasm, or as discussed above, it may occur together with a pelvic tilt, when the legs are of unequal length. When due to the former, it is sometimes only seen on forward flexion, whereas with the latter this movement usually causes it to disappear.

Wasting of the muscles

It should also be noted whether there is any wasting of the muscles. Wasting of the paraspinal muscles, for example, often occurs with chronic inflammatory conditions of the spine.

Movements of the spine

The movements of the spine should next be tested, including forward flexion, lateral flexion, extension and rotation. In the case of non-mechanical pain due to inflammatory or neoplastic conditions there is often a generalized restriction of all lumbar movements. When pain is of a mechanical type and therefore likely to be suitable for treatment with acupuncture, only certain movements are likely to be limited, and observing which these are gives helpful guidance as to where trigger points are likely to be found. Trigger points are also often more readily palpable when muscles are put on the stretch. And following treatment with acupuncture, it is wise to re-test the spine's range of movements as in this way attention may be drawn to trigger points which have been overlooked.

Examination of the patient lying down

For the second part of the examination the patient lies face upwards on the examination couch in order that the abdomen may be examined for evidence of visceral disease. The femoral pulses should also be palpated at this stage.

This should be followed by an assessment of hip and knee movements; a neurological examination; and the carrying out of the straight-leg raising test (Lasègue's sign). A vaginal or rectal examination should then be performed when indicated.

The search for trigger points

The final part of the examination and one which should be carried out especially carefully is a search for trigger points. This is of particular importance when the pain is found to be of the mechanical type and due to some relatively benign structural disorder because it would seem that it is from activated trigger points that much of this pain emanates. The reason for saying this is that pressure applied to these points aggravates the pain and relief from it may often be obtained simply by deactivating these points by means of the acupuncture technique of inserting dry needles into them. This search has to be conducted in an unhurried and systematic manner because, unlike the trigger points responsible for similar pain in the neck, which are always to be found at identical sites in everyone, the distribution of trigger points in the lower back has no fixed pattern and is in fact widely variable from person to person.

The patient should first be placed in the prone position, and the muscles of the back from the lower thoracic region downwards should be palpated by placing the examining hand flat on the back and rolling the skin and subcutaneous tissue over the underlying muscle by means of flexing fingers in a manner similar to that used in kneading dough.

Trigger points in the lower back occur as focal areas of exquisite tenderness either in muscle which otherwise feels normal, or in elongated fibrous bands of muscle (palpable bands) or in so-called 'fibrositic' nodules.

It is a good rule to start the search by palpating along the length of the spine in the midline from the level of the 10th dorsal vertebra above, to the coccyx below, and then systematically to examine every part of the musculature on each side of the back in turn, by palpating along lines about 1 cm apart and parallel to the spine, from a similar level above, to the upper border of the buttocks below. The muscles of the buttocks should next be palpated, first using light pressure, and then deep pressure, and this should be followed by palpation of the muscles along the back of the leg.

The patient should then roll on to each side in turn so that the muscles of the flank can be palpated from the iliac crest above to the greater trochanter below, with special attention being paid to the area around the latter structure as it is surprising how often there is a crop of trigger points in muscles near to their sites of attachment to it. The outer side of the thigh should then be palpated because it is common to find trigger points along the length of the tensor fasciae latae.

The examination should be completed by getting the patient to lie in the supine position and the search for trigger points continued by palpating the muscles of the anterior abdominal wall and the inner side of the thigh, with special attention being paid to sites where the adductor muscles of the leg become attached to the pelvis.

Back pain referred from trigger points in the abdominal wall musculature is discussed in Chapter 20. It is important to remember that trigger points in and around the pubic region and the upper inner part of the thigh, at or near to the site of the attachment of the adductor muscles to the pelvis, may not only be associated with low-back pain, but on occasions are responsible for pain being referred to the hip region, to the scrotum, or to the vagina. It should also be noted that it is activation of these trigger points that sometimes makes a person with low-back pain complain that the pain is worse on sitting down. The following case is a typical example.

A housewife (62) was referred to me with persistent pain in the lower back and buttocks which was made worse both by certain movements and on sitting down. Dry-needle deactivation of many trigger points in the lower back relieved her of much of the pain but the pain on sitting persisted. There was no trigger point in the region of the ischial tuberosity to account for this but there were some exquisitely tender ones at the sites of insertion of the adductor muscles into the pubis, and once these were deactivated the sitting position became comfortable.

An account of some of the commoner sites where trigger points are to be found in the muscles of the lower back, and their specific patterns of pain referral, will be given towards the end of this chapter. It is remarkable how often they coincide in position with traditional Chinese acupuncture points, and, as Gunn & Milbrandt (1976) have shown, they also often coincide with the motor points of muscles.

Investigations of assistance in distinguishing between the mechanical and non-mechanical types of low-back pain

Erythrocyte sedimentation rate (ESR)

The erythrocyte sedimentation rate, using the standard Westergren technique, is one of the most reliable means of distinguishing between these two types of low-back pain in view of the fact that with mechanical type low-back pain the rate is usually not above the upper limit of normal of 25 mm in the first hour, whereas with disorders responsible for non-mechanical type pain the rate is in general well above this. One important exception is early ankylosing spondylitis when the rate in about 20% of cases may for a time remain normal.

Plain radiographs

As will be seen when chronic low-back pain is considered in detail later, there is no clearly defined relationship between its development and the radiographic changes of disc or facet joint degeneration. Also, with acute disc prolapse, the plain X-ray appearances are normal. In the assessment of low-back pain of the mechanical type, therefore, there is little to be learnt from plain radiographs of the spine. The main importance of having them is to exclude non-mechanical causes of low-back pain including infective, inflammatory, and neoplastic lesions. It is essential to bear in mind, however, that in the early stages of such disorders the radiographic appearances may be normal, and therefore at times it is wise to have a technetium scan. It is believed that an increased uptake of this radioisotope is dependent on an increased bone blood flow and metabolism, and as this is common to all these various diseases, it necessarily follows that a positive result does not distinguish between them, but does serve to rule out the possibility of the pain being only mechanical in type (McKillop & McDougal 1980).

Computerized axial tomography (CAT scanning)

CAT scanning also has an important place in the assessment of lumbar spine problems. It is particularly valuable in the assessment of intervertebral disc herniation, spinal stenosis, paravertebral spinal infection and neoplastic disease, and in excluding retroperitoneal and pelvic disease as a cause of referred back pain (Isherwood & Antoun 1987).

It also provides extremely clear visualization of the facet joints thus allowing an accurate assessment of the extent of apophyseal joint disease including the extent and direction of osteophytes, and the shape and size of the spinal canal. However, as will be discussed later, the role of facet joint disease in the causation of low-back pain remains highly speculative and therefore it is unlikely that this particular diagnostic innovation will significantly contribute to advances in the treatment of mechanical type low-back pain.

Some causes of mechanical type low-back pain and their management

There are many potential causes of low-back pain of the mechanical type, both psychological and physical, and, frequently, several of them contribute to the condition simultaneously. The situation is further complicated by the fact that the exact manner in which some of the factors operate remains obscure. There can be no doubt that it is because of such difficulties that the management of this type of pain remains far from satisfactory, and why the effects of most forms of treatment for it, including acupuncture, are notoriously unpredictable.

It was because of this that Nachemson (1979) was prompted to say,

Having been engaged in research in this field for nearly 25 years and having been clinically engaged in back problems for nearly the same period of time and as a member and scientific adviser to several international back associations, I can only state that for the majority of our patients, the true cause of low-back pain is unknown . . . since the cause is unknown there is only symptomatic treatment available.

This undoubtedly is true, so the remainder of this chapter will be devoted to reviewing the clinical characteristics of the various structural disorders in the lower back considered to be capable of giving rise to pain of the mechanical type, and examining the various neurological mechanisms thought to be responsible for this. An attempt will also be made to evaluate the various forms of symptomatic treatment available, in order to assess which of them in the light of our present knowledge seem to be based on sound physiological principles. The purpose of this is to show that acupuncture may be included amongst these, and that there is much to be gained by using it, either in conjunction with, or at times instead of, some of these other so-called more orthodox forms of treatment.

During the course of this review it will be observed how often with many of these structural disorders, myofascial trigger points are an important source of pain. The activation of points is sometimes a primary event and at other times a secondary one. There is a need for wider recognition of this phenomenon now that it has been shown that deactivation of these points by the acupuncture technique of dry needle stimulation is not only frequently effective in alleviating low-back pain, but also is both simple to apply and safe to use, this being more than can be said for some of the more complex forms of treatment in current use.

ACUTE LOW-BACK PAIN

The description of Mixter & Barr in 1934 of the symptoms and signs of a prolapsed intervertebral disc (PID) and how the pain from this condition can often be relieved by a laminectomy was undoubtedly of considerable importance. However, as already explained (Ch. 14), since the chemistry of the intervertebral disc has become better understood (Urban & Maroudas 1980), it is now recognized that PID as a cause of acute low-back pain must be a comparatively rare event. The reason for this is that the central nucleus pulposus of a disc, over the years, becomes increasingly inspissated, and it is only possible for it to bulge through a ruptured annulus fibrosus and impinge on a nerve root, whilst it still remains in a relatively fluid state. This is approximately up to the age of 50, and during this earlier part of adult life, rupture of an annulus fibrosus is uncommon because the degenerative changes are still at an early stage.

As Dixon (1980) rightly points out, disc prolapse is probably the most overdiagnosed cause of low-back pain, and goes on to state that 'indeed the whole myth of the "slipped disc" is one of the deep rooted weeds that have sprung up in this area. Discs do not "slip" in the way in which laymen and not a few doctors imagine'. He believes that this over-diagnosis may be due to the fact that most patients with proved prolapse give a history of past episodes of acute low-back pain without nerve root compression, and that the diagnosis is often one of convenience. Wyke (1980) in support of this view estimates that 'contrary to popular impression ... less than 5% of patients with backache have prolapsed intervertebral discs', but at the same time agrees that 70% of those with PID have backache as the initial symptom.

It is now generally accepted that acute mechanical type low-back pain is most commonly due to some primary disorder of muscle, for example,

such as when the tendinous attachments of muscles become avulsed, or muscle fibres and their fascial sheaths become torn as a result of the lower back muscles being suddenly overloaded as a result of a heavy object being lifted in the stooping position; or, for example, when the muscles become strained by being overloaded for some considerable time. Alternatively it may occur when the back is exposed to draughts or damp, or at times for no obvious reason. Formerly its development under such circumstances led to a diagnosis of fibrositis or myositis, or more recently to one of myofasciitis. As previously explained (Ch. 5) all such terms are no longer acceptable as inflammatory changes in the muscle have never been demonstrated.

Acute low-back pain also commonly occurs when the nociceptive receptor systems in either the fibrous capsules of the facet joints or the lumbosacral ligaments become stimulated as a result of the spine being subjected to persistent postural stress. The clinical picture, irrespective of the structure or structures involved, is one of acute localized pain with reflex spasm of the paravertebral muscles, and the presence of exquisitely tender trigger points. This picture is identical to that seen with the much rarer acute disc prolapse at a stage before pain extends down the leg. With regard to the activation of trigger points, the only difference is that with disorders of the muscle or ligaments the activation is a primary event, but with facet joint strain or disc prolapse it is a secondary one.

It therefore follows that with the development of acute low-back pain, because of the difficulty in distinguishing clinically between these various causes, it is impossible to make a precise diagnosis, and it is better, in my opinion, to refer to all such cases as being examples of the acute lumbar myofascial trigger point pain syndrome. This at least helps to guard against the all too frequent error of assuming that acute low-back pain must be due to a 'slipped disc', and for this reason alone, automatically subjecting the person concerned to a period of strict bed rest without first of all carrying out a detailed examination. Admittedly acute low-back pain may require bed rest but it is essentially the severity of the pain that dictates when this is necessary. Bed rest should certainly never be prescribed without there first being a systematic search for trigger points, because, when present, the deactivation of these by acupuncture by alleviating the pain may obviate the need for bed rest, or it may shorten the period for which it is required, as is illustrated by the following case:

A housewife (38) suddenly developed severe pain in the left lower back after bending for some time doing some strenous gardening. She therefore took to her bed and called the doctor. After listening to the story, he told her she must have 'slipped a disc', and that she would have to lie flat on her back for 2–3 weeks. This immediately created a domestic crisis as she and her family had planned to drive to Switzerland 2 days later. The husband therefore persuaded the general practitioner to let me see her.

On examination she was lying very still, and reluctant to move because of the pain it caused. When, after a certain amount of persuasion, she rolled over sufficiently for her back to be examined, one focal area of exquisite tenderness in the left flank was found, with pressure on this considerably aggravating the pain. After deactivating this trigger point with a dry needle, the patient was more comfortable. When seen the next day, she reported that the pain relief had only lasted for about 2 hours, and on re-examination the trigger point was as tender as before. It was therefore once again deactivated with a dry needle, and this time the pain relief was longer lasting, so that 24 hours later she was able to set off on the journey to Europe without any discomfort.

Spontaneous resolution of acute low-back pain

It could be argued that in the case just quoted the pain might have resolved spontaneously within a few days, but from its severity and the degree of muscle spasm present, this would seem to have been unlikely.

Nevertheless, it is important to remember in assessing the effects of any form of treatment for acute low-back pain that most of those who suffer from it become symptom-free in 4–6 weeks irrespective of treatment (White 1966, Rowe 1969) and as Waddell (1982) says in discussing the subject 'frequently treatment simply takes the credit for natural history and the pasage of time'.

This no doubt is true but acute low-back pain that persists for 4–6 weeks can often seriously interfere with a person's ability to work or to carry out sporting activities, and if it can be shown, as my everyday clinical experience would lead me to believe, that acupuncture by its direct action on trigger points is capable of alleviating the pain more quickly than might be expected if left to resolve spontaneously, then such treatment is obviously well worth using. The difficulties of proving this statistically, however, are formidable as with a condition with such as relatively short natural history, the numbers of cases required both for the treatment and control groups would be extremely large, and in order that such a trial could be completed in a reasonable time, many centres would have to participate.

ACUTE SCIATICA

Following Mixter & Barr's important contribution to the subject of acute disc prolapse in 1934, it became generally assumed that the diagnosis of this condition, and that of acute sciatica were synonymous, and moreover it was also widely believed that the sciatic pain was invariably due to the disc exerting pressure on a nerve root.

In recent years it has been found necessary to modify these concepts because, although it is undoubtedly true that acute sciatica may occur when a disc is sufficiently badly prolapsed as to exert pressure on a nerve root, it is now realized that acute pain along the course of the sciatic nerve is more often due to it being referred down the back of the leg from trigger points in the muscles of the lower back. These trigger points become activated either as a result of a partially prolapsed disc causing the back muscles to go into spasm but even more frequently as a result of the muscles being subjected to strain during the course of some physical activity.

Firstly, therefore, a description will be given of the clinical picture that arises when acute sciatica is caused by a badly prolapsed disc pressing on a nerve root, and following this, acute sciatica of the referred type will be discussed.

Acute prolapse of a disc with 'sciatica' due to pressure on a nerve root

The discs most likely to prolapse are the ones between the 4th and 5th lumbar vertebrae with involvement of the 5th lumbar nerve root, and the one between the 5th lumbar vertebra and the sacrum with involvement of the 1st sacral nerve root. Much less commonly, the disc between the 3rd and 4th vertebrae prolapses with involvement of the 4th lumbar nerve root.

With involvement of the 5th lumbar nerve root, pain is felt in the buttock, down the postero-lateral aspect of the thigh and leg, and over the inner half of the foot; dorsi flexion of the toes is weak; the tendon reflexes are normal.

With involvement of the 1st sacral nerve root, pain is felt in the buttock, down the back of the thigh and leg and along the outer side of the foot. Planter flexion of the foot is weak; and the ankle jerk diminished. With the less common involvement of the 4th lumbar nerve root there is pain down the outer side of the thigh, and the inner side of the leg. There is weakness of knee extension and a diminished knee jerk. The pain in the buttock and thigh, no matter which root is involved, is associated with widespread muscle tenderness and the spasm of paravertebral muscles leads to the spine becoming rigid with a loss of the normal lumbar lordosis and the development of a scoliosis.

Straight leg-raising test (Lasègue's sign)

This test involves the passive flexion of the leg at the hip with the knee straight. The test is said to be positive when there is a restriction of movement to 45° or less.

This test is positive with compression of the 5th lumbar or 1st sacral nerve roots, and for many years subsequent to Mixter & Barr's original paper in 1934 it was thought that limitation of straight leg-raising only occurs when there is pressure on a nerve root by a prolapsed intervertebral disc. Nobody was therefore surprised when Edgar & Park (1974) found the straight leg-raising test to be positive in 94% of patients with a surgically confirmed prolapse pressing on a nerve root, or that in 95% of such cases, pain could be induced in the affected leg by raising the opposite leg (the well leg-raising test). Such teaching, however, has had to be revised since King & Lagger (1976) have shown that a positive Lasègue's sign also occurs with acute sciatica of the referred type and

that in such cases it can be reversed by interrupting the arc between the posterior primary division, the cord, and the anterior primary division of a root segment. This no doubt explains why Spangfort (1972), in a computer-aided analysis of 2504 operations, found that of those patients with acute sciatica shown not to have a prolapsed disc at operation, 88.8% of them had a positive Lasègue's sign pre-operatively.

It therefore now has to be accepted that the restricted straight leg-raising that occurs with acute sciatica is not necessarily indicative of nerve root entrapment as it also occurs when the pain is of the referred type.

Trigger points

Activation of trigger points in the muscles of the back and leg is a prominent feature in all cases of acute disc prolapse.

When the disc prolapse is of sufficient degree to exert direct pressure on a nerve root, it is the trigger points in muscles which happen to be situated in areas affected by pain from this, that become activated as a secondary phenomenon.

When the disc prolapse is of a lesser degree, myofascial trigger points, as mentioned previously, become activated as a primary event, and are responsible for pain being referred along the course of the sciatic nerve.

Radiographic examination

A plain X-ray of the spine is never of help in the diagnosis of acute disc prolapse because, as explained earlier, it always takes place at a time of life when disc degeneration is at an early stage, and therefore before there has been time for narrowing of the intervertebral space to take place.

One means of demonstrating a prolapsed disc radiographically is by performing a myelogram. As this investigation is occasionally associated with side-effects, it is at times difficult to interpret; and because, in the vast majority of cases of disc prolapse, the pain responds to conservative measures, it should only be carried out in those cases (approximately 10%) that prove refractory to this, in order to assess whether or not, a laminectomy might be helpful.

Formerly the contrast medium widely used in Britain and America was the iodized oil, iophendylate (Myodil; Pantopaque). Unfortunately this oil, even when completely removed following the examination, may give rise to an arachnoiditis, a cause of severe intractable pain. In recent years in the investigation of lumbar disc prolapse the contrast medium has been superseded by water soluble metrizamide. Metrizamide has so far been shown to be safe (Hansen et al 1976) and whereas oil myelography correctly predicts surgical findings in only 75–80% of cases, the water soluble contrast medium improves this to 90%.

It is essential to remember that myelography may have an up to 10% negative rate, and up to 10% false positive rate (Hansen et al 1976) and that therefore no decision concerning surgery can ever be made from the myelographic appearance alone, without at the same time taking into consideration the clinical findings. CAT scanning is now proving to be a more sensitive means of confirming the presence of this lesion (Haughton et al 1982).

Acute sciatica of the referred type

From what has been said it is clear that a confident diagnosis of disc prolapse with acute sciatica due to the entrapment of a nerve root can only be made with any degree of confidence when there are objective neurological signs including motor weakness followed later by muscle wasting; sensory impairment; and suppression of tendon reflexes; and particularly if, in addition, it is possible to obtain confirmatory evidence of nerve root compression electromyographically, and in cases where laminectomy is contemplated by the carrying out of a myelogram.

With most cases of acute sciatica, however, there is no neurological deficit and the pain is referred from trigger points in the muscles and ligaments of the lower back. King & Lagger (1976) believe that this occurs when a partially prolapsed disc impinges on the sinu-vertebral nerve causing the paravertebral muscles and adjacent ligaments innervated by posterior rami to go into acute spasm, with this, in turn, causing trigger points in these structures to become activated. The consequence of this to quote King & Lagger is that 'pain

impulses initiated in these posterior rami areas are referred to areas innervated by the anterior rami of the same and juxtaposed spinal roots'. In support of their hypothesis is their ability to alleviate this type of pain and at the same time to render negative the Lasègue's sign by interrupting this arc between the posterior rami, the cord, and the anterior rami, by deactivating these trigger points. It is only a pity that the methods they chose to use in order to achieve this were somewhat unnecessarily complicated and included radio-frequency percutaneous rhizotomy (Shealy et al 1974) and multiple bilateral percutaneous rhizolysis (Rees & Slade 1974).

The concept, however, that radiation of pain down the leg, in patients with low-back, is not necessarily due to nerve root entrapment and that sometimes it may occur as a result of it being referred down the leg from trigger points in the muscles and ligaments of the back, is not a recent one. It was first put forward by Steindler & Luck (1938), over 40 years ago, when they showed that it is possible to alleviate not only the pain in the back, but also the pain down the leg simply by injecting procaine into a trigger point in the lumbar region. It was their observations concerning this that led them to develop their procaine hydrochloride test for use in patients with both low-back and leg pain. The test consists of injecting procaine into a trigger point situated in a lumbar muscle or ligament in order to prove whether or not it is from that point that both the low-back and leg pain emanates. Such proof, according to them, required the following five postulates to be fulfilled:

1. The insertion of the needle into the trigger point must aggravate the local pain in the back.
2. It must also elicit or aggravate the pain referred down the leg.
3. The injection must suppress the referred pain.
4. The injection must suppress local tenderness.
5. Limited lumbar flexion or straight leg-raising must return to normal following the injection.

It is of course now recognized that with referred leg pain from trigger points in the back it is possible to fulfil these criteria of Steindler & Luck even more simply just by inserting an acupuncture needle into the appropriate point. This, however, in no way detracts from the importance of their work, and it is only very much to be regretted that until recent years such little attention has been paid to the basic principles propounded by them.

It is clear from what Steindler & Luck had to say on the subject that they believed that with most cases of sciatica of the referred type, the pain stems from trigger points activated by what they termed deep ligamentous injuries and myofasciitis, and the possibility, as suggested by King & Lagger, that such activation may also develop as a result of partial prolapse of a disc does not seem to have occurred to them.

There is not doubt that this type of referred pain may be produced by either of these means but, because for reasons already given, a prolapsed disc is somewhat of a rarity, the commonest cause would seem to be an acute primary strain of the muscles and ligaments.

Treatment of acute sciatica

With acute sciatica, irrespective of whether the pain is due to nerve root entrapment from a severe disc prolapse or occurs because of being referred along the sciatic nerve, either as the result of partial prolapse of a disc, or most commonly of all because of a primary muscle lesion, the sheet anchor of treatment is bed rest. The pain is usually so severe that there is no alternative but for this to be carried out or up to 3–6 weeks. And, in the vast majority of cases, no other form of treatment is required.

The important question, however, that has to be answered is whether any other form of treatment is likely to help ease the pain during this period of bed rest or even more importantly foreshorten the length of time for which it is required.

Analgesics

Some suitable analgesic such as a non-steroidal anti-inflammatory drug is often helpful.

Traction

The simplistic idea that the pain of acute sciatica can be relieved by taking pressure off the disc by widening the intervertebral foramen has for many years led to the use of traction in those cases in which bed rest alone does not appear to be affording relief. The weight applied is usually about 10–15 lb as anything heavier cannot be tolerated for long. This, however, is certainly not sufficient, for even when the weight is increased to 50–100 lb the effects on the spine seem only to be transient (Youel 1967, Mathews 1968). Finneson (1980) believes that the effects of traction are merely to 'alleviate the monotony of bed rest, and be of some psychological advantage in imparting to the patient a sense of active therapy'. Certainly it would seem that the treatment, whilst no doubt impressing the patient, is of very doubtful efficacy.

Corticosteroids

The marked inflammation and oedema around a compressed nerve root often observed whilst removing a prolapsed disc is the reason for using a corticosteroid during the initial conservative phase of treatment. This can either be injected extradurally (Yates 1978) or administered orally in the form of dexamethasone (Green 1975). Such treatment of course is only likely to be helpful when acute sciatica is due to nerve root entrapment and, as it takes time for the neurological signs of this to develop, it is not always possible soon after the onset of acute sciatica to pick out which cases in particular are likely to be suitable for this form of treatment. This is probably one of the reasons why, in practice, a small number of patients respond dramatically — some appear to obtain transitory relief — whilst others are not helped at all.

Acupuncture

Extremely tender trigger points, often coinciding with the motor points of muscles (Gunn & Milbrandt 1976), are frequently found in cases of acute sciatica, both when this is caused by nerve root entrapment and when it is of the referred type. Also, pressure on one of these trigger points, or the insertion of a needle into it, often evokes pain in the distribution of the spontaneously occurring pain; and the straight leg-raising test may be rendered negative by injecting trigger points with a local anaesthetic (Steindler & Luck 1938) or by inserting a dry needle into the tissues overlying them (Cailliet 1977a). These facts imply that acupuncture should be of benefit in alleviating this type of pain. And certainly it does seem clinically that with acute sciatica, where there is no neurological deficit, the use of acupuncture may well be helpful in giving some symptomatic relief, but as in such cases, bed rest is usually also necessary, it is very difficult to determine exactly how much acupuncture influences the outcome. As was said in discussing the response of acute low-back pain to acupuncture, in any clinical situation where fairly rapid spontaneous recovery is the rule, it is essential to guard against giving credit to some form of treatment undeservedly.

Acupuncture is also of use in those cases where persistent pain following a laminectomy is mainly due to the activation of myofascial trigger points but it is unlikely to be helpful where it is due to chronic irreversible nerve damage having taken place prior to the operation (p. 273). It is also of value in those cases where pain following a post-laminectomy spinal fusion is coming from activated myofascial trigger points.

Laminectomy

Laminectomy is obviously only likely to be of benefit when a disc has herniated sufficiently to exert pressure on a nerve root, and even then it should never be contemplated until 4–6 weeks of conservative treatment has failed to alleviate the pain, or until such a time as it becomes clear that repeated periods of conservative treatment are only giving relief from pain for short periods.

Rapid deterioration of neurological signs, however, will necessitate earlier intervention in order to exclude the possibility of an underlying spinal tumour. The rarer form of central protrusion with cauda equina compression, which gives rise to bilateral sciatic pain and involvement of the bladder, also requires urgent surgery.

The difficulties so often encountered in diagnosing nerve root entrapment from the usual posterolateral disc protrusion have already been touched upon when discussing the indications for and limitations of myelography. Physical signs

seem to be the most reliable guide to diagnosis. Matthews (1975) in discussing this goes so far as to say:

a myelogram is not essential and can be positively misleading but surgeons vary considerably in their requirements . . . no clear guidance can be given as I have watched experienced surgeons repeatedly surprised at both negative and positive findings.

The general consensus, however, would seem to be that, although a diagnosis of nerve root compression should be mainly clinical, a myelogram or CAT scan is helpful in so much as precise pre-operative localization is of considerable assistance to the surgeon.

It is also generally agreed that surgery should never be performed solely because pain fails to respond to conservative treatment. As Waddell (1982) said in referring to this 'because of pressure to "do something" there is a strong temptation to proceed to myelography and if that shows a bulge then the trap is complete and it is almost impossible to withhold the knife'. It is essential to regard nerve entrapment from a disc prolapse as a specific anatomical and pathological diagnosis based on clearly defined diagnostic criteria.

It is clear that this fundamental principle is not always strictly adhered to because for example as Loeser (1980) points out:

. . . 78% of the Labor and Industries sponsored patients with low-back pain in Washington State had no signs of nerve root entrapment, and yet 25% of the total group had surgery. Therefore a major fraction of the operations performed could not have been warranted.

Post-laminectomy pain syndrome

One of the main reasons for disc pain not being relieved by a laminectomy is because the operation is all too often carried out for sciatica of the referred type, but nevertheless, even when strict criteria for surgery are adhered to, there is no certainty that removal of the disc will alleviate the pain. Spangfort (1972) in a review of the results of 2504 laminectomies selected for surgery because of clear-cut neurological signs of nerve root entrapment found that complete relief of both leg and back pain occurred in only 60% of cases.

Failure to relieve pain in those with nerve root entrapment is usually attributed to one or other of the following causes:

— the exploration being carried out at the wrong site
— a second disc prolapse being overlooked;
— the nerve root continuing to be compressed by the posterior intervertebral joints
— spinal stenosis causing pressure on the nerve root
— or, rarely, because of an extraforaminal lateral disc herniation (Nelson1980).

It may also be due to chronic irreversible nerve damage having developed (p. 273) prior to the operation being carried out (Wynn Parry 1989).

What, however, is not sufficiently recognized is that pain in the back and down the leg that persists in spite of successful decompression of a nerve root often emanates from myofascial trigger points. Certainly in all such cases referred to me there have been readily identifiable trigger points, and, with most of them, repeated deactivation of these points by the acupuncture technique of dry needle stimulation at weekly intervals for a varying number of weeks has eventually brought the pain under control.

It would seem that these trigger points may become activated either before the operation, or as a direct result of it.

Loeser (1980), in recognizing that surgical trauma may sometimes be the cause of post-laminectomy pain, suggests that microsurgical techniques might help to reduce the incidence of this. Any operation by temporarily damaging the tissues is liable to give rise to short-term pain, but one of the reasons for it becoming persistent in my opinion is that iatrogenically induced trauma activates trigger points. Certainly it is not uncommon in cases of persistent pain following spine surgery to find exquisitely tender trigger points in the midline scar as well as in the muscles of the lower back.

There is also no doubt that myofascial trigger points which have become activated preoperatively, as result of them being situated in areas of the back and leg affected by the pain of nerve root entrapment, are likely to remain active and therefore likely to continue to cause pain long after

the nerve root has been satisfactorily decompressed (Travell & Simons 1983b). And what is particularly confusing is that the pattern of distribution of this pain is similar to that of the original radicular pain.

It is obvious that when radicular compression is so severe as to necessitate an operation to relieve it that any attempt to deactivate myofascial trigger points preoperatively is not likely to have any lasting effect but nevertheless, it is always worthwhile making a note of their distribution at that stage in order to ensure that their presence is not overlooked and that they get deactivated after the disc has been removed should persistent pain continue to be a problem.

It has to be remembered that trigger point activation is not only an important cause of musculoskeletal pain but is also responsible for generalized muscle stiffness. This stiffness commonly affects the muscles of the lower back, both before and after disc surgery, and must be an important factor in causing pain postoperatively to persist, because by restricting normal movements of the back, it interferes with the important low-threshold mechanoreceptors A-beta nerve fibre-pain modulating mechanism responsible for 'closing the dorsal horn gate' (see Ch. 6). It is for this reason that Rubin (1981) stresses how important it is with the post-laminectomy pain syndrome not only to deactivate trigger points but also to overcome this muscle stiffness by stretching the muscles and applying a vapocoolant spray to them.

The following case shows how failure to recognize the importance of trigger points as a source of post-laminectomy pain nearly resulted in the patient being subjected to a spinal fusion.

A housewife (41), after 3 months of much heavy lifting while nursing her husband, developed acute low-back pain and was put into a plaster jacket for 2 months. Three years later she had a similar episode of pain but this settled spontaneously fairly quickly. Six months later, however, she developed acute sciatica for which she was kept in bed for 10 weeks. Even so the pain persisted. As there were objective neurological signs and a positive myelogram, her back was explored and a badly prolapsed disc removed.

Whilst being mobilized postoperatively, widespread pain in the back and leg recurred and she was advised to have an opeation to 'strengthen' her spine. On refusing this she was discharged home. Her general practitioner then referred her to me for assessment as to whether acupuncture might help. There were readily identifiable trigger points in the midline scar; also, scattered throughout the muscles of the lower back on the affected side, along the iliotibial tract, and around the external malleolus at the ankle.

Deactivation of these with a dry needle on several occasions at weekly intervals eventually brought much of the widespread aching type of pain under control. She was, however, left with a persistent burning sensation in the calf. Myelography was once again carried out and this showed evidence of some residual nerve root entrapment.

Spinal fusion

When pain due to a prolapsed disc is not relieved by laminectomy it is not uncommon to attempt to provide structural support for the spine by means of fusing together several vertebrae. The results of this operation in such circumstances have however been very disappointing leading Loeser (1980) somewhat tersely to remark:

the greatest folly of all in the management of low-back pain is the use of fusion of the vertebrae in the absence of demonstrated instability due to a congenital or acquired lesion. There simply is no good evidence that fusion is ever beneficial to the patient with only a herniated lumbar disc; there is considerable evidence that it may be deleterious. Why patients are subjected to a major operative procedure with no evidence of efficacy is beyond my comprehension.

There can be not doubt that one of the major disadvantages of the operation is that by rendering the spine rigid it seriously interferes with the low-threshold mechanoreceptor pain inhibiting mechanism (Ch. 6), as the action of the latter is entirely dependent on an ability to carry out normal movements. Also, the rigidity of the back seems to put an abnormal strain on the paravertebral muscles and this in itself must encourage the activation of myofascial trigger points. In addition, it is not uncommon to find iatrogenically induced trigger points in the midline surgical scar.

Patients who have come under my care with persistent pain in spite of having had a spinal fusion following failed laminectomy, have not unnaturally been very depressed, particularly as most of them have been told that other than the long-term use of analgesics there is nothing more that can be done. Each one without exception, however, has been found on examination to have readily demonstrable trigger points and it has been possible to improve the quality of life by repeatedly deactivating these points with a dry needle. Unfortunately, and probably mainly because of the mechanical disadvantage to which the operation puts the spine, the pain relief from acupuncture is seldom long-lasting and the necessity of having to continue with treatment on a long-term basis has to be explained to the patient at the outset in order to avoid any undue disappointment.

In conclusion, it has to be said that when pain persists following a laminectomy it is firstly essential to ascertain that it is not due to residual nerve root compression, but once this has been excluded, it is better to attempt to alleviate the pain by the acupuncture technique of deactivating trigger points rather than to embark on a spinal fusion which leaves the spine permanently rigid and rarely relieves the pain.

CHRONIC MECHANICAL TYPE LOW-BACK PAIN

The pathogenesis of chronic mechanical type low-back pain is poorly understood, and as a consequence of this both the manner in which the condition is investigated, and its treatment are far from satisfactory (Flor & Turk 1984, Turk & Flor 1984). The greatest obstacle to the rational treatment of chronic low-back pain is the difficulty of deciding in any particular case the primary source of the pain. The main possibilities are that the pain comes either from degenerative changes in the intervertebral discs and facet joints, or from a disorder of the muscle. Each of these will therefore be considered in turn.

Pain arising from degenerative changes in the intervertebral discs and facet joints

There can be no doubt that degenerative changes in the spine are potentially capable of causing low-back pain for, as Wyke (1987a) has pointed out, the structures in the vicinity of the spine in which nociceptive receptor systems are present include the spinal ligaments, the periosteum, the duramater, the walls of the blood vessels, and also the fibrous capsules of the facet joints.

It is generally believed that the degenerative changes in the spine start first in the discs, and that it is the reduction in the vertical height of the lumbar spine occurring as a result of this that encourages the development of arthritic changes in the facet joints (Vernon-Roberts & Pirie 1977). It should be noted, however, that disc degeneration itself cannot be responsible for pain as there are no nerve endings either in the nucleus pulposus or the annulus fibrosus. It can therefore only occur once degenerative changes in the facet joints lead to the stimulation of the nociceptive receptor system in their capsules.

Hirsch et al (1963) were among the first to show that the facet joint is a potential source of chronic back pain by showing that pain in the back and leg can be artificially induced by injecting 11% hypertonic saline around it.

Mooney & Robertson (1975) studied the matter more specifically by injecting 5% hypertonic saline into a facet joint in 5 normal individuals and 15 patients with chronic pain in the back and leg. They first ensured that the needle was directly in the joint by means of inserting it under fluoroscopic control and then injected sufficient contrast medium into the joint to outline its capsule. In each case, within about 5 seconds of injecting the hypertonic saline, pain was felt in the lower back, and within 20 seconds, this had increased in intensity and had spread to the greater trochanter and down the posterolateral part of the thigh. Such pain patterns however are in no way specific. Similar ones have been produced, as discussed in Chapter 4, by Kellgren, and also by Inman & Saunders, by injecting hypertonic saline into muscles and ligaments, and the possibility cannot be excluded that Mooney & Robertson's hypertonic saline did not remain confined to the facet joints, and, by diffusing into the tissues, it may have also stimulated other structures in the vicinity.

Fairbank et al (1981) have also studied the effects of injecting a local anaesthetic into facet joints for the purpose of ascertaining whether or not this procedure might act as a diagnostic aid. In their study, 25 adults suffering for the first time from severe low-back pain, were given an injection into a facet joint under X-ray control. The facet joints selected for injection were situated at points of maximum tenderness. Their results were that 14 obtained immediate relief (the responders) and 11 did not (the non-responders). They concluded that this might suggest that the responders had pain of mechanical origin possibly arising in the facet joint, and that the non-responders' pain may have originated from one of the many other possible sources in the back.

The reason for their conclusions being so tentative was that they were aware that the anaesthetic may not have remained confined to the facet joint but may have diffused out into the tissues to involve the nerve root or the posterior primary ramus, and that this in turn may have affected other structures with a common innervation. It is of course possible that by using points of maximum tenderness for their injections that the anaesthetic was acting on nerve endings at trigger points because, for as they admitted, Lewit (1979) had alleviated pain of this type simply by inserting dry needles into such points.

It may therefore be seen that various experimental studies aimed at showing whether or not facet joints are an important source of low-back pain have been somewhat inconclusive, and certainly observations by pathologists and above all by radiologists, would seem to suggest that the widely-held view that chronic mechanical type low-back pain, from middle age onwards, is mainly due to degenerative changes in the lumbar discs and facet joints, is almost certainly erroneous.

It was in 1932 that Schmorl & Junghanns, from their classic autopsy studies of over 4000 spines, established that degenerative changes in the lumbar spine are present in 50% of the population by the end of the 4th decade, in 70% at the end of the 5th decade, and in 90% at the age of 70. And since then, numerous comparative studies by radiologists have shown that the radiographic features of disc degeneration including the narrowing of intervertebral spaces, osteophyte formation, disc calcification, and Schmorl's nodes, as well as those of facet joint arthrosis, are found as commonly in asymptomatic controls as they are in those with low-back pain (Splithoff 1952, Hult 1954, Hussar & Guller 1956, Horal 1969, Magora & Schwartz 1976).

Furthermore, there is also no evidence to suggest that the intensity of lumbar pain is in direct proportion to the amount of degenerative changes seen on a radiograph. It is not uncommon for a person with only slight changes to have severe pain; and conversely for a person with advanced changes to be symptomless.

It would therefore seem that whilst degenerative changes in the spine may make some contribution towards the development of chronic low-back pain there is no direct correlation between the two, and in everyday clinical practice it would seem important not to assume just because there is radiographic evidence of disc and facet joint degeneration that this is necessarily the cause of the pain, as often this is not more than a chance investigatory finding in someone whose pain can be shown to be primarily muscular in origin. Waddell (1982), with considerable wisdom, comments,

the case for degenerative disc disease as the explanation of backache must still be regarded as not proven. It is important to treat patients and not X-rays of spines.

Pain primarily of muscular and ligamentous origin

Those currently responsible for teaching medicine, when considering the causes of mechanical type low-back pain, tend to dismiss pain of muscular origin as being of little or no consequence, and hardly worthy of their attention. This is no doubt, in part, due to the pathology of the underlying condition continuing to remain so singularly elusive; but also because, now that it is generally agreed that it is not of an inflammatory nature, and that therefore, diagnoses such as fibrositis and myofasciitis, are no longer acceptable, there is even difficulty in knowing what to call the condition!

Everyday clinical experience, however, leads me to agree with Wyke (1987b) that irritation of the nociceptive receptor system in the lumbar muscles, their fascial sheaths, their tendinous insertions, and in the ligaments of the spine is a common cause of chronic low-back pain. This occurs either directly as a result of various factors to be discussed (p. 269) acting locally on the muscle or ligaments, or indirectly, as a result of anxiety causing them to be held in a state of persistent tension. There can be no doubt that mechanical type low-back pain that is primarily muscular in origin is frequently both severe and incapacitating; and it may affect not only adults but also children (Bates & Grunwald 1958, Grantham 1977). It is however reasonable to suppose that the nociceptive receptor system in lumbar muscles may also become irritated as a result of pain from a degenerative lesion in the spine causing them to go into spasm.

Trigger points

Careful examination of the lumbar muscles and the supraspinous ligament in someone with chronic mechanical type low-back pain, irrespective of whether the pain is primarily from degenerative changes in the spine, or is primarily muscular in origin, reveals the presence of focal points of exquisite tenderness. In the lower back these points may be found in muscle that otherwise feels normal but often they are present in palpable bands or fibrositic nodules that develop in the substance of the muscles. And of particular significance is the fact that pressure applied to these points exacerbates any pain felt locally in the back, and at times causes pain to radiate down the leg in the same distribution as that occurring spontaneously. This of course is no recent observation for, as explained earlier, Kellgren first drew attention to the significance of 'tender spots' in muscles as progenitors of musculoskeletal pain nearly half a century ago, and once Janet Travell shortly after this, for obvious reasons, called them trigger points she and others have written extensively about them.

Unfortunately, when the idea that trigger points might be an important source of low-back pain was first put forward, the climate of opinion was against it due to the medical profession in the Western world at that time being firmly wedded to the belief that acute 'lumbago' and sciatica are principally caused by the prolapse of an intervertebral disc, and that chronic 'lumbago' and sciatica occur as a result of degenerative changes in the discs and facet joints.

This for many years was to remain one of the deeply entrenched beliefs of medical orthodoxy. It is therefore very much to the credit of St Claire Strange that in his Presidential address to the section of orthopaedics of the Royal Society of Medicine, London, in 1966, he had the boldness to question the validity of this view by stating that whilst he had no doubt that such lesions may at times be the cause of low-back pain, he was certain from his everyday clinical experience that they were not the only ones, and that, in investigating such pain, more attention should be paid to examining the muscles for points of maximum tenderness in what he termed 'muscle bundles in spasm' that are, 'sometimes "as slender as the shaft of a pin" and at other times "as thick as a pencil" ' or in other words to look for what today would be called trigger points in palpable bands. His insistence on the importance of such an examination stemmed from his belief that it is from these structures that much of the pain emanates, for, as he said, when you press on one of these tender spots 'the patient knows you have "found the spot", found the site of the pain from which he is complaining. And you can see it in his face'.

Since the 1930s, therefore, a succession of people have drawn attention to the importance of trigger points in the aetiology of musculoskeletal pain including that which affects the lower back, and yet those currently engaged in research into the problems of low-back pain still pay scant attention to them. There is, for example, no reference to these structures, either in the first, second or third edition of such an authoritative textbook as *The Lumbar Spine and Back Pain* (Jayson 1976, 1980, 1987); or in the report of the Working Group on Back Pain set up by the Department of Health in 1979.

However, now that such leading authorities on the neurophysiology of pain as Melzack & Wall (1982) have come to recognize the importance of trigger points in the genesis of musculoskeletal pain in general, those engaged in investigating and managing chronic mechanical type low-back pain can no longer afford to ignore the part played by these structures in its development.

In view of this and because our understanding concerning the various mechanisms responsible for chronic mechanical type low-back pain remains so limited, it seems to me that rather than continuing to use some of the currently fashionable diagnostic terms such as lumbar 'arthritis' or 'spondylitis', the specificity of which implies a certainty concerning the underlying pathological cause of this type of pain that is seldom justified, it would be better to employ a more non-commital term, but one that nevertheless emphasizes the importance of trigger points in its pathogenesis. The term suggested is the chronic lumbar myofascial trigger point pain syndrome.

Chronic lumbar myofascial trigger point pain syndrome

There is, as yet, no adequate explanation as to why some people more than others are prone to activate trigger points in their lumbar muscles, and for this reason to be particularly liable to suffer from chronic low-back pain. Certainly there is no definite evidence that structural disorders of the spine make any significant contribution to this. Admittedly it is theoretically possible for myofascial trigger points to become activated as a result of structural disorders of the spine causing the lumbar muscles to go into spasm, but, as has already been discussed, so far as degenerative changes are concerned, a number of well-controlled studies have failed to show any direct relationship between the presence of radiographically observable degenerative changes in the discs and facet joints, and the development of intermittently recurrent low-back pain.

There is in addition no definite evidence that other structural disorders such as sacralization of the spine, spondylolisthesis, or various abnormal curvatures of the spine are associated with the activation of trigger points. It has, for example, been generally assumed that the abnormal fusion that sometimes occurs between the 5th lumbar vertebra and the sacrum — so-called sacralization of the spine — is a cause of chronic low-back pain but Magora & Schwartz (1978) from their extensive survey were unable to confirm this.

Similarly, although the forward shift of one vertebra or another — so-called spondylolisthesis

— has been said to contribute to the development of chronic low-back pain, the evidence for this is conflicting with some observers such as Hult (1954), Horal (1969), and Torgerson & Dotter (1976) supporting this belief, but with others, including Splithoff (1952) and Rowe (1965), being unable to demonstrate such a relationship.

Furthermore, although congenital or acquired abnormalities such as scoliosis, kyphosis, exaggerated lordosis, and spina bifida occulta have all been assumed to cause chronic low-back pain, several studies including those of Hult (1954), Horal (1969), Torgerson & Dotter (1976), and Magora & Schwartz (1978) have failed to confirm this.

Before leaving the subject of the possible activation of trigger points in response to structural disorders in the spine, the following observations will be made concerning the most common of these, namely degenerative changes in the discs and facet joints.

Myofascial trigger points are to be found in every case of mechanical type low-back pain but in those cases, where degenerative changes are demonstrable radiographically, there is no correlation between the number of trigger points present and the amount of degenerative change in the spine; furthermore, distribution of the trigger points in the back often bears no relationship to the part of the spine affected by degenerative changes; and when one comes to consider the treatment of low-back pain by the acupuncture technique of dry needling trigger points, experience shows that it is wrong to assume that the chances of a good response diminish in proportion to the amount of degenerative disease present. On the contrary, a patient with little or no degenerative changes in the spine may, for reasons to be discussed later, have a poor response to this type of treatment, whereas conversely a patient with advanced degenerative disease may respond well.

A woman (89), who had had episodes of low-back pain since the age of 35, and had experienced severe pain in the left buttock for a year, asked her doctor if she might try acupuncture, only to be told that this would be a waste of time as the X-ray of her lumbar spine showed that the pain was due to severe arthritis. However, she finally got her own way! And,

on examination, there were only two trigger points to be found, which were in muscles situated in the postero-inferior part of the chest wall at the level of the 10th and 11th ribs. The pain in the buttock must clearly have been referred from these (Fig. 15.3) as it disappeared after deactivating them with a dry needle on only two occasions. Following this she remained free from pain for 18 months in spite of the advanced 'arthritic changes' in the spine.

It is from having had a similarly good response to acupuncture in a large number of cases of chronic low-back pain with equally advanced degenerative changes on X-rays of the spine, that leads me to believe that such changes in the discs and facet joints are often no more than a chance radiographic finding in someone whose pain is primarily due to the activation of trigger points by factors acting directly on the muscles themselves.

Those who treat chronic low-back pain by manipulating the spine might not agree with this but, nevertheless, it would seem reasonable to postulate that any success they may have with this form of treatment may be due more to their manipulative procedures exerting traction on muscles than to any effect these procedures may have on the spine itself. This would certainly be in keeping with Travell's observation (1968) that it is possible to inactivate myofascial trigger points by passively stretching affected muscles.

Moreover, it has to be admitted that this belief that chronic low-back pain is possible mainly due to the primary activation of trigger points in muscles is entirely at variance with the views of Nachemson (1980a) who has spent very many years carrying out research into this subject, and who as a result puts more emphasis on degenerative processes in the discs as being the principal cause.

His work has included the use of an ingeniously contrived miniaturized pressure transducer with which he has been able to measure the pressure on the intervertebral disc, and to calculate the approximate loads exerted on the lumbar spine during the course of commonly performed movements. He, together with others, has also studied biological and biochemical changes in the discs and has shown that avascularity and a defective diffusion mechanism are conducive to early degeneration of both the annulus fibrosus and nucleus pulposus, and further that this process is likely to be accelerated by the considerable mechanical forces intermittently imposed upon these structures. Their contention is that it is a combination of progressive degenerative changes in the disc, together with tensile stresses exerted on the posterior part of the annulus fibrosus that renders the latter vulnerable to becoming ruptured, and that when this occurs it is possible that various chemicals, including lactic acid and histamine-like substances, leak into the surrounding tissues and by stimulating nearby nociceptive receptor systems give rise to pain.

Nevertheless, all those engaged in such work are agreed that it still lies in the realm of speculation and as Nachemson (1980b), in spite of years of work investigating chronic low-back pain, so honestly admits,

it is pertinent to remember that with most of our patients we are uncertain of the true cause of this pain, and that present day methods of treatment suffer from this lack of knowledge.

This undoubtedly being true, it is only possible for me as a physician to express my views concerning the aetiology of chronic low-back pain in a tentative manner, and with the only justification for expressing them at all being that they are based on my own personal everyday clinical observations, and supported by those of others with a similar approach to the subject. It is therefore necessary now to turn to various physical and psychological factors which, because of their ability to activate trigger points, seem to me to have considerable importance in the causation of low-back pain.

Physical and psychological factors capable of activating myofascial trigger points

Some of the physical factors capable of activating myofascial trigger points in the lumbar muscles include, as Travell & Simons (1983c) point out, the sudden overloading of the muscles as when lifting objects whilst in an awkward position such as with the back twisted and flexed; or when, for one or another reason, they are subjected to sustained overloading, as may occur during the pursuit of athletic activities, or at work, particularly when this involves much heavy lifting, or stooping, or

the adoption of awkward standing or sitting postures.

Surgeons should also note that the putting of patients into unusual postures such as the Trendelenburg or lithotomy positions for prolonged periods, particularly when the muscles are particularly relaxed due to the effects of a general anaesthetic, is liable to cause the activation of myofascial trigger points with the development of chronic postoperative low-back pain.

Magora (1970), who has extensively investigated the relationship between low-back pain and occupational factors has found that this type of pain is more frequent in those whose work forces them to sit for prolonged periods, than in those who constantly move about. And that heavy lifting, particularly when this is only occasional, is a frequent cause of this type of pain. He also found that low-back pain occurs with about the same frequency in those with sedentary occupations as in those doing heavy labour, but the sedentary worker's symptoms come on more after weekend athletic activities.

It is interesting to note, too, that although he found a high incidence of absence from work amongst manual workers because of the pain preventing them from carrying out their duties, the incidence of back pain correlated best with how physically demanding workers perceived their work to be rather than how objectively demanding it was. And as he pointed out, its incidence is also more closely related to whether there are psychological problems at the workplace or at home rather than to objective physical factors. Westrin (1973) has also recently studied low-back pain and concluded that its incidence is especially high in those not happy with their job situation, or who are divorced, or have problems with alcohol.

This therefore leads to a consideration of psychological factors which so far as chronic low-back pain is concerned seem to be of particular importance as trigger point activators. Turk & Flor (1984) state that 'chronic back pain is increasingly viewed as a psychophysiological and psychosocial problem stemming from the interaction of physical, psychological and social factors'. It has in fact to be accepted that the condition is often multifactorial and this reflects itself in its treatment which not infrequently has to include therapeutic procedures directed both to the mind and the body.

There is a large group of patients who hold the muscles of their scalp, neck, or lower back in a state of persistent tension in response to nervous strain, and as discussed on pages 55 and 76, this leads to the activation of trigger points in these muscles with, as a result, of this, the development of either persistent headaches, or chronic pain in the neck, or chronic low-back pain, or a combination of these.

Some people come to recognize that their attacks of pain coincide with times of particular stress. One young executive, for example, told me that public speaking terrified him, and that his low-back pain always came on about 2 weeks before having to address a business conference. Others can date the onset of recurrent low-back pain to some specific time when they were subjected to some particularly distressing experience. One housewife, for example, told me that her attacks of neck and low-back pain started the year that both her husband and only daughter died within 6 months of each other.

It obviously cannot be assumed that either an anxiety state or an agitated depressive one (reactive depression), occurring in association with chronic low-back pain, has necessarily contributed to the development of this, because often such mood changes develop some months after the onset of the pain, and in such circumstances have to be considered to have arisen as a result of it.

It is important to realize that so-called psychological low-back pain is in reality psychosomatic because, as he already been explained, there are almost invariably trigger points to be found in the muscles usually in the form of foci of maximum tenderness in palpable bands or 'fibrositic' nodules. This has considerable diagnostic and therapeutic implications because when an overtly anxious person with low-back pain is found to have no abnormality on X-rays of the spine, no evidence of disease in the pelvis, and the trigger points in the muscles, as all too often happens, are overlooked, there is a tendency for the assumption to be made that the pain must be entirely psychological in origin, and for the patient concerned to be referred to a psychiatrist. This, in my experience, is rarely helpful, not because of any lack of expertise on the part of the latter but because in such a case it does not matter how much psychotherapy is given, it will in no way influence the course of the pain unless at the same time the trigger points are deactivated. The converse, however, is also true, that when psychological factors contribute to low-back pain no amount of trigger point deactivation by acupuncture or by any other means will give any lasting relief from the pain, unless at the same time some form of therapy is given to reduce the nervous tension.

It is my belief that, whenever possible, it is preferable for the patient to receive both these forms of treatment from the same physician, and it is for this reason that the patients with psychosomatic low-back pain under my care receive from me a combination of hypnotherapy and acupuncture.

An even more serious error, and one which not infrequently occurs because of a general lack of understanding concerning the significance of trigger points, and therefore a failure to look for them, is to conclude that a patient with normal X-ray appearances of the lumbar spine is in need of psychological help, or even is frankly malingering, when in fact the pain is entirely of organic origin.

An example of this is that of a housewife who at the age of 35 was referred to an orthopaedic surgeon because of persistent low-back pain, only to be told that the pain could not be coming from her back because the X-ray of her spine was normal. She was then referred to a gynaecologist, who finding no abnormality on physical examination, carried out a dilatation and curettage. This operation was complicated 10 days later by a near fatal pulmonary infarct. The patient then continued to be quite markedly incapacitated by persistent pain for another 2–3 years, and, as during this time certain marital difficulties had arisen, it was assumed that the pain must be of psychological origin and she was referred to a psychiatrist. It was very much to his credit that he frankly admitted he could find no psychiatric cause for the pain, and the patient in desperation then asked her doctor whether she could try acupuncture.

On examination, there were some trigger points in quite enormous, exquisitely tender fibrositic nodules and palpable bands. Once these trigger points had been deactivated with a dry needle at weekly intervals on four occasions, she obtained lasting relief from pain for the first time for many years.

It has to be admitted that some people, whose low-back pain has occurred as a result of injury at work or in a traffic accident, and who are claiming compensation for this, do exaggerate their symptoms. Unfortunately, however, a litigant is sometimes unjustifiably assumed to be doing this, often for no better reason than that the X-ray of the spine is normal, when a careful examination of the back would show a sound physical basis for the pain in the form of activated trigger points in the muscles.

A self-employed heating engineer, very anxious to keep his business going but unable to do so because of persistent low-back pain following a car accident, very much resented being told by an orthopaedic surgeon that his symptoms would not improve until his claim for compensation had been settled, particularly as when he eventually decided to try acupuncture, it only required dry needle stimulation of trigger points to be carried out on three occasions before his pain was sufficiently alleviated for him to return to quite hard physical work.

Finally, before leaving the subject of the influence of psychological factors on chronic low-back pain, it has to be said that, in my experience, acupuncture often fails to relieve this type of pain in those who because of long-standing neuroticism persistently hold their lumbar muscles in a state of tension, and similarly is rarely helpful in those who develop low-back pain as a manifestation of conversion hysteria in order to escape from seemingly intolerable domestic, marital or occupational obligations.

A prison officer, who had complained of low-back pain for many years, was finally persuaded by his general practitioner to come to me for treatment with acupuncture. During the course of taking the history it seemed obvious that for some time he had found the pain to be extremely useful to him in so much that it enabled him to avoid some of the more arduous duties associated with his job. It therefore came as no surprise to me when after two sessions he failed to attend for any further treatment. He told his doctor that this was because the treatment had made him worse but almost certainly it was because, perhaps unknowingly, he was afraid it might eventually make him better!

CHRONIC SCIATICA

As acute sciatica has already been dealt with earlier in this chapter, it now remains necessary to consider pain that is similar in distribution but which has a more insidious onset and takes a more protracted course. This chronic type of sciatica always requires to be extensively investigated as it is essential to exclude any form of underlying malignant disease, degenerative spondylolithesis, central spinal stenosis or lateral root canal stenosis.

When the pain is due to long-term compression of a nerve root by a disc, there is usually well-marked evidence of weakness and wasting of leg muscles. This however is not necessarily so because at times myelography and subsequent surgery somewhat surprisingly reveal the presence of a prolapsed disc of sufficient size to cause nerve entrapment without there having been any objective evidence of this on clinical examination.

In most cases, however, in which there are no neurological signs of nerve root compression, the pain is of the referred type, and occurs as the result of the primary activation of trigger points in the muscles of the lower back. As chronic sciatica, when due to this, is likely to respond well to acupuncture, it will be discussed in detail.

Chronic sciatica occurring as a result of the referral of pain from lumbar myofascial trigger points

The narrowing of the gap between adjacent vertebrae, that occurs as a result of degenerative changes in the intervertebral discs, leads to a loss of alignment and abnormal movements in the facet joints and because of this to the development of arthritic changes in these joints. As stated earlier, it could be argued that it is the stimulation of the nociceptive receptor system in the capsules of these joints when they become arthritic that is the cause of pain in the back and down the leg. This is not a new concept for, as long ago as 1941, Badgley put forward the idea that facet joint degeneration can be a cause of chronic sciatica. Then more recently, Rees (1971) and Rees & Slade (1974), believing that a displaced intervertebral disc leads to mechanical derangement of the facet joints and that it is this that is the cause of sciatica, tried to alleviate such pain by attempting to denervate these joints with a scalpel. However, because this procedure is liable to cause much uncontrolled bleeding, Shealy et al (1974) decided to alleviate the pain by denervating the facet joints with a temperature controlled radio-frequency cautery.

Both of these techniques achieved their purpose, but, as King & Lagger (1976) have shown, they did so for entirely different reasons to those put forward by either Rees or Shealy. King & Lagger's views on the subject are based on observations made during the course of a prospective study of 60 patients with chronic sciatica, and who, in addition, had readily identifiable trigger points in muscles in the paravertebral gutter. They divided the 60 patients into three groups. One group was treated in a manner similar to that employed by Shealy et al, that is to say at a point of maximum tenderness, or trigger point, an electrode was inserted, under radiographic control, into the part of the facet joint where the posterior ramus is located, proximal to the branch that innervates the joint. They then proceeded to denervate the joint by applying a radio-frequency cautery to the posterior ramus for 2 minutes at 80°C.

The second group was treated in a manner similar to that used by Rees but using a cautery rather than a knife; at a point of maximum tenderness, or trigger point, an electrode was inserted into the tissues for a distance of $1\frac{1}{4}$", it having been established that this was the depth reached by the blade used by Rees. They then applied heat to the tissues at that site in exactly the same manner as with the first group. The heat-induced lesion was clearly some distance from the facet joint and essentially its effect was to destroy the trigger point.

With the third group, which served as a control, the treatment consisted of inserting an electrode into the tissues some distance from a trigger point, and then applying a stimulating rather than a coagulating current.

The result of this controlled experiment was that, of the patients in the first group treated by having posterior primary rami destroyed, 72%

obtained immediate pain relief, and of the patients in the second group, treated by having trigger points destroyed, 71% achieved this.

From this study, King & Lagger came to the conclusion that chronic referred sciatic pain, like acute referred sciatic pain, already discussed (p. 260), occurs as a result of nociceptive impulses being generated in myofascial trigger points, and then being conducted along posterior primary rami to the cord, and from there to areas innervated by the anterior primary rami of the same and juxtaposed spinal roots. They put forward the idea that the activation of these trigger points occurs because of muscle spasm developing as a result of the acute rupture or chronic degeneration of an intervertebral disc, but from what is known about the activation of myofascial trigger points in general, it would seem rasonable to suppose that this activation occurs even more frequently as a primary event in response to one or other of various factors acting directly on the muscles.

It is interesting to note that although 72% of the group that underwent cauterization of the posterior primary rami achieved immediate pain relief, only 27% were still free from pain at follow-up 6 months later. This is as one might expect because it is now known that all forms of nerve destruction have the disadvantage that they are based 'on a unidimensional, sensory model of pain pathways and pain transmission ... and disregard the multidimensionality of the pain experience, and especially the importance of pain inhibition via afferent stimulation' (Flor & Turk 1984).

By contrast, of those in the second group, treated by destroying trigger points by means of heat coagulation, 71% experienced initial relief and at the end of 6 months this had only fallen to 53%. The second of these two methods is therefore to be preferred as at least it leaves the sensory nervous system intact, but nevertheless it necessitates using a somewhat sophisticated type of apparatus for the purpose. Fortunately, there are good reasons for believing that similar results may be obtained simply by deactivating the trigger points by the far more straightforward non-destructive technique of inserting dry needles into the tissues overlying them.

The importance of distinguishing between nocigenic and neurogenic chronic low-back and leg pain

It is important to realize that the insidious development of combined low-back and 'sciatic-type' leg pain may be either nocigenic or neurogenic or a mixture of both. For all too long there has been a belief that pain in this distribution, particularly when it is accompanied by restricted straight leg raising, must be due to nerve root entrapment. However, from what has already been said and as will be seen when trigger point pain referral patterns from individual muscles in the lower back are considered, it is evident that chronic 'sciatica', even when it is associated with restricted straight leg raising, may be entirely nocigenic and occur as the result of the primary activation of myofascial trigger points. At the same time, it has to be clearly understood that myofascial trigger points may become activated as a secondary event in areas affected by pain from nerve root entrapment.

It therefore follows that in all cases a systematic search for trigger points is essential. Also, in those cases where the history or physical signs suggest that the pain might be neurogenic, further investigations, including plain radiography, computed axial tomography (CAT scanning), myelography and in certain cases electromyographic studies should be carried out.

Pain in this distribution occurring as the result of the primary activation of myofascial trigger points is readily relieved by acupuncture. If, however, there is any suggestion that the pain might be due to nerve root entrapment then it is better not to embark upon acupuncture until this has been fully investigated. The reasons for this are that, should nerve root entrapment be present, not only will the deactivation of trigger points with dry needles do no more than temporarily alleviate the pain, but also the longer the nerve root remains compressed the more likely is it to become irreversibly damaged so that even if surgical decompression is eventually carried out, the operation may not relieve the pain.

Wynn Parry (1989) has recently reviewed experimental studies carried out by various people over the past fifteen years showing that compression of a nerve ultimately leads to the development of irreversible pain-producing degenerative changes both in the nerve itself and in the central nervous system. As he points out, it is this peripheral and central damage that is the main reason for surgery failing to relieve symptoms from nerve root compression and why, when this happens, further operations are also doomed to failure.

As, therefore, it is essential to be able to recognize the clinical manifestations of the various causes of chronic nerve root entrapment in the lower back these will now be considered.

Spondylolisthesis

Spondylolisthesis, the forward displacement of a vertebra relative to the one below it, may either be congenital or acquired. The diagnosis and management of five separate types have recently been reviewed by Nelson (1987) but only the degenerative type which affects adults from the age of 40 onwards will be discussed.

Symptoms and signs

Degenerative spondylolisthesis affects mainly females and occurs predominately at the L 4/5 level. The back pain is aggravated by activity, relieved by resting and is commonly made worse by standing. The pain in the leg is in the distribution of a nerve root with physical examination revealing the presence of a motor and sensory deficit. In addition, bilateral paraesthesiae and muscle weakness may be present in those cases in which degenerative changes have led to the development of spinal stenosis.

Investigations

Plain radiography, myelography and CAT scanning are necessary in order to confirm the diagnosis.

Treatment

Conservative treatment may be all that is necessary in mild cases, but surgery is required for the relief of severe pain with evidence of nerve root compression.

Spinal stenosis

Eisenstein (1977), from a comparison of negro and caucasoid skeletons, showed that it is when a congenitally narrowed spinal canal becomes further narrowed as a result of the development of degenerative changes in the posterior facet joints that symptoms develop. The clinical manifestations depend on whether the stenosis is of the central canal, or of the lateral root canal.

Central canal stenosis (neurogenic claudication)

The patient, usually a middle-aged male, gives a long history of low-back pain and a more recent one of a vice-like claudication type pain with feelings of numbness, tingling and heaviness affecting one or both legs. The pain, as when due to vascular disease, is brought on by walking and relieved

a

b

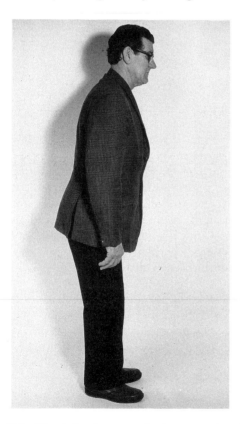

Fig. 17.1   The simian stance — a classic posture adopted by patients with neurogenic claudication, with flexed hips and knees. Reproduced with Professor Porter's permission from *The Lumbar Spine and Back Pain*, Churchill Livingstone 1987

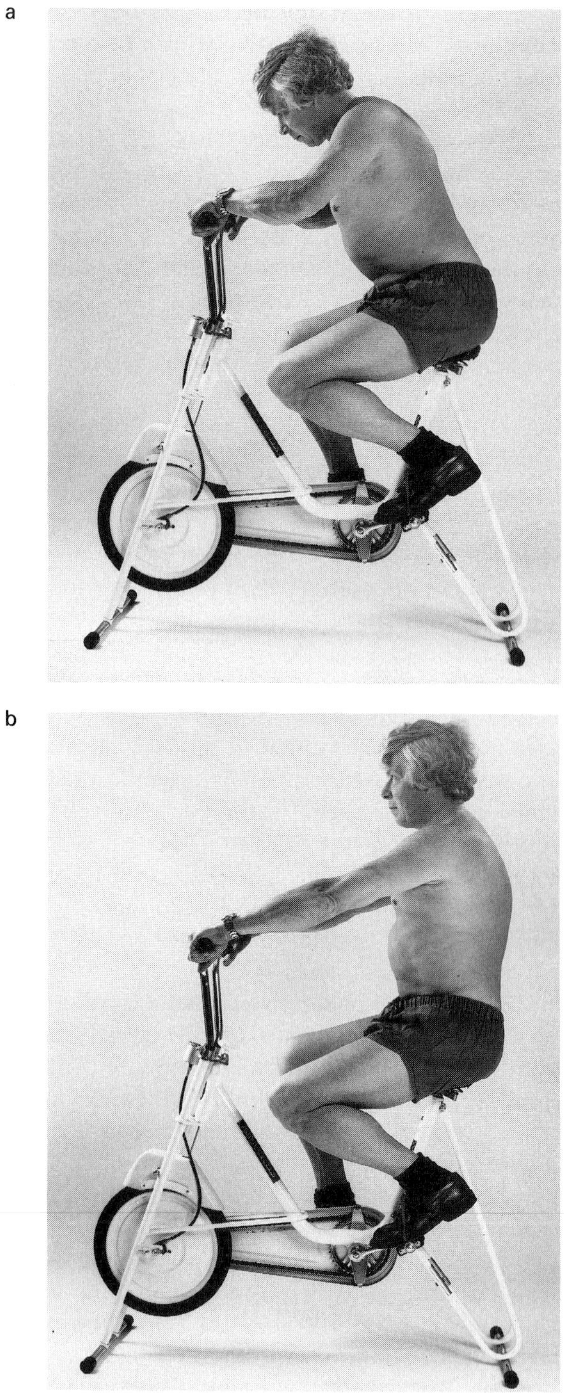

Fig. 17.2   The cycle test. The cycling distance is the same in vascular intermittent claudication whether the spine is flexed (a) or upright (b). The extended spine in (b) limits the cycling distance in neurogenic claudication. Reproduced with Professor Porter's permission from *The Lumbar Spine and Back Pain*, Churchill Livingstone 1987

by resting. Characteristically, relief from the pain is obtained by bending forwards. It is for this reason that patients with this disorder adopt an ape-like posture with both hips and knees flexed — the so-called simian stance (Simkin 1982). It is also because bending forwards relieves the pain that patients have less pain walking up a hill than down a hill and continue to be able to cycle long distances even when it is too painful to walk more than short distances on the flat (Figs 17.1 and 17.2).

Clinical examination

Physical signs are widely variable. In some cases there is some limitation of straight leg raising and evidence of a lower motor neurone lesion but with others their straight leg raising is normal and there are no abnormal neurological signs.

Peripheral pulses may or may not be palpable depending on whether arterial occlusion is or is not also present. The provisional diagnosis therefore mainly comes from the history.

Investigations

Plain radiographs of the lumbar spine frequently show diffuse degenerative changes; a myelogram shows segmental filling defects or a total block and ultrasound measurements confirm the reduced diameter of the vertebral canal.

Treatment

When symptoms are relatively mild, conservative measures may be helpful, but in those cases where there is severe pain and walking is restricted to short distances in association with a progressive neurological deficit, it is essential to carry out some form of surgical decompression.

Lateral root canal stenosis

In this condition pain in the back with radiation down one leg occurs as a result of stenosis at this site causing entrapment of a nerve root — usually the 5th lumbar or 1st sacral. The stenosis may occur as the result of bony encroachment from osteophytes or ossified spinal ligaments, or from soft tissue changes including facet joint capsule hypertrophy, posterior longitudinal ligament thick-ening and scar tissue developing around a ruptured annulus fibrosus or extruded nucleus pulposus.

Symptoms

The sciatic pain is in the same distribution as with a disc lesion but, unlike the latter, it is not relieved by lying down and remains severe and unremitting both day and night. Fortunately, however, unlike with disc pain, coughing and sneezing does not make it worse. In a series of 78 cases reported by Getty et al (1981) 58% also had numbness and paraesthesiae in the leg and 17% had claudication.

Physical signs

These are widely variable. In the series of patients reported by Getty et al (1981), only 49% showed evidence of a motor deficit and only 38% had impairment of sensation to light touch and pin-prick. Perhaps most surprising of all, most had a normal straight leg raising test.

It is probably because patients with lateral canal stenosis are liable to have bizarre sensory symptoms together with a paucity of physical signs, and frequently have unrestricted straight leg raising despite complaining of severe sciatica that the diagnosis in the past was frequently overlooked and patients suffering from it ran the risk of being considered to be neurotic.

Investigations

Plain radiographs may show a reduction of the L4/S1 disc space. A CAT scan will usually reveal the presence of degenerative changes in the facet joints but similar changes may also be evident in patients who do not suffer from back pain.

It is not possible to demonstrate the presence of nerve root entrapment in a stenosed lateral canal on a myelogram. Fortunately Leyshon et al (1981) have shown that the diagnosis may be confirmed by electromyographic studies.

Management

Porter et al (1984) have shown that the root pain not infrequently gradually subsides spontaneously However, as Wynn Parry (1989) points out, the difficulty is that whilst waiting for this to happen a proportion of patients develop irreversible pain-producing changes both in the entrapped nerve and in the central nervous system. It is obvious therefore that any decision concerning if and when surgical decompression should be carried out requires considerable clinical experience.

Indications for acupuncture and TENS

There is an important place for acupuncture and TENS as part of the conservative treatment of lumbar chronic nerve root entrapment pain and also post-operatively in those cases where surgery has failed to relieve this.

Acupuncture is of particular value in those cases where the nerve root is not severely compressed and much of the pain is coming from secondarily activated myofascial trigger points.

TENS is likely to be more helpful in cases where the pain is predominately neurogenic but it must be remembered that the electrodes should never be placed on anaesthetic skin but always on skin where the sensation is normal in order that the high-frequency low-intensity stimulus provided by this form of therapy may be enabled to recruit A-beta nerve fibres.

MANAGEMENT OF CHRONIC LOW-BACK PAIN

It is a measure of the general public's disillusionment with all the various conventional methods of treating chronic low-back pain that it is ever increasingly turning to alternative forms of therapy including acupuncture.

It is not possible, however, to come to any conclusions concerning the possible place of acupuncture in the treatment of chronic low-back pain without first of all critically appraising some of the other more widely used forms of treatment, including drugs, physiotherapy, spinal supports, cryoanalgesia, facet joint injections and steroid injections.

Drugs

Analgesics

Variosu non-narcotic pain-killing drugs such as aspirin, phenacetin, paracetomol and pentazocine,

together with a number of non-steroidal anti-inflammatory drugs, and even at times narcotic ones such as pethidine, are prescribed for chronic back pain. Although they are all capable of relieving pain for short periods, this is more than offset by the disadvantages of using them on a long-term basis including tolerance, habituation and side-effects, many of which are liable to be of a serious nature.

Antidepressants

Patients with chronic low-back pain are sometimes sufficiently depressed as to require a tricyclic antidepressant, but in addition a drug of this type may also be used for its analgesic effect.

The evidence that tricyclic antidepressants have an analgesic action independent of their anti-depressive properties includes Monks (1981) finding that the onset of analgesia in chronic pain conditions with this group of drugs is more rapid (3–7 days) than that of their antidepressant effect (14–21 days). Also Couch & Hassanein (1976) show that they are capable of producing chronic pain relief in the absence of an antidepressant response; and Couch et al (1976) report that this may also occur in patients in which there is no detectable evidence of depression.

It would seem that the analgesic and anti-depressant effects of this group of drugs are due to their ability to increase the concentration in the brain and spinal cord of amine transmitters such as serotonin (Sternbach et al 1976). Controlled trials comparing a tricyclic antidepressant with a placebo in chronic low-back pain have given somewhat equivocal results with Sternbach et al (1976) showing that amitriptyline, and Jenkins et al (1976) showing that imipramine, are no better than a placebo, but with Sternbach et al (1976) showing that clomipramine (Anafranil) is more effective than a placebo.

Muscle relaxants

As nervously holding muscles tense aggravates musculoskeletal pain it might be thought that diazepam would be helpful in the management of chronic low-back pain but Hingorani (1966), from the results of a double-blind controlled trial, was unable to confirm this.

Physiotherapy

Ultrasound

Sclapbach (1991) has pointed out that despite the fact that ultrasound is probably one of the most frequently used physiotherapeutic modalities for the relief of musculoskeletal pain, there have been remarkably few controlled studies to assess its effectiveness for this purpose.

During the past 35 years there have only been 9 such trials and of these only one has been in patients with low-back pain. This was a study carried out by Nwuga (1983) who compared bed rest and ultrasound, bed rest and sham ultrasound, and bed rest alone for the relief of acute low-back pain from intervertebral disc prolapse. Unfortunately, as bed rest was used in all three groups and is known to be effective itself in relieving acute low-back pain (Deyo et al 1986, Wiesel et al 1980), the results of the trial are difficult to interpret.

Sclapbach, from a review of these 9 studies, is of the opinion that, 'based on the results of the few available controlled trials, it must be concluded that we are far from being able to judge either the efficacy or inefficacy of therapeutic ultrasound'.

Exercises

Exercises are sometimes advocated but there is no good evidence that increasing the strength of the lumbar muscles reduces the frequency with which low-back pain recurs, and indeed Nachemson (1980c) warns against them in view of the fact that they may increase the load on the lumbar spine to unacceptable levels.

Manipulation

This highly specialized form of physical therapy has many advocates and is widely practised by doctors and others but, having no personal experience of its use, it would be wrong for me to express any opinion concerning its efficacy other than to say that from a study of the literature it would seem that whilst it is of undoubted value in the treatment of acute low-back pain (Berquist-Ullman & Larsson 1977), its place in the management of chronic low-back pain is far less certain (Doran & Newell 1975, Glover et al 1974, Evans et al 1978, Sims-Williams et al 1982).

Spinal supports

Corsets are widely prescribed but in spite of the fact that, at times, they are incredibly elaborate there is little or no evidence that they are of any benefit. A corset may in fact do harm because by limiting the movements of the back, it may lead to wasting of the muscles, and in addition is liable to suppress the action of the low-threshold mechanoreceptor large diameter fibre pain modulating mechanism (Ch. 6). Furthermore, a corset sometimes aggravates low-back pain by exerting pressure on trigger points. Quinet & Hadler (1979) in referring to these devices remark:

The widespread use of these gimmicks ought to be curtailed until we have data suggesting that our patients are more likely to profit from their continued use than are orthopaedic supply houses.

Cryoanalgesia

An ingenious technique that has been widely used in the alleviation of chronic pain since Amoils (1967) developed the enclosed gas expansion cryoprobe is one in which a reversible nerve block is achieved by the application of intense cold (Evans 1981).

It was Lloyd et al (1976) in their preliminary report on the use of this technique in a number of different painful conditions, who first referred to it as cryoanalgesia. Cryoanalgesia, a procedure carried out under direct vision or by a closed technique, is one in which the cryoprobe is inserted through the tissues via an introducer. In order that the cryoprobe may be accurately positioned, it is coupled to a nerve stimulator, and then, when it is correctly placed, an iceball is generated at its tip.

With regard to chronic low-back pain Lloyd et al (1976) stated that:

17 patients with low-back pain, in which the sciatic distribution of pain was predominant, were treated with closed application via the sacral hiatus or the relevant sacral foramina. The median duration of pain relief achieved was 10 days with a range of up to 49 days. 5 patients obtained no relief.

The relatively prolonged but reversible nerve block obtainable with this procedure offers great advantages over methods that destroy nerves such as crushing or sectioning. It is particularly useful in the alleviation of postoperative pain, and, so far as chronic pain is concerned, has proved to be surprisingly helpful in the alleviation of pain around the face (Barnard 1980), but in the treatment of chronic low-back pain it cannot be said that the results have been particularly impressive. Moreover, although in skilled hands it is a relatively straightforward technique, it relies on the use of somewhat complex apparatus and therefore can only be used in specially equipped units.

Facet joint injection

Mooney & Robertson (1975), having shown that it is possible to alleviate pain (artificially induced by injecting hypertonic saline into a facet joint) by injecting a local anaesthetic into this structure, were then prompted to treat 100 consecutive patients with pain the lower back and leg by injecting a steroid-local anaesthetic mixture into it. Because of difficulties in deciding from which joint or joints the pain might be coming, most patients were given injections into all three lower facet joints.

The technique could not be said to have been particularly successful as long-term relief was only obtained in one-fifth of the patients and partial relief in another third. Yet in spite of this, many physicians are beginning to adopt this form of treatment in the routine management of chronic low-back pain. Such treatment, however, can only be carried out in units equipped with fluoroscopic screens and there would seem to be no good grounds for advocating its routine use especially as a recent placebo-controlled trial, involving large numbers of patients with chronic low-back pain confirmed that it is of little value (Carette et al 1991). Therefore, this type of treatment is certainly not superior to other simpler and more readily carried out techniques.

Injections of a corticosteroid and/or local anaesthetic into points of maximum tenderness

Since Kellgren, nearly 50 years ago, started injecting Novocain into 'tender spots' in order to alleviate musculoskeletal pain, this type of treatment has been commonly employed in the treatment of low-back pain. Then once corticosteroids became available, the injection of a steroid/local anaesthetic mixture has been used (Bourne 1979). And in order to decide whether there was any advantage in using a steroid, Bourne (1984) decided to compare the effects of injecting, on repeated occasions, either, a corticosteroid-lignocaine mixture, or lignocaine by itself, into points of maximum tenderness in the lower back, in the treatment of chronic back pain. He concluded that the mixture gave better results.

It should be noted that the injection was sometimes given under the deep fascia but at other times into the periosteum, and, also, that amongst the transient side-effects were menstrual irregularities, flushing of the face, and glycosuria. Bourne ascribed the good results obtained with a steroid to certain softening and stretching effects on the collagen, together with the growing of new fibrocytes, and a consequent reduction in tissue tension described by Ketchum et al (1968) and Ketchum (1971). If indeed this type of tissue reaction does contribute to pain relief, it is bound to take time and hardly accounts for the immediate relief from pain so often observed when tender 'spots' are needled.

The alternative explanation is that a corticosteroid, when introduced into the tissues, and particularly when injected around the periosteum, has a powerful irritant effect on peripheral nerve endings, and in a similar manner to stimulating nerve endings with a dry needle, evokes activity in pain-modulating mechanisms in the central nervous system.

Acupuncture

From what has just been said in reviewing some of the present methods of treating chronic low-back pain, it is clear that none of them are particularly effective, some are associated with undesirable side-effects, and some can only be carried out in specially equipped centres. Few would disagree with Waddell (1982) when he says,

Future improvements in treatment for backache and the creation of a truly scientific basis for treatment depend on better biochemical understanding, more accurate identification and localization of the source of pain, recognition of specific clinical syndromes within mechanical backache, and critical evaluation of the effectiveness of treatment. While awaiting such developments it is best to use the simplest, safest, and cheapest treatment possible.

Acupuncture certainly fulfils these criteria, and there is therefore much to be said for exploring its use in everyday clinical practice and, above all, by the setting up of statistically controlled clinical trials. In my view, because of its simplicity, it is best to employ it as a first line of treatment, and then to turn to other more complex therapeutic procedures in those cases not helped by it.

The trigger points from which chronic neck pain is referred are situated in much the same muscles in everyone, but this certainly is not so with the trigger points responsible for chronic low-back and leg pain, and for this reason the task of finding them is that much more difficult. However, the task is facilitated by having a knowledge of specific patterns of pain referral from trigger points in individual muscles.

Paraspinal musculature

Trigger points in the paraspinal musculature may occur either in the superficial group of muscles known collectively as the erector spinae, or in muscles deep to this such as the multifidus and rotatores.

The two muscles in the superficial group (the erector spinae) most likely to develop trigger points are the longissimus thoracis and lateral to this, the iliocostalis lumborum muscle (Fig. 17.3).

Referred pain from trigger points in these muscles is mainly felt locally in areas immediately adjacent to these points, but sometimes it is felt at a distance. As King & Lagger (1976) have shown, trigger points in the erector spinae muscles may cause pain to be referred down the course of the sciatic nerve. And, as Travell &

Simons (1983d) have stated, trigger points in the iliocostalis lumborum muscle at the upper lumbar level, and in the longissimus thoracis at the lower thoracic level, cause pain to be referred to the buttock (Figs 17.4 and 17.5). It is because of this that earlier in this chapter it was stressed that the search for trigger points must always start some distance above the 12th rib.

The two muscles in the deep group likely to develop trigger points are the multifidi and rotatores. Pain from these trigger points is referred to the midline with the development of exquisite tenderness on palpating the spinous processes (Fig. 17.6A). Deep trigger points low down in the sacral region may also refer pain in a downwards direction to the coccyx and cause it to become very tender (Fig. 17.7).

It should also be noted, as stated by Travell & Simons (1983d), that trigger points in the iliocostalis muscle in the lower part of the thorax and in the multifidus muscle anywhere along the length of the lumbar spine may refer pain anteriorly to the abdomen, and that such pain may readily be misinterpreted as being visceral in origin (Fig. 17.6B).

Examination to locate trigger points in these muscles

The examination to locate trigger points in the paraspinal muscles should be conducted either with the patient seated and leaning forwards to flex the spine or with the patient in the semi-prone position with the painful side uppermost, and the knees brought up towards the chest. The full prone position should be avoided because, if the muscles are allowed to become too relaxed, it is difficult to identify palpable bands.

Trigger points in the superficial erector spinae muscles are readily felt by palpating down the length of the paravertebral gutter.

In order to identify a trigger point in one of the deeper muscles it is necessary to apply firm pressure immediately lateral to the spine in a postero-medial direction towards the body of a vertebra at the level of a tender spinous process.

Deactivation of trigger points

Trigger points in the superficial paraspinal muscles should be deactivated with needles inserted at

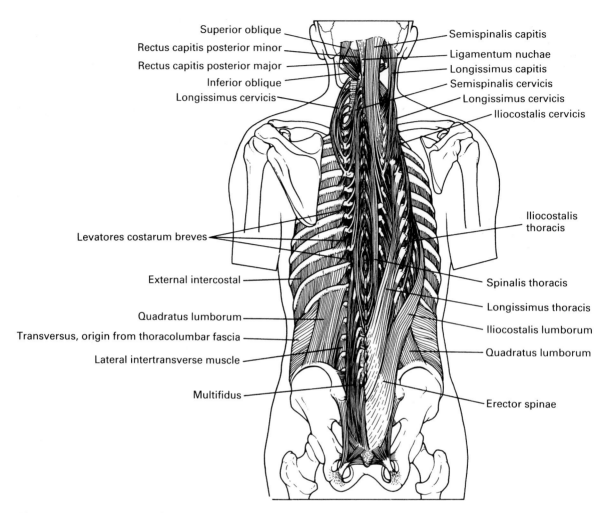

Fig. 17.3   The deep muscles of the back. On the left side the erector spinae and its upward continuations (with the exception of the longissimus cervicis, which has been displaced laterally) and the semispinalis capitis have been removed.

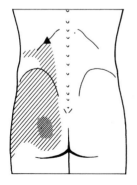

Fig. 17.4   The pattern of pain referral from a trigger point (▲) in the iliocostalis lumborum muscle.

Fig. 17.5   The pattern of pain referral from a trigger point (▲) in the longissimus thoracis muscle.

right angles to the skin, except in the lower thoracic region where, to avoid any chance of penetrating the pleura, it is wiser to insert them tangentially.

In deactivating trigger points in the more deeply situated paraspinal muscles, the needles have to be inserted lateral to the midline and in a diagonal direction towards the vertebral bodies.

The supraspinous ligament connecting the apices of the lumbar vertebral spines

Trigger points in the paraspinal muscles are often accompanied by trigger points in the midline supraspinous ligament, and when present these should also be deactivated.

Traditional Chinese acupuncture points

As will be seen from Figure 17.8 traditional Chinese acupuncture points are located down the midline in the so-called 'Du' channel, and in the paravertebral region in the so-called 'Urinary Bladder' channel. There is therefore a close spatial correlation between points in the Chinese system and the trigger points just described.

Other muscles in which the activation of trigger points may lead to the development of chronic low-back pain are the quadratus lumborum, the iliopsoas and the glutei.

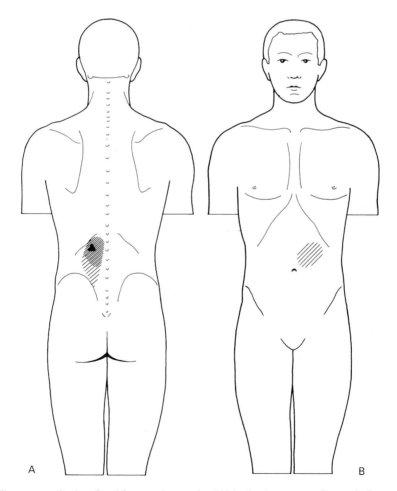

A   B

Fig. 17.6 A & B   The pattern of pain referral from a trigger point (▲) in the deep group of paraspinal muscles (multifidi and rotatores) in the upper lumbar region.

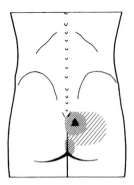

Fig. 17.7   The pattern of pain referral from a trigger point (▲) in the deep group of paraspinal muscles (multifidi and rotatores) in the sacral region.

Quadratus lumborum muscle (Fig. 17.9)

It is relatively common for trigger points to become activated in this muscle but because it lies deep to the paraspinal muscles they tend to get overlooked (Travell 1976). Sola & Williams in 1956 reported it to be a frequent cause of unilateral low-back pain amongst young adults in the American Air Force.

Activation of trigger points

Trigger points in this muscle become activated either when, because of a sudden twisting or stooping movement, an acute strain is put on the muscle, or when because of bending for long periods the muscle is subjected to sustained or repeated overload. The patient may then complain of pain on walking, but particularly on stooping or twisting such as when turning over in the bed, also on rising from a chair, and with sharp respiratory movements such as coughing or sneezing.

Specific patterns of pain referral

The pattern of pain referral depends on whether the trigger points are in the superficial lateral part or the deeper medial part of the muscle. When trigger points are located in the lateral part, the pain is referred down to the outer side of the iliac crest and over the greater trochanter (Fig. 17.10). It may also extend anteriorly towards the groin. When they are located in the medial part, the pain is referred to the region of the sacroiliac joint and buttock (Fig. 17.11). According to Sola & Williams (1956) trigger point activity in this

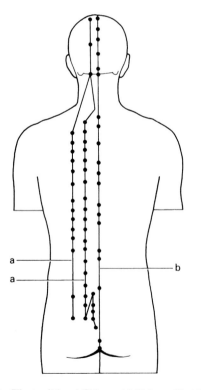

Fig. 17.8   The traditional Chinese (a) Urinary Bladder and (b) Du acu-tracts

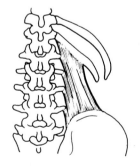

Fig. 17.9   The quadratus lumborum muscle

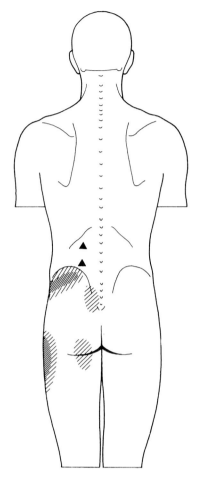

Fig. 17.10 The pattern of pain referral from trigger points (▲) in the lateral part of the quadratus lumborum muscle.

muscle is also a frequent cause of anterior abdominal pain.

Trigger point examination

Trigger points in this muscle, particularly in its deeper medial part, are liable to be overlooked unless care is taken to put the muscle on the stretch. The patient whilst lying on the un-affected side, as during the examination of the paraspinal muscles, should separate the 12th rib from the iliac crest, by reaching upwards with the free arm whilst at the same time drawing down the pelvis by dropping the uppermost thigh back-wards on to the couch. This manoeuvre brings the muscle nearer to the surface whilst at the same time tensing it.

Trigger points in the superficial lateral part of the muscle tend to be found, either where it inserts into the 12th rib, or into the iliac crest.

Trigger points in the medial deeper part of the muscle may be located by exerting firm pressure directed medially towards the transverse processes of the vertebrae. Again trigger points in this part of the muscle tend to cluster in the upper part around the 12th rib or in the lower part at the level of the 4th lumbar vertebra.

Glutei muscles (Fig. 18.6)

Trigger points in the gluteus maximus may occur at any of a variety of sites in the belly of this muscle. They become activated as a primary event or secondarily when pain is referred to the

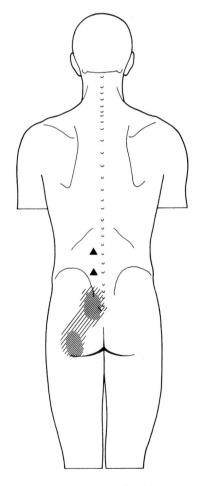

Fig. 17.11 The pattern of pain referral from trigger points (▲) in the medial part of the quadratus lumborum muscle.

buttock from trigger points in muscles situated in the postero-inferior part of the chest wall.

Pain from trigger points in this muscle is referred locally to the buttock itself and the coccyx (Fig. 17.12).

Trigger points in the gluteus medius and minimus are often found near to their insertions into the greater trochanter. The referral of pain from these is into the buttock; also sometimes down the outer side of the thigh along the length of the iliotibial tract, and when this happens it is often associated with the secondary activation of trigger points in this structure (Fig. 17.13).

With trigger points situated more posteriorly in one or other of these muscles, the pain is referred down the back of the thigh when it may be misdiagnosed as sciatica (Fig. 17.14).

Deactivation of trigger points in the glutei and iliotibial tract with a dry needle usually presents no difficulties, providing it is carried out systematically and no trigger points are overlooked.

Piriformis muscle (Fig. 17.15)

Trigger point activation in the piriformis muscle may also cause pain to be referred to the buttock, to the hip, and down the back of the leg in the distribution of the sciatic nerve (Fig. 17.16).

This muscle, an external rotator of the hip, arises from the internal surface of the sacrum, and then passes outwards and downwards through the sciatic notch to become inserted into the greater trochanter of the femur (Fig. 18.6).

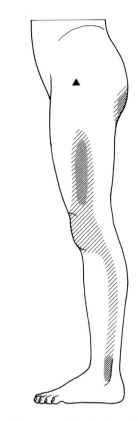

Fig. 17.13   The pattern of pain referral from a trigger point (▲) in either the gluteus medius or minimus near to the attachment of these muscles to the greater trochanter.

The sciatic nerve on leaving the pelvis is normally situated behind the muscle (Fig. 17.15) but in more than 10% of people the peroneal part of the nerve passes through the belly of the muscle (Grant 1978), and in less than 1% of people the entire sciatic nerve passes through the muscle (Beaten & Anson 1937). In those patients in which part or the whole of the sciatic nerve takes this course, increased tension in the muscle as a result of trigger point activation may cause entrapment of the nerve and the development of 'sciatica' — the so-called piriformis syndrome.

Piriformis syndrome

For some unexplained reason, this syndrome occurs six times more often in women than in men (Cailliet 1977b). On examination there is marked tenderness over the sciatic notch, and the pain is made worse by attempting to abduct and

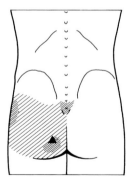

Fig. 17.12   The pattern of pain referral from a trigger point in the gluteus maximus muscle.

externally rotate the thigh against resistance. This test is most readily carried out by applying resistance to the outside of the thigh whilst the patient in the sitting position attempts to abduct the leg (Pace & Nagle 1976).

Trigger point tenderness may be elicited by exerting deep pressure on the lateral part of the muscle through the overlying gluteal muscles.

Pain in and around the sacroiliac joint

Pain in the region of the sacroiliac joint in a young man may herald the onset of ankylosing spondylitis and should be investigated with this in

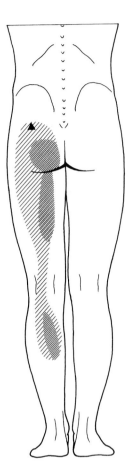

Fig. 17.14   The pattern of pain referral from a trigger point (▲) in the posterior part of either the gluteus medius or minimum muscles.

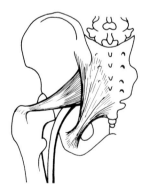

Fig. 17.15   The outer part of the piriformis muscle with its attachment to the greater trochanter. The sciatic nerve is shown in its normal position behind this muscle.

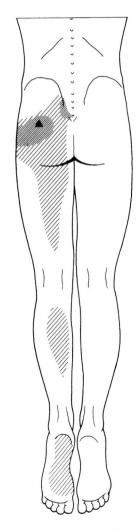

Fig. 17.16   The pattern of pain referral from a trigger point in the piriformis muscle.

mind (p. 252). Pain from sacroiliac strain may also occur during the last few months of pregnancy and in the postpartum period, but it is doubtful whether it is possible to subject this joint to strain at any other time of life.

During the later stages of pregnancy, hormonally-induced laxity of the ligaments of the joint takes place, and this is sometimes associated with pain both in the region of this joint and the hip, and on occasions down the front of the thigh. On examination, there is often quite marked tenderness over one or both sacroiliac joints but the temptation to attempt to relieve this pain by inserting dry needles into points of maximum tenderness should, in my opinion, be resisted. This is because now that it has been shown that it is possible to induce labour at full term by stimulating nerve endings in the pelvic region, it might be difficult to defend oneself in a court of law if acupuncture carried out near to term for the treatment of low-back pain appeared to be responsible for labour starting prematurely. It was as well that my policy of not carrying out acupuncture during pregnancy was adhered to in the case of the 8 months pregnant woman who was particularly anxious for me to alleviate some persistent sacroiliac pain by means of this technique, because 2 days after advising her against having acupuncture in view of her being pregnant, she spontaneously went into labour!

Pain in the region of the sacroiliac joint may also occur following pregnancy when the joint, having opened during delivery, fails to close properly. Radiographic investigation may also show evidence of misalignment of the pubic rami. The sacroiliac pain may be relieved by inserting a dry needle into a point of maximum tenderness along the line of the joint but, in my experience, this usually, even when repeated, only gives temporary relief, and if the pain becomes chronic, there is a case for strengthening the ligaments by injecting a sclerosing agent into them.

Sacroiliac strain unrelated to pregnancy

Low-back pain occurring without any relationship to pregnancy is often diagnosed as being due to sacroiliac strain, particularly by osteopaths,

but the joint normally has such little movement, due to it being held in position by particularly strong ligaments, that other than during pregnancy it seems very unlikely to be subjected to strain, and also it seems equally unlikely that it is amenable to manipulative procedures. However, it has to be admitted that in cases of chronic low-back pain there is often exquisite tenderness on applying pressure to the 'dimple' overlying the joint, and the insertion of an acupuncture needle into the point of maximum tenderness is often very helpful.

Iliopsoas muscle (Fig. 17.17A)

In the investigation of chronic low-back pain no examination for trigger points is complete without finally turning the patient into the supine position to check for trigger points in the anterior abdominal wall and in the groin.

The activation of a trigger point immediately below the inguinal ligament, in the tendon of the iliopsoas muscle where it lies in close relationship to the femoral artery, just before it becomes inserted into the lesser trochanter of the femur, is a cause of pain being referred up a line immediately lateral to the spine in the paravertebral gutter, and also in some cases down the front of the thigh (Fig. 17.17A and B). Deactivation of the trigger point with a dry needle is best carried out with the thigh abducted and externally rotated, and with care being taken not to damage the femoral nerve.

Trigger point activity in the iliopsoas muscle may be associated with similar activity in muscles in the lower back such as the quadratus lumborum, but occasionally it is present on its own. It is important to examine the groin routinely for trigger points in all cases of low-back pain as otherwise they can easily be overlooked.

A physical training instructor (34), whilst playing football, twisted his left leg and shortly after developed pain in the left lower back, and down the back of the leg a far as the calf; any stretching movement of the trunk made the pain worse. An osteopath manipulated his spine on several occasions but without any improvement in the pain, and after this had persisted for 12 months, he was sent to me for possible treatment with acupuncture. In view of the

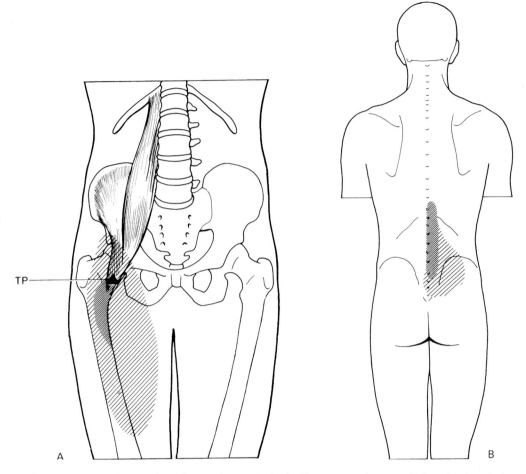

Fig. 17.7 A & B   Patterns of pain referral from a trigger point in the iliopsoas muscle near to its insertion into the lesser trochanter.

history there was no doubt in my mind that trigger points would be readily demonstrable in the muscles of the lower back, and it came as a great surprise to me when this proved not to be so. However, on getting him to lie on his back, trigger points were found in the groin, in the iliopsoas and adductor tendons. It is interesting to note that, as so often happens, in spite of them being exquisitely tender, he was quite unaware of their presence until pressure was put on them at the time of the examination. Also of particular interest was the fact that the insertion of a needle into one of them evoked a transient sensation of pain in the back and down the leg in exactly the same distribution as that occurring spontaneously. Furthermore, the importance of the part played by these trigger points in provoking the pain was further confirmed by the latter being alleviated quite dramatically once they were

deactivated with dry needles. The first time that this was done he was pain-free for 3 days, and although the pain had been present for over a year, it was only necessary to repeat the procedure on two further occasions at weekly intervals before he obtained lasting relief.

Electrical stimulation in the alleviation of low-back pain

Electroacupuncture, the technique in which needles, inserted either into traditional Chinese acupuncture points, or into trigger points, are stimulated by means of a low-frequency, high-intensity current for a relatively short period of 10 to 20 minutes, and transcutaneous electrical nerve stimulation (TENS) in which electrodes are placed on the skin over similar points, and stimulated by a high-frequency, low-intensity current for a prolonged period (Ch. 9), are now well-established methods of alleviating chronic pain in various parts of the body including the lower part of the back.

As stated previously, in the symptomatic treatment of chronic musculoskeletal pain, including that which affects the lower back, some people such as myself use manual acupuncture almost exclusively, some employ electroacupuncture or TENS when the response to manual acupuncture is disappointing and still others use nothing else but electrical methods of stimulation. There is therefore no uniformity of approach to this subject and any differences of opinion concerning the merits of and indications for these various techniques can only eventually be resolved by carefully conducted clinical trials. In the meantime the position has become further complicated by Melzack in 1975 showing that perhaps it is even better to use yet another method of electrical stimulation that combines some of the advantages of both electroacupuncture and conventional TENS.

It will be remembered (see Ch. 9) that Melzack (1975) was led to do this because high-frequency, low-intensity TENS applied via electrodes attached to the skin for many hours often causes a dermatitis, and because low-frequency, high-intensity electroacupuncture using needles can only be administered by medical practitioners. He therefore decided to investigate the use of an acupuncture-type low-frequency, high-intensity stimulation of brief duration delivered through skin electrodes, rather than via needles.

Melzack found this acupuncture-like type of TENS to be so effective in giving symptomatic relief in a number of different types of pain including that which affects the lower back that he and Elizabeth Fox (Fox & Melzack 1976) carried out a cross-over type trial in order to compare it with manually performed acupuncture in the treatment of chronic low-back pain. The trial included 12 patients, with 6 of these given two treatments with manual acupuncture and then two treatments with acupuncture-like TENS; the other 6 were given these treaments in

the reverse order. The treatments were given at weekly intervals. The manual acupuncture consisted of needles being inserted into three arbitrarily chosen traditional Chinese acupuncture points and each needle rotated strongly for 1 minute. The TENS took the form of a low-frequency, high-intensity current being applied for 10 minutes at each of the same points in succession, with an indifferent electrode placed at a distant site.

It was found that manual acupuncture gave moderate to good pain relief in 75% of patients, and acupuncture-like TENS in 60% of cases. The mean duration of this pain relief was 40 hours and 23 hours respectively.

It is difficult, however, to draw conclusions from this trial owing to the small numbers in the groups; also, the cross-over design of the trial, which, because the effects of all types of acupuncture are sometimes delayed, is best avoided; and the fact that the only assessment measure used was a self-rating questionnaire.

Laitinen's (1976) trial carried out about the same time in which he quite independently used two similar types of treatment also showed them to be equally effective in alleviating low-back pain. This trial admittedly was on a larger scale with 50 patients in each group but again the methods of evaluating pain relief were somewhat unsophisticated and it is possible that a more detailed analysis using more sensitive assessment measures (Ch. 11) might have revealed greater differences between the two groups.

Clinical trials to assess the effectiveness of acupuncture in the treatment of chronic low-back pain

The general consensus of opinion among those with much experience of using acupuncture in the treatment of chronic low-back pain is that it provides worthwhile symptomatic relief in about 70% of cases. This however can be considered to be no more than a clinical impression as the number of statistically controlled trials so far conducted has been small, and of those that have been carried out, most have been poorly designed and have lacked sufficient numbers of patients in them.

It has to be admitted that the objective assessment of the effectiveness of acupuncture, or any other type of treatment, in relieving chronic low-back pain is particularly difficult because the considerable uncertainty concerning the aetiological factors responsible for this type of pain in any particular individual, makes it virtually impossible to divide cases into clearly definable sub-groups. It is because of this that the Working Group on Back Pain, set up by the Minister of Health in 1976, considered that in order to be certain that randomization ensured that all the various factors likely to influence the outcome of treatment are equally distributed amongst the actively treated group and the control group in any such trial, it might well be necessary to study up to 500 pairs or more. The Working Group, however, being well aware of the very considerable practical problems associated with conducting trials of such magnitude, suggested that initially it might be more expedient to settle for less than that which might be considered to be ideal.

Some of the problems related to statistically controlled trials designed to assess the effectiveness of acupuncture in relieving musculoskeletal pain including that which affects the lower back have already been considered in Chapter 11, and so at this stage nothing more need to be said other than to draw attention to some personal observations made during the course of using this form of treatment in a large number of cases of chronic low-back pain that seem to me to be of relevance when planning, carrying out, and assessing the results of such trials.

Firstly, it is my belief that the response to acupuncture seems to bear little or no relationship to the amount of degenerative changes a person has in the lumbar discs or facet joints, but it does seem to be very much influenced by his or her psychological state. By this is meant that at one end of the spectrum psychologically stable people with low-back pain often respond well to acupuncture, in spite of having advanced degenerative changes in their spine, whereas at the other end of the spectrum, the response to this form of treatment in people who hold their lumbar muscles in a state of persistent tension because of chronic anxiety is liable to be poor, even when the X-rays

of their spines are normal. The implication of this, with respect to clinical trials, might seem to be that so far as psychosocial factors and degenerative changes in the spine are concerned, that of the two, it is particularly important that randomization ensures that neuroticism is evenly spread between the treatment and control groups. It was no doubt considerations such as these that led Mendelson et al (1983) in their statistically controlled study of the use of acupuncture in low-back pain to carry out a detailed pre-trial psychological assessment in all their patients. And there are many who now believe that psychosocial factors are of such importance both in the aetiology of chronic low-back pain, and in causing it to persist, as to make it essential with some patients to employ various psychological forms of relaxation therapy such as hypnosis (Crasilneck 1979) or biofeedback (Keefe et al 1981), in addition to physical measures applied locally to the back, such as acupuncture. Trials in anxious low-back pain patients to assess whether or not the use of acupuncture and a relaxation technique give better results than those obtained by the use of one of these treatments on its own have not as yet been carried out.

Before leaving the subject it must be admitted that the belief that unrelieved chronic anxiety tends to nullify the effects of acupuncture is not held by everyone, with, for example, Levine et al (1976) finding that a high score on psychometric indicators of anxiety and depression is a significant predictor of successful needle puncture analgesia in patients with chronic pain. It is clear therefore that with such diversity of views on this subject there is much scope for clinical trials specifically designed to resolve this issue.

The other matter that has to be considered when discussing the design of clinical trials to assess the efficacy of acupuncture in relieving chronic low-back pain, and for that matter all other forms of musculoskeletal pain, is that responders to acupuncture may be divided into a group consisting of those who obtain long-lasting relief from chronic pain after a comparatively few treatment sessions, and another group consisting of those who benefit from acupuncture but require ongoing treatment over a long period in order to keep chronic pain adequately suppressed.

These differences in people's reaction to acupuncture so far as low-back pain is concerned again seem to bear little or no relationship to the type or extent of any pathological changes that may happen to be present in their spines, but, as with musculoskeletal pain anywhere in the body, it does seem to depend on the varying manner in which individuals' endogenous pain-modulating mechanisms respond to peripheral nociceptive stimulation.

The ability of acupuncture in some people at times not only to give symptomatic relief, but to cut short a long-standing episode of pain is well recognized, and a possible explanation for this phenomenon is given in Chapter 10. However, it has to be realized that such a response may on occasions be more apparent than real and be due to the acupuncture treatment being given coincidentally with the onset of a natural remission. If by chance this should happen to occur with a number of patients in a clinical trial, then of course it might seriously interfere with the results. And it was in an attempt to safeguard against this as much as is possible that Macdonald et al (1983), in their statistically controlled trial of acupuncture in the relief of chronic low-back pain, only included patients whose pain had persisted for at least 1 year. Their reasoning behind this was of course that the longer chronic pain persists, the less likely it is to undergo a spontaneous remission.

Many chronic low-back pain sufferers only obtain relatively short periods of symptomatic relief from acupuncture and because of this have to be given it at fairly frequent intervals on a long-term basis. Such relief, however, is clearly of great benefit to them, and repeated treatment with a procedure so free of side-effects as acupuncture is of course a small price to pay for it. Fox & Melzack (1976) clearly had this in mind when during the course of commenting on the results of their comparative trial of transcutaneous electrical stimulation and acupuncture in the treatment of chronic low-back pain, they stated,

transcutaneous stimulation and acupuncture, however, are not 'cures' and repeated treatments are usually necessary to provide continuing periods of relief. When it is recalled that many of the patients in this study had suffered pain for years, and several had undergone

major surgery without relief, the value of a technique which brings partial relief for a few hours or days at a time is especially evident. It makes the difference between unbearable and bearable pain, between a sedentary, sometimes bed-ridden life and one that, for at least several hours or days a week, allows a normal social, family, or business life. Even a few hours or days of pain at tolerable levels permits some of these patients to live with more dignity and self-assurance, so that life in general becomes more bearable.

These differing effects of acupuncture on chronic low-back pain, with at times it being capable of giving long-lasting relief but at other times of only giving short-term, but nevertheless much appreciated, relief, have to be taken into account when evaluating the results of clinical trials.

Furthermore, when planning such trials it has to be remembered that individuals vary widely as to how much peripheral nerve stimulation they require in order to obtain optimum response, and also as to how many times treatment has to be given in order to bring the pain under control. It would therefore seem expedient, when drawing up protocols for these trials, to allow for these varying treatment requirements, by permitting the rules governing the administration of the acupuncture and the control type of therapy to be more flexible than those governing the prescribing of pharmacological substances in drug trials.

Such considerations of course apply to acupuncture trials in general and have already been referred to in Chapter 11, but it is appropriate to draw attention to them again here because it would seem that up to now only Macdonald et al (1983) have realistically taken them into account when drawing up the protocol for their trial in patients with chronic low-back pain. In that trial the effect of inserting needles superficially through the skin to an approximate depth of 4 mm at trigger point sites was compared with that obtained by a placebo treatment consisting of the placing of electrodes on the skin at similar points and then attaching them to a non-functioning TENS machine. The protocol for this trial laid down that treatment both in the acupuncture group and in the placebo control group should be given once a week. For the acupuncture group, it was decreed that each treatment should take the form of needles being left in situ, without any form of rotation, for 5 minutes, and that if, on any occasion, such treatment failed to produce beneficial results, then at the next treatment the needle insertion time had to be doubled, and if necessary on a further occasion doubled again up to a maximum of 20 minutes. If there was still no response, electroacupuncture had to be used. It was laid down that, initially, impulses of 700 µs. duration should be obtained at a frequency of 2 hertz, with the amplitude being increased approximately every 2 minutes to maintain the stimulation just above the pain threshold. Again if 5 minutes of this treatment produced no effect, the duration had to be doubled at each treatment up to a maximum of 20 minutes. The number of treatments given could be varied according to an individual's response with an arbitrarily defined upper limit of 10. The number of treatments was reduced, however, if further improvement failed to occur, or indeed if the pain continued to progress.

The rules governing the application of elec-

trodes to the skin over the trigger points in the control group were exactly similar, including that if the patient reported a worsening of the pain immediately following 'treatment' as happened in three cases, then in exactly the same way as with the needle insertion time in the acupuncture group, the electrode application time was reduced.

The trial was small, but nevertheless, largely due to its design, it was possible to show a statistically significant superiority of acupuncture over placebo in the alleviation of chronic low-back pain.

There remains a pressing need for larger scale statistically-controlled randomized trials, with in my opinion protocols similar to the one just described, in order to determine the relative indications for manual acupuncture, electroacupuncture, conventional transcutaneous electrical stimulation (TENS) and acupuncture-like TENS. And, also to compare the efficacy to these types of therapy with that of all other forms of treatment currently in use for chronic low-back pain.

REFERENCES

Amoils S P 1967 The Joule Thompson cryoprobe. Archives of Ophthalmology 78: 201–207
Badgley C E 1941 The articular facets in relation to low back pain and sciatic radiation. Journal of Bone and Joint Surgery 23: 481–496
Barnard D 1980 The effects of extreme cold on sensory nerves. Annals of the Royal College of Surgeons of England 62: 180–187
Bates T, Grunwald E 1958 Myofascial pain in childhood. Journal of Pediatrics 53: 148–209
Beaton L E, Anson B J 1937 The relation of the sciatic nerve and of its subdivision to the piriformis muscle. Anatomical Record 70: (suppl. 1) 1–5
Berquist-Ullman M, Larsson U 1977 Acute low-back pain in industry. A controlled prospective study with special reference to therapy and confounding factors. Acta Orthopaedica Scandinavica Supplement 170
Bourne I H J 1979 Treatment of backache with local injections. The Practitioner 222: 708–711
Bourne I H J 1984 Treatment of chronic back pain comparing corticosteroid-lignocaine injections with lignocaine alone. The Practitioner 228: 333–338
Cailliet R 1977a Soft tissue pain and disability. F A Davis, Philadelphia, p 32; 1977b: p 99
Calin A, Porta J, Fries J F F 1977 The clinical history as a screening test for ankylosing spondylitis. Journal of the American Medical Association 273: 2613–2615
Carette S, Marcoux S, Truchon R et al 1991 A controlled trial of corticosteroid injections into facet joints for chronic low back pain. New England Journal of Medicine 325 (14) 1002–1007
Couch J R, Hassanein R S 1976 Migraine and depression: effect of amitriptyline prophylaxis. Transactions of the

American Neurological Association 101: 1–4
Couch J R, Ziegler D K, Hassanein R S 1976 Amitriptyline in the prophylaxis of migraine. Effectiveness and relationship of anti-migraine and anti-depressant effects. Neurology 26: 121–127
Crasilneck H B 1979 Hypnosis in the control of chronic low-back pain. American Journal of Clinical Hypnosis 22: 71–78
Deyo R A, Diehl A K, Rosenthal M 1986 How many days of bed rest for acute low-back pain? A randomized clinical trial. New England Journal of Medicine 315: 1064–1070
Dixon J St J 1980 Introduction. In: Jayson M I V (ed) The lumbar spine and back pain, 2nd edn. Pitman, London, p XI & 147
Doran D M L, Newell D J 1975 Manipulation in the treatment of low-back pain, a multicentre study. British Medical Journal 2: 161–164
Edgar M A, Park W M 1974 Induced pain patterns in passive straight-leg raising in lower lumbar disc protrusion. Journal of Bone and Joint Surgery 56B: 658–667
Eisenstein S 1977 The morphometry and pathological anatomy of the lumbar spine in South African negroes and caucasoids with special reference to spinal stenosis. Journal of Bone and Joint Surgery 59B: 173–180
Evans P J D 1981 Cryoanalgesia. Anaesthesia 36: 1003–1013
Evans D P, Burke M S, Lloyd K N, Roberts G M 1978 Lumbar spinal manipulation on trial. Part I Clinical assessment. Rheumatology and Rehabilitation 17: 46–53
Fairbank J C T, Park W M, McCall I W, O'Brien J P 1981 Apophyseal injection of local anaesthetic as a diagnostic aid in primary low-back pain syndromes. Spine 6: 598–605
Finneson B 1980 Low-back pain. Lippincott, Philadelphia, pp 202–203

Flor H, Turk D C 1984 Etiological theories and treatments for chronic back pain. Part I Somatic models and interventions. Pain 19: 105–121

Fox E, Melzack R 1976 Transcutaneous electrical stimulation and acupuncture — a comparison of treatment for low-back pain. Pain 2: 141–148

Getty C J M, Johnson J R, Kirwan E O'G et al 1981 Partial undercutting facetectomy for bony entrapment of the lumbar nerve root. Journal of Bone and Joint Surgery 63B: 330–335

Glover J R, Morris J G, Khosla T 1974 Back pain — a randomized clinical trial of rotational manipulation of the trunk. British Journal of Industrial Medicine 31: 59–64

Grant J C 1978 An atlas of human anatomy, 7th edn. Williams & Wilkins, Baltimore

Grantham V A 1977 Backache in boys — a new problem? The Practitioner 218: 226–229

Green L N 1975 Dexamethasone in the management of symptoms due to herniated lumbar disc. Journal of Neurology Neurosurgery and Psychiatry 38: 1211–1217

Gunn C C, Milbrandt W E 1976 Tenderness at motor points: a diagnostic and prognostic aid for low back injury. Journal of Bone and Joint Surgery 58A (6): 815–825

Hansen E B, Praestholm J, Fahrenkrug A, Bjerrium J 1976 A clinical trial of Amipaque in lumbar myelography. British Journal of Radiology 49: 34–38

Haughton V M, Eldevik O P, Magnaes B, Amunsdon P 1982 A prospective comparison of computed tomography and myelography in the diagnosis of herniated lumbar disks. Radiology 142: 103–110

Hingorani K 1966 Diazepam in backache. A double blind controlled trial. Annals of Physical Medicine 8: 303–306

Hirsch C, Ingelmark B, Miller M 1963 The anatomical basis for low-back pain. Acta Orthopaedica Scandinavica 33: 1–17

Horal J 1969 The clinical appearance of low-back pain disorders in the city of Gothenberg, Sweden. Acta Orthopaedica Scandinavica supplement 118: 8–73

Hult L 1954 Cervical dorsal and lumbar spinal syndromes. A field investigation of a non-selected material of 1200 workers in different occupations with special reference to disc degeneration and so-called muscular rheumatism. Acta Orthopaedica Scandinavica supplement 17: 1–102

Hussar A E, Guller E J 1956 Correlation of pain and the roentgenographic findings of spondylosis of the cervical and lumbar spine. American Journal of Medical Science 232: 518–527

Isherwood I, Antoun N M 1987 C T scanning in the assessment of lumbar spine problems. In: Jayson M I V (ed) The lumbar spine and back pain, 3rd edn. Churchill Livingstone, Edinburgh, p 269–285

Jayson M I V 1976 The lumbar spine and back pain. Pitman, London

Jayson M I V 1980 The lumbar spine and back pain, 2nd edn. Pitman, London

Jayson M I V 1987 The lumbar spine and back pain, 3rd edn. Churchill Livingstone, Edinburgh

Jenkins D G, Ebbutt A F, Evans C D 1976 Imipramine in treatment of low-back pain. Journal of International Medical Research 4: (Suppl 2) 28–40

Keefe F J, Schapira B, Williams R B, Brown C, Surwet R S 1981 EMG assisted relaxation training in the management of chronic low-back pain. American Journal of Clinical Biofeedback 4: 93–103

Ketchum L D 1971 Effects of triamcinolone on tendon healing and function. A laboratory study. Plastic and Reconstructive Surgery 47: 471–482

Ketchum L D, Robinson D W, Masters F W 1968 The degradiation of mature collagen. A laboratory study. Plastic and Reconstructive Surgery 40: 89–91

King J S, Lagger R 1976 Sciatica viewed as a referred pain syndrome. Surgical Neurology 5: 46–50

Laitinen J 1976 Acupuncture and transcutaneous electric stimulation in the treatment of chronic sacrolumbalgia and ischialgia. American Journal of Chinese Medicine 4 (2): 169–175

Lamerton A J, Banninster R, Wittington R, Seifert M H, Eastcott H H G 1983 'Claudication' of the sciatic nerve. British Medical Journal 286: 1785–1786

Levine J, Gormley J, Fields H L 1976 Observation on the analgesic effects of needle puncture (acupuncture) Pain 2: 149–159

Leyshon A, Kirwan E O, Wynn Parry C B 1981 Electrical studies in the diagnosis of compression of the lumbar root. Journal of Bone and Joint Surgery 63B: 51–75

Lewit K 1979 The needle effect in the relief of myofascial pain. Pain 6: 83–90

Lloyd J W, Barnard J D W, Glynn C J 1976 Cryoanalgesia. Lancet 2: 932–934

Loeser J D 1980 Low-back pain. In: Bonica J J (ed) Pain. Raven Press, New York, p 363–377

Macdonald A J R, Macrae K D, Master B R, Rubin A P 1983 Superficial acupuncture in the relief of chronic low-back pain. Annals of the Royal College of Surgeons of England 65: 44–46

McKillop J H, McDougal I R 1980 The role of skeletal scanning in clinical oncology. British Medical Journal 281: 407–410

Magora A 1970 Investigation of the relation between low-back pain and occupation to age, sex, community, education and other factors. Industrial Medicine and Surgery 39: 465–471

Magora A, Schwartz A 1976 Relation between the low-back pain syndrome and X-ray findings. 1. Degenerative osteoarthritis. Scandinavian Journal of Rehabilitation Medicine 8: 115–175

Magora A, Schwartz A 1978 Relation between the low-back pain syndrome and X-ray findings. 2. Transitional vertebra (mainly sacralization). Scandinavian Journal of Rehabilitation Medicine 10: 135–145

Mathews J A 1968 Dynamic discography: a study of lumbar traction. Annals of Physical Medicine 9: 275–279

Matthews W B 1975 Practical neurology, 3rd edn. Blackwell Scientific, Oxford, p 142

Melzack R 1975 Prolonged relief of pain by brief intense transcutaneous somatic stimulation. Pain 1: 357–373

Melzack R, Wall P D 1982 The challenge of pain. Penguin Books, Harmondsworth, p 249–254

Mendelson G, Selwood T S, Kranz H, Loh T S, Kidson M A, Scott D S 1983 Acupuncture treatment of chronic back pain: a double blind placebocontrolled trial. American Journal of Medicine 74: 49–55

Mixter W J, Barr J S 1934 Rupture of the intervertebral disc with involvement of the spinal canal. New England Journal of Medicine 211: 210–215

Monks R C 1981 The use of psychotropic drugs in human chronic pain. A review. 6th World Congress of the International College of Psychosomatic Medicine, Montreal, Canada, Sept 15

Mooney V, Robertson J 1975 The facet syndrome. Clinical Orthopaedics and Related Research 115: 149–156

Nachemson A 1979 A critical look at the treatment for low-back pain. Scandinavian Journal of Rehabilitation Medicine 11: 143–149

Nachemson A 1980a A critical look at conservative treatment for low-back pain. In: Jayson M I V (ed) The lumbar spine and back pain, 2nd edn. Pitman, London, p 458; 1980b: p 453; 1980c: p 459

Nelson M A 1980 Surgery of the spine. In: Jayson M I V (ed) The lumbar spine and back pain, 2nd edn. Pitman, London, p 477

Nelson M A 1987 Indications for spinal surgery in low back pain. In: Jayson M I V (ed) The Lumbar Spine and Back Pain 3rd edition. Churchill Livingstone, Edinburgh, p 321–352

Nichols P J R 1960 Short-leg syndrome. British Medical Journal 1: 1863–1865

Nwuga V C B 1983 Ultrasound in treatment of back pain arising from prolapsed intervertebral disc. Archives of Physical Medicine and Rehabilitation 64: 88–89

Pace J Blair, Nagle D 1976 Piriform syndrome. The Western Journal of Medicine 124: 435–439

Porter R W 1987 Spinal stenosis in the central and root canal. In: Jayson M I V (ed) The lumbar spine and back pain, 3rd edn. Churchill Livingstone, Edinburgh, p 383–400

Porter R W, Hibbert C, Evans C 1984 The natural history of root entrapment syndrome. Spine 9: 418–422

Porter R W, Wicks M, Ottewell D 1978 Measurement of the spinal canal by diagnostic ultrasound. Journal of Bone and Joint Surgery 60B: 481–487

Quinet R J, Hadler N M 1979 Diagnosis and treatment of backache. Seminars in Arthritis and Rheumatics 8: 261–287

Rees W S 1971 Multiple bilateral subcutaneous rhizolysis of segmental nerves in the treatment of the intervertebral disc syndrome. Annals of General Practice 26: 126–217

Rees W S, Slade H W 1974 Multiple bilateral percutaneous rhizolysis in the treatment of the slipped disc syndromes. Paper delivered before the American Association of Neurological Surgeons meeting in St Louis, Missouri, April 22–25, 1974

Rowe M L 1965 Disc surgery and chronic low-back pain. Journal of Occupational Medicine 7: 196–202

Rowe M L 1969 Low back pain in industry. A position paper. Journal of Occupational Medicine 11: 161–169

Rubin D 1981 Myofascial trigger point syndromes. An approach to management. Archives of Physical Medicine and Rehabilitation 62: 107–110

Schmorl G, Junghanns H 1932 Die gesunde und kranke Wirbelseule im Roentgenbild. Thieme, Leipzig

Schumaker T M, Genant H K, Korobkin M, Bovill T R 1978 Computerized tomography — its use in space-occupying lesions of the musculoskeletal system. Journal of Bone and Joint Surgery 60A: 600–607

Sclapbach P 1991 Ultrasound. In: Schlapbach P, Gerber N J (eds) Physiotherapy: Controlled Trials and Facts, Rheumatology. Karger, Basel, vol. 14 p 163–170

Shealy C N, Prieto A Jr, Burton C, Long D M 1974 Radiofrequency percutaneous rhizotomy of the articular nerve of Luschka — an alternative approach to chronic low-back pain and sciatica. Paper delivered before the American Association of Neurological Surgeons' meeting, Los Angeles, California, April 9th 1974

Simkin P A 1982 Simian stance: a sign of spinal stenosis. Lancet 2: 652–653

Sims-Williams H, Jayson M I, Young S M, Baddeley H, Collins E 1982 Controlled trial of mobilization and manipulation for patients with low-back pain in general

practice. British Medical Journal 2: 1338–1340

Sola A E, Williams R L 1956 Myofascial pain syndromes. Neurology (Minneapolis) 6: 91–95

Spangfort E V 1972 The lumbar disc herniation. A computer-aided analysis of 2504 operations. Acta Orthopaedica Scandinavica supplement 142: 1–95

Splithoff C A 1952 Lumbosacral junction. Roentgenographic comparison of patients with and without backaches. Journal of the American Medical Association 152: 1610–1613

Steindler A, Luck J V 1938 Differential diagnosis of pain low in the back. Journal of the American Medical Association 110: 106–112

Sternbach R A, Janowsky D S, Huey I Y, Segal D S 1976 Effects of altering brain serotonin activity on human chronic pain. In: Bonica J J, Albe Fessard D (eds) Advances in pain research and therapy 1. Raven Press, New York, p 601–606

Strange F G St Clair 1966 Debunking the disc. Proceedings of the Royal Society of Medicine 59: 952–956

Torgerson W R, Dotter W E 1976 Comparative roentgenographic study of the asymptomatic and symptomatic lumbar spine. Journal of Bone and Joint Surgery 58A: 850–853

Travell J 1968 Office hours: day and night. The World Publishing Company, New York

Travell J G 1976 The quadratus lumborum muscle, an overlooked cause of low-back pain. Archives of Physical Medicine and Rehabilitation: 57: 566

Travell J G, Simons D G 1983a Myofascial pain and dysfunction. The trigger point manual. Williams & Wilkins, Baltimore, p 105–109; 1983b: p 645; 1983c: p 644; 1983d: p 637

Turk D C, Flor H, 1984 Etiological theories and treatments for chronic back pain II. Psychological models and interactions. Pain 19: 209–233

Urban T, Maroudas A 1980 In: Graham R (ed) Clinics in rheumatic diseases vol 6, no 1. Saunders, Philadelphia, p 51

Vernon-Roberts B, Pirie C J 1977 Degenerative changes in the intervertebral discs and their sequelae. Rheumatology and Rehabilitation 16: 13–21

Waddell G 1982 An approach to backache. British Journal of Hospital Medicine 28 (3): 187–219

Westrin C G 1973 Low back sick-listing. A sociological and medical insurance investigation. Scandinavian Journal of Social Medicine Supplement 7

White A W M 1966 Low-back pain in men receiving workmen's compensation. Canadian Medical Journal 95: 50–56

Wiesel S W, Cuckler J M, De Luca F et al 1980 Acute low back pain: an objective analysis of conservative therapy. Spine 5: 324–330

Working Group on Back Pain 1979 Department of Health and Social Security. Her Majesty's Stationery Office, London

Wyke B 1980 The neurology of low-back pain. In: Jayson M I V (ed) The lumbar spine and back pain, 2nd edn. Pitman, London, p 307

Wyke B 1987a The neurology of low-back pain. In: Jayson M I V (ed) The lumbar spine and back pain, 3rd edn. Churchill Livingstone, Edinburgh, p 59; 1987b: p 74

Wynn Parry C B 1989 The failed back. In: Wall P D, Melzack R (eds) Textbook of pain, 2nd edn. Churchill Livingstone, Edinburgh, p 341–353

Yates D W 1978 A comparison of the types of epidural

injection commonly used in the treatment of low-back pain and sciatica. Rheumatology and Rehabilitation 17: 181–186

Youel M A 1967 Effectiveness of pelvic traction. Journal of Bone and Joint Surgery 41A: 2051

18. Pain in the lower limb

INTRODUCTION

As pain in the leg from entrapment of lumbar nerve roots and from trigger points in the muscles of the lower back and buttocks has been dealt with in the previous chapter, and as pain in and around the hip, knee, and ankle joints will be discussed in Chapter 19, this chapter will be restricted to a consideration of pain in the lower limb occurring as a result of the activation of trigger points in muscles of the lower limb itself.

Investigations to ascertain the cause of persistent pain in the leg are usually directed at excluding diseases of the bones or joints, circulatory disorders, and neuropathies, but the possibility that such pain might occur as a result of the activation of trigger points in the muscles is all too frequently passed over, with the result that it is often allowed to continue for much longer than it need.

A man (75) began to get pain in the calves, ankles, and the soles of the feet on climbing stairs, together with troublesome cramps in the calves at night disturbing his sleep. After the symptoms had been present for 4 weeks, he sought medical advice. As investigations at that time showed no evidence of arthritis, no circulatory disturbance, and no evidence of a diabetic neuropathy, he was treated symptomatically with paracetamol for the pain on exertion, and quinine sulphate for the nocturnal cramps. These, however, had little or no effect and after a further 3 months he was referred to me as a case of persistent pain in the legs of unknown cause.

On taking this history, it became apparent that the patient spent much time cruising on the river. This involved frequently opening heavy lock gates, and to assist with this he was in the habit of pressing hard with his legs against concrete blocks. It would seem that this must have strained the muscles of his calves for, on examination, there were numerous exquisitely tender trigger points in the gastrocnemius and soleus muscles. Deactivation of these with dry needles on only one occasion gave him relief from the symptoms for 3 days, and after repeating the procedure a further three times at weekly intervals they disappeared altogether. A state of affairs of course that could have been achieved both more quickly and at an earlier stage if only the diagnosis had been made more promptly.

The muscles in the leg which, in my experience, most often develop active trigger points are the adductor longus, the quadriceps femoris group of muscles, the hamstrings, the tibialis anterior, the gastrocnemius, the soleus, the peronei and the dorsal interossei.

Adductor longus muscles (Fig. 18.1)

Trigger points in the adductor longus commonly develop near to its insertion into the pubis, and as referral of pain from these is predominantly into the groin, as well as down the inner side of the thigh, consideration will be given to pain from trigger points in this muscle when discussing pelvic pain in Chapter 20.

Quadriceps femoris group of muscles (Fig. 18.1)

Trigger points may become activated in any of the quadriceps group of muscles (the rectus femoris, the vastus medialis, the vastus intermedius, and the vastus lateralis), when these muscles become strained either as a primary event, or secondarily to walking badly because of some painful disorder in the foot, ankle or knee.

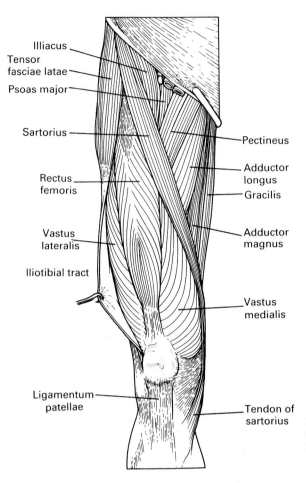

Fig. 18.1   Superficial muscles of the thigh. Extensor aspect.

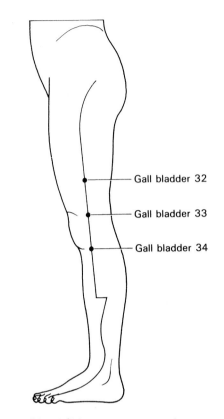

Fig. 18.2   Some traditional Chinese acupuncture points along the Gall Bladder meridian in the region of the knee joint.

With arthritis of the knee it is the vastus medialis that most commonly develops trigger points. The vastus medialis is the main muscular support of the knee, and as pointed out by Travell (1952), the development of trigger point activity in it, whether this be due to a primary muscle strain, or to arthritis in the knee, is liable to cause the knee to become unstable and for it suddenly to give way. This often occurs before this trigger point activity is a cause of pain. It therefore follows that a history of painless buckling of the knee is an indication for examining this muscle for a trigger point, and, if present, for it to be deactivated by means of inserting a dry needle into the tissues overlying it.

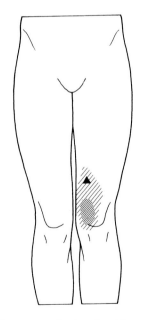

Fig. 18.3   The pattern of pain referral from a trigger point (▲) in the vastus medialis muscle.

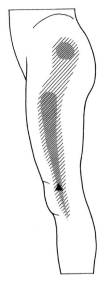

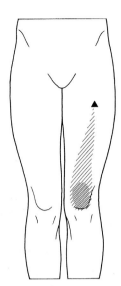

Fig. 18.4   The pattern of pain referral from a trigger point
(▲) in the vastus lateralis muscle.

Fig. 18.5   The pattern of pain referral from a trigger point
(▲) in the rectus femoris muscle.

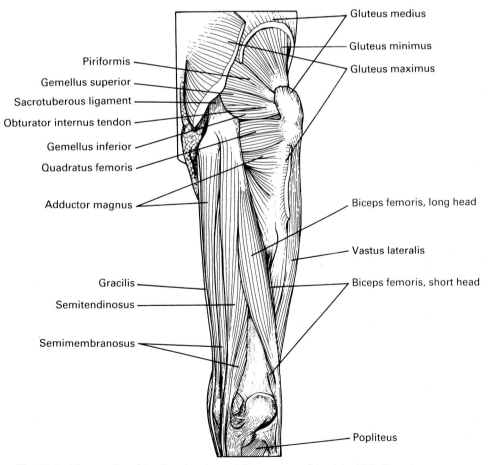

Fig. 18.6   The muscles of the gluteal region and flexor aspect of the right thigh. Posterior aspect.

For those interested in comparing positions of trigger points with those of traditional Chinese acupuncture points, it should be noted that the trigger point in the vastus medialis just above the knee is in close relationship to the traditional Chinese point Spleen 10 (Fig. 16.1) and one in the vastus lateralis, just above the knee, occurs close to the Chinese point Gall Bladder 33 (Fig. 18.2).

Pain from a trigger point just above the knee in the vastus medialis, is felt around the inner side of the knee (Fig. 18.3).

Pain from a trigger point just above the knee, in the vastus lateralis, is referred up the side of the thigh, from the trigger point below, up as far as the greater trochanter above (Fig. 18.4).

Trigger points in the vastus intermedius and rectus femoris are usually to be found in the upper third of the thigh, and pain from these is referred down the anterior surface of the thigh (Fig. 18.5).

Hamstrings (Fig. 18.6)

Trigger points in the hamstring muscles — the biceps femoris, the semimembranosus and the semitendinosus — are liable to become activated either in the bellies of these muscles high up on the posterior surface of the thigh or in their tendons at their sites of attachment just below the knee. It will be remembered that the lower attachment of the biceps femoris, the lateral hamstring, is by a tendon inserted into the fibula; the semimembranosus is inserted into the medial condyle of the tibia; and the semitendinosus, together with the gracilis and sartorius muscles, are inserted by a conjoined tendon — the pes anserinus (the goose's foot) — into the upper part of the medial surface of the tibia (Fig. 18.7).

Pain from trigger points in the bellies of these muscles is referred mainly to the region of the popliteal fossa (Fig. 18.8). Pain from trigger

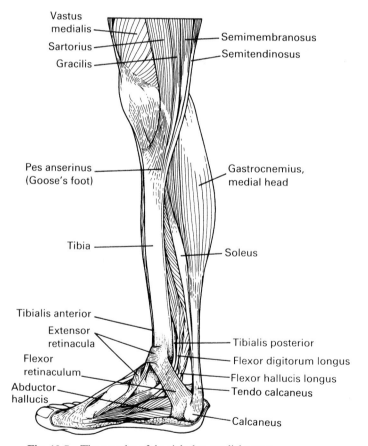

Fig. 18.7 The muscles of the right leg, medial aspect.

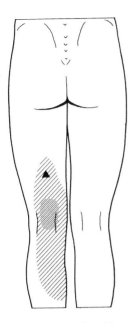

Fig. 18.8   The pattern of pain referral from a trigger point (▲) in the belly of the biceps femoris muscle.

points at their insertions is felt locally in the areas immediately adjacent to these sites.

When trigger points are widespread throughout the bellies of the hamstrings, they cause these muscles to become shortened with, as a consequence of this, restricted flexion of the hip and a positive straight-leg raising test (Simons & Travell 1984).

Tibialis anterior muscle (Fig. 18.9)

The tibialis anterior muscle which arises mainly from the upper two-thirds of the lateral surface of the tibia is a thick fleshy muscle that ends in a tendon attached on the medial side of the foot to the medial cuneiform bone and the first metatarsal bone.

Active trigger points usually occur in the belly of the muscle, with pain from this being referred down the front of the shin, the medial side of the ankle and foot, and sometimes extending as far as the big toe (Fig. 18.10).

Trigger point activity in this muscle is liable to develop in athletes and, as Sola & Williams (1956) point out, in members of the armed services who do much marching. The pain is quickly brought under control by deactivating the

trigger point with a dry needle, but is liable to recur if any activity responsible for the trigger point activation is persisted with.

Gastrocnemius muscle (Fig. 18.11)

Trigger points become activated in the belly of the muscle in the centre of the calf as a result of the muscle becoming strained either, as a primary event, or when a limp develops as a result of a painful disorder occurring in the heel or foot, and also when, because of a circulatory disorder, the muscle becomes ischaemic (Fig. 18.12).

The pain from trigger points in this muscle is felt in the calf and the sole of the foot. It is often worse on walking uphill, and may be associated with the development of nocturnal cramps. As may be seen from the case quoted at the beginning of the chapter, nocturnal cramps should not be treated with quinine sulphate until a search for trigger points in this muscle has been carried out, for if these are present, the cramps will not be brought under control until they have been deactivated.

Soleus muscle (Figs 18.9 and 18.11)

The soleus, a broad flat muscle situated immediately anterior to the gastrocnemius, and which together with the latter, is inserted into the calcaneus by means of the Achilles tendon, is liable to develop trigger points in its distal third for the same reasons as they do in the gastrocnemius.

Pain from these trigger points is referred distally along the Achilles tendon to the heel (Fig. 18.13). Simons & Travell (1983) state that the pain may also be referred upwards to the sacroiliac joint. No case with this particular pattern of referral has, as yet, come under my care. They also point out that the ankle jerk may be decreased or absent in patients with trigger point activity in the soleus. And that the deactivation of the trigger points restores this reflex to normal.

Activation of trigger points in the gastrocnemius and soleus as a consequence of lower leg ischaemia

Intermittent claudication (L. *claudicatio*, limping

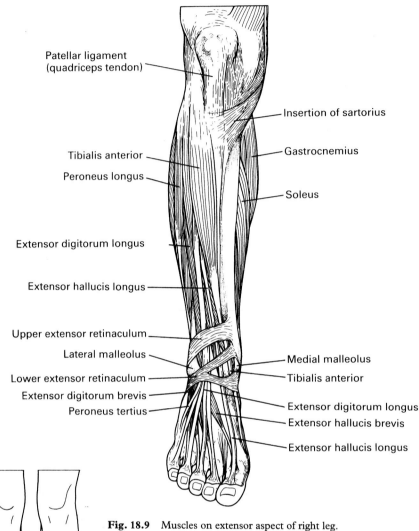

Fig. 18.9 Muscles on extensor aspect of right leg.

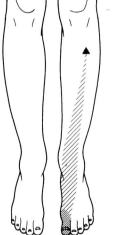

Fig. 18.10 The pattern of pain referral from a trigger point (▲) in the tibialis anterior muscle.

or lameness), a condition characterized by calf pain brought on by exertion and relieved by resting (angina cruris), is primarily due to femoro-popliteal artery occlusion. However, Dorigo et al (1979) have shown that another factor contributing to the pain is the activation of trigger points in the gastrocnemius and soleus when these muscles become ischaemic as a result of an impaired arterial blood supply to the leg. They further showed that deactivating these trigger points, by injecting procaine into them, increases the exercise capacity of the limb in spite of the blood flow to the limb remaining the same. Deactivation of trigger points in these two

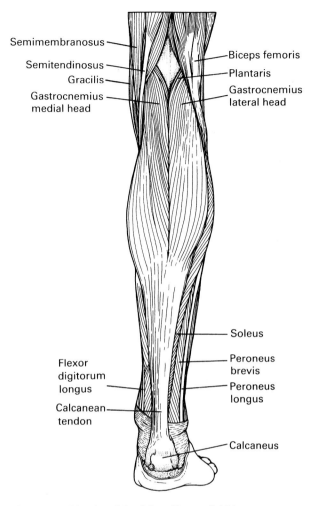

Semimembranosus

Semitendinosus

Gracilis

Gastrocnemius
medial head

Biceps femoris

Plantaris

Gastrocnemius
lateral head

Soleus

Peroneus
brevis

Peroneus
longus

Flexor
digitorum
longus

Calcanean
tendon

Calcaneus

Fig. 18.11 Muscles of the right calf; superficial layer.

muscles is therefore a worthwhile symptomatic therapeutic procedure in this condition and one that can be carried out even more readily and just as effectively by inserting dry needles into the tissues overlying these trigger points.

Painful heel

Persistent pain may develop in the heel, either by being referred from trigger points in the soleus muscle, or from an inflammatory reaction occurring in either the Achilles tendon, or the plantar fascia. This inflammatory reaction in both Achilles tendinitis and plantar fasciitis may develop as a result of some underlying disease such as ankylosing spondylitis, psoriatic

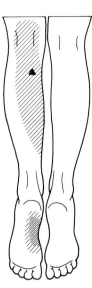

Fig. 18.12 The pattern of pain referral from a trigger point (▲) in the gastrocnemius muscle.

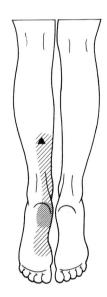

Fig. 18.13 The pattern of pain referral from a trigger point (▲) in the soleus muscle.

arthropathy, or Reiter's disease. More commonly, however, it occurs as a result of an injury to the heel or pressure from an ill-fitting shoe. At times it seems to occur for no apparent cause.

Achilles tendinitis

It is particularly important to distinguish between

pain developing in the base of the heel as a result of an inflammatory lesion in the tendon and pain referred to that site from trigger points in the soleus muscle. In Achilles tendinitis, the tendon is liable to be slightly swollen and there may be crepitus over it when the foot is moved. Also, on examination, exquisitely tender trigger points are to be found in the tissues around the tendon.

The pain may be relieved by inserting dry needles into the tissues overlying these trigger points. Admittedly this usually has to be repeated three or more times at weekly intervals in order to obtain any lasting benefit but it is certainly preferable to injecting hydrocortisone into them. Not only is hydrocortisone associated with the development of much post-injection pain but should it inadvertently be injected into the tendon itself, this structure may rupture and then need to be repaired surgically.

Plantar fasciitis

The plantar fascia is attached by a tendon inserted into the periosteum of the calcaneus. Trauma, with tearing or stretching of the plantar tendon fibres, causes the periosteum to become detached from the calcaneus, with, as a consequence of this, the development of subperiosteal inflammation, the laying down of fibrous tissue, the deposition of calcium and the formation of a calcaneal spur. It is thought that the initial pain and discomfort is probably due to the soft tissue inflammation and that at a later stage it is due to the spur (Cailliet 1977). However, not infrequently, there is radiographic evidence of a calcaneal spur in people who are asymptomatic. Furthermore, plantar fasciitis may occur without the development of a spur. Radiographically a calcaneal spur in traumatic fasciitis has smooth borders in contrast to one occurring in association with a seronegative arthropathy when they are fuzzy.

Plantar fasciitis leads to the development of severe pain under the heel, and also in some cases in the sole of the foot. It is a condition that most often occurs in those whose work requires much standing. On examination, there is a point of maximum tenderness close to where the plantar tendon attaches to the calcaneus. It is

standard practice to inject hydrocortisone plus a local anaesthetic into this point. It is often necessary to carry out this procedure more than once. It is also possible to control the pain simply by inserting into the point of maximum tenderness a dry needle and then leaving it in situ for 3–5 minutes. There is no need to carry out any twirling movements, particularly as at this particular site, it is liable to cause considerable pain. If the needle is left in place for a sufficient length of time, with this varying according to the needs of the individual patient, it will be found on withdrawing it, that the original exquisite tenderness has disappeared, and that weight bearing can be carried out far more comfortably. For long-term pain relief, however, it is usually necessary to repeat this procedure on several occasions. In addition strain should be taken off the plantar fascia by the wearing of a sorbo rubber heel pad with the centre cut out.

Metatarsalgia

Metatarsalgia, a condition characterized by the development of pain and tenderness in the region of the metatarsal heads, may be either congenital or acquired.

Congenital metatarsalgia (Morton's syndrome)

The underlying abnormality consists of a congenitally short first metatarsal bone and a relatively long second one (Morton 1952, 1955). This makes the foot unstable with a tendency for the ankle to rock inwards on standing. It is because of this that the ankle often becomes recurrently sprained. Calluses are liable to form under the prominent second metatarsal head. Also, on examination, the second toe is seen to protrude. The diagnosis is readily confirmed by an X-ray of the foot taken with the patient standing. The structural instability of the foot, and the pain in the sole occurring as a result, causes the patient to hobble. This, in turn, puts a strain on muscles throughout the whole of the leg and because of this pain frequently becomes widespread due to the activation of trigger points in various muscles.

The instability of the foot is liable to result in

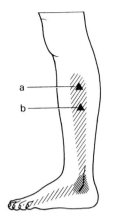

Fig. 18.14   The pattern of pain referral from a trigger point (▲) in (a) the peroneus longus muscle (b) the peroneus brevis muscle.

the hip being held in an adducted and internally rotated position; the knee being internally rotated; and the ankle pronated, with, as a consequence of this, trigger points becoming activated in the glutei muscles, particularly the gluteus medius (p. 284), the vastus medialis (p. 312), and the peroneus longus and brevis (Travell 1975).

Trigger points in the peroneus longus are to be found on the lateral surface of the leg about a hand's breadth below the head of the fibula. Trigger points in the peroneus brevis occur lower down the outside of the leg about two hand breadths above the external malleolus. Pain from trigger points in both these muscles is referred down the outer side of the leg and foot often as far as the little toe, with it being felt particularly strongly on the outer side of the ankle (Fig. 18.14).

The pain in the foot is best combated by placing a pad in the shoe under the head of the first metatarsal bone. Widespread pain throughout the leg necessitates careful examination of the muscles from the hip downwards for trigger points and any that are exquisitely tender should then be deactivated by means of inserting needles into them.

Acquired metatarsalgia

An anatomical abnormality such as claw-toes or an equinus deformity of the foot leads to stretch-

ing of the interosseous ligament and depression of the transverse arch so that instead of, as normally, most of the weight being placed on the first and fifth metatarsal heads, it is transferred to the 2nd, 3rd and 4th heads causing them to become painful and tender.

Treatment is directed at elevating the arch by inserting a pad inside the shoe under the second and third metatarsal bones *proximal* to the heads. It should not be placed under the heads themselves as this aggravates the pain.

Another cause for pain developing in the sole of the foot is a neuroma on the digital nerve between the 3rd and 4th toes, or occasionally between the 2nd and 3rd ones (Morton's neuroma). This condition, for some reason, most often occurs in middle-aged women who characteristically find when affected by it that taking off their shoes and massaging the soles of their feet gives them comfort.

On examination, the pain is aggravated by pressing between the metatarsal heads rather than over them. The pain is relieved by wearing broader shoes and by elevating the transverse arch by suitably padding the inside of the shoe. It is also sometimes necessary to attempt to suppress the pain by inserting a dry needle into a point of maximum tenderness. If this fails to give relief, a hydrocortisone-local anaesthetic mixture should be injected into it. And in particularly stubborn cases the neuroma may have to be excised. It also has to be remembered that metatarsalgia may also herald the onset of rheumatoid arthritis, long before the disease manifests itself by the development of a polyarthritis.

Finally, it is important to bear in mind that metatarsalgia, no matter how it is caused, may, by placing a strain on the muscles of the leg, lead to trigger points becoming activated in them, with as a result of this, pain developing over a wide area. Such widespread pain is best brought under control by deactivating these trigger points by means of the acupuncture technique of inserting dry needles into the tissues overlying them.

Pain in a toe

Pain in a toe is clearly most often due to some

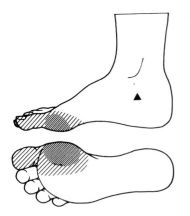

Fig. 18.15   The referral of pain to the big toe from a trigger point near to the medial malleolus.

obvious local pathology, but occasionally the pain persists in spite of the tissues in and around the toe having a normal appearance. In such a case it is likely that the pain is being referred to that site from a trigger point some distance away.

Trauma may cause trigger points to become activated in a dorsal interosseous muscle. When this occurs, pain is referred to the side of the toe

to which the muscle is attached. In relation to this it will be remembered that the 1st dorsal interosseous muscle is attached to the medial side of the 2nd toe. The 2nd, 3rd and 4th dorsal interosseous muscles are attached to the lateral side of the 2nd, 3rd and 4th toes.

Pain in the big toe may be referred from a trigger point high up on the outer aspect of the leg in the tibialis anterior muscle, or from a trigger point in the region of the medial malleolus (Fig. 18.15).

A schoolgirl (14) complained bitterly of pain in the big toe. Her doctor was at a loss to account for this as the appearances of the toe were normal and an X-ray of the foot showed no abnormality.

When, 6 months later, she was seen by me, the only abnormality to be found was an exquisitely tender point on the inside of the foot just in front of the medial malleolus. Long-term relief from the pain was obtained by deactivating this trigger point with a dry needle on two occasions. On going back over the history it seems likely that she had activated the trigger point some months previously at a time when she wrenched her ankle in the gymnasium.

REFERENCES

Cailliet R 1977 Soft tissue pain and disability. F A Davis, Philadelphia, p 288–290
Dorigo B, Bartoli V, Gristillo D, Beconi D 1979 Fibrositic myofascial pain in intermittent claudication. Effect of anaesthetic block of trigger points on exercise tolerance. Pain 6: 183–190
Morton D J 1952 Human locomotion and body form. A study of gravity and man. Williams & Wilkins, Baltimore
Morton D J 1955 Foot disorders in women. Journal of the American Medical Women's Association Feb 10: 41–46
Simons D G, Travell J G 1983 Myofascial origins of low back pain. Postgraduate Medicine 73: 66–108
Simons D G, Travell J G 1984 Myofascial pain syndromes. In: Wall P D, Melzack R (eds) Textbook of pain. Churchill Livingstone, Edinburgh, p 271
Sola A E, Williams R L 1956 Myofascial pain syndromes. Neurology (Minneapolis) 6: 91–95
Travell J 1952 Pain mechanisms in connective tissue. In: Ragan C (ed) Connective Tissues, Transactions of the Second Conference, 1951, Josiah Macy Jnr Foundation, New York, p 86–125
Travell J 1975 Pain and the Dudley J Morton foot (long second toe). Archives of Physical Medicine and Rehabilitation 56: 566

19. Pain in and around joints

It is now necessary to discuss pain in and around various joints that have not already been considered in previous chapters, and in particular to give a detailed account as to how acupuncture may be used to alleviate the pain of osteoarthritis, and also the pain in and around a non-arthritic joint that occurs as a result of trauma to its periarticular soft tissue. Brief reference will also be made to its limited application of rheumatoid arthritis.

OSTEOARTHRITIS

In order to be able to give a rational explanation as to how acupuncture may be used, either alone, or in conjunction with other forms of treatment, in the alleviation of osteoarthritic pain, it is first necessary to give a short summary of present-day knowledge concerning the aetiology and pathology of the disorder, and in particular to consider the various mechanisms thought to be responsible for the development of its characteristic type of pain.

Modes of presentation

The manner in which this condition presents and the course it takes are widely variable depending on whether it affects one joint alone, or many, and in the case of the latter, depending on which joints in particular are involved. Its presentation and natural history are also influenced by whether it occurs as a separate entity or as part of some systemic disease.

Primary generalized osteoarthritis

It would seem that by far the commonest form of

the condition is so-called primary generalized osteoarthritis (Huskisson et al 1979), a disorder that is most often seen in middle-aged women and one that mainly affects the knees and small joints of the hands and feet. The latter includes the carpo-metacarpal joint of the thumb, the terminal interphalangeal joints of the fingers (sometimes in association with Heberden's nodes), occasionally the proximal interphalangeal joints (sometimes in association with Bouchard's nodes), and also the metatarsophalangeal joint of the big toe (poor man's gout).

It is, however, the knees that are most often the dominant source of pain, and, as will be discussed later, it is in the relief of this that acupuncture is particularly useful. Other joints that may occasionally be affected are the hips, shoulders and elbows. The cervical and lumbar facet joints are usually also included amongst the joints affected in generalized osteoarthritis, but, as already discussed in Chapter 14 and 17 the part played by osteoarthritis of these joints in conjunction with degenerative disc disease in the condition known as spondylitis in the causation of chronic cervical and lumbar pain would seem to be far from clear.

It is generally agreed that genetic factors play a major role in the development of generalized osteoarthritis (Stecher 1955, Kellgren et al 1963) but, as Harper & Nuki (1980) point out, the nature of these remain poorly understood.

This genetic predisposition is of particular importance because for a long time osteoarthritis was considered to be more likely to occur in joints repeatedly subjected to trauma. It was said, for example, to be more common in miners working underground, particularly in confined spaces. Huskisson (1985), however, points out that this apparent, somewhat simplistic, link between osteoarthritis and trauma is not confirmed by recent studies which show, for example, that osteoarthritis of the knee is no commoner in parachute jumpers or footballers, except in those who have had a meniscectomy, and then there would seem to be some genetically determined underlying biochemical predilection in addition to the mechanical insult to the joint.

Monarticular hip disease

Osteoarthritis of the hip joint sometimes occurs alone, and would then seem to be a separate entity if for no other reason than, unlike generalized osteoarthritis, it is commoner in men (Wood 1976). The clinical course is also different with pain in generalized osteoarthritis tending to be episodic but with the pain in monarticular hip disease usually being persistent with a slow or, at times, rapid increase in intensity. This is a distinction of some importance considering how essential it is to take into account the natural history of pain from any particular joint when attempting to assess the effectiveness of some treatment, such as acupuncture, in relieving it.

Primary and secondary osteoarthritis

Osteoarthritis is traditionally divided into two groups, a primary one, and another in which it occurs secondary to some underlying disorder. This, however, is far from satisfactory because although, admittedly, examples of the latter include congenital, traumatic, and inflammatory conditions acting locally and various metabolic diseases such as alkaptonuria and haemochromatosis affecting the body in general, it is often by no means clear why so-called secondary osteoarthritis should develop as a result of, for example, some relatively minor congenital disorder of a joint. The term primary is also somewhat of a misnomer. Idiopathic or cryptogenic would be far more appropriate, for there is no doubt that the more that becomes known about the condition, the smaller this group will become.

Biochemical and mechanical factors in the aetiology of the disease

As stated earlier, the long-held concept that primary osteoarthritis is entirely mechanical in origin and due to 'wear and tear' of the cartilage is no longer tenable. It is true that a mechanical factor plays a part in its development, but there are now good reasons for believing that biochemical factors, yet to be identified, must also contribute.

Inflammation of the synovium

In recent years it has become apparent that chronic inflammation of the synovium is an important feature in the pathology of the disease. This is a finding of considerable significance as it has led to a better understanding of the mechanisms responsible for the pain, and as a direct result of this to a more rational approach to methods of alleviating it.

The disease in fact was originally known as osteoarthritis but in order to emphasize what was considered to be its mechanistic nature, it became fashionable not so long ago to call it osteoarthrosis. However, with recent recognition (Dieppe 1978) that inflammation of the synovium is an important part of the pathological process it is clearly preferable to revert to the original terminology. The tissue first to be affected and ultimately destroyed in osteoarthritis is cartilage, and fragments of this floating in the joint space are known to cause an inflammatory reaction in the synovium (George & Chrisman 1968). In addition, various chemical substances, such as pyrophosphates (McCarty 1976) and hydroxyapatite (Dieppe et al 1976, Schumacher et al 1977), found on occasions in crystal form in osteoarthritic joints, may also contribute to this inflammatory response in some patients.

The realization that an inflammation of the synovium similar to that seen in rheumatoid arthritis occurs in osteoarthritis has come from observations made both by clinicians and pathologists.

Clinically, it has now become widely recognized that an osteoarthritic joint may not only be painful but may also show evidence of warmth, swelling, redness, and stiffness on waking and after prolonged sitting. These are, as Ehrlich

(1975) points out, all classical symptoms and signs of inflammation. It is interesting to note with respect to this that Huskisson et al (1979), in comparing and contrasting the clinical features of 100 consecutive cases of rheumatoid arthritis and 100 consecutive cases of osteoarthritis, frequently found evidence of inflammation in those with osteoarthritis. Such evidence included morning stiffness, redness of distal interphalangeal joints, warmth, and effusion in the knees. And as they said,

the absence of morning stiffness has often been suggested as a helpful diagnostic feature of osteoarthritis, but it was noted by almost as many of our patients with osteoarthritis as those with rheumatoid arthritis. Synovial fluid also provided evidence for a low-grade inflammation with greater than normal number of cells.

Evidence for an inflammatory reaction being present has also recently been obtained by thermography confirming that osteoarthritic joints are warm (Collins et al 1976), although not to the same degree as in rheumatoid arthritis, thus confirming the clinical impression that the reaction is less severe.

Recently reported pathological evidence of an inflammatory reaction in the synovium includes Cooper et al (1981) finding this as commonly in synovial tissue taken from patients with osteoarthritis as from those with rheumatoid arthritis; Schumacher et al (1981) finding it in a large proportion of osteoarthritic knees examined at autopsy; and Goldenberg et al (1982) finding it in a majority of synovial specimens taken from osteoarthritic patients during the course of surgical operations.

Much space has been devoted to discussing this inflammatory change, because, as Fassbender (1975) has said, and as will be seen from the following discussion, it is in general only when synovitis occurs in an osteoarthritic joint that it becomes painful.

The pathological changes in an osteoarthritic joint, and the relationship of these to the production of pain

As has already been stated, the primary change in osteoarthritis is the destruction of the articular cartilage, and with the narrowing of the joint space that occurs as a result of this, changes take place fairly quickly in the underlying bone (Radin et al 1976). These include microfractures, sclerosis, and remodelling of the bone with the formation of osteophytes and the development of cysts.

When attempting to understand how pain may arise in an osteoarthritic joint, it is important to appreciate that there are no receptor nerve endings in the articular cartilage, synovium, or the menisci (Wyke 1981). Pain therefore cannot arise directly from the cartilage itself.

Subchondrial bone, however, is well supplied with nerves and therefore it would not be unreasonable to assume that the various changes just described that take place in it, and which start to develop at an early stage in the disease, are likely to generate pain. It is therefore somewhat surprising to find that there is no good evidence for this. For example, Lawrence et al (1966), in studying the relationship between symptoms and X-ray changes in an extensive population survey, found that bone cysts in the metacarpophalangeal joints and hip joints were seen no more frequently in those with pain than in those without pain. And Danielsson's (1964) 10 years' prospective study of patients with osteophytes in the region of the hip showed that they contributed little to the evolution of the osteoarthritic process or to the development of pain.

This therefore explains the seeming paradox that it is possible to have extensive osteoarthritic changes in a joint including a well-marked loss of joint space, sclerosis, cysts, and osteophytes, demonstrable radiographically, and yet for the joint not to be painful. And, as a corollary to this, it can never be assumed just because an X-ray shows changes of the disease in a joint that any pain from which a person may be suffering necessarily comes from this source. It is only possible to make a decision about this following a careful clinical examination.

Although it is true that at rest pain in the knee or hip may occur as a result of intramedullary venous stasis and hypertension both in patients with osteoarthritis of these joints and in those without (Arnoldi et al 1980), most of the various forms of pain that often occur episodically in osteoarthritis including the morning stiffness, and the aching type of discomfort that initially comes on with movements, but subsequently occurs at rest and also at night, would seem to develop only if and when there is inflammation of the synovium.

The synovium itself, as stated earlier, is devoid of nociceptive receptors but when it becomes inflamed and because of the effect this has on other tissues, pain occurs as a result of stimulation of nerve endings in the synovial blood vessels, the joint capsule, the fat pads, the collateral ligaments, and the adjacent muscles. There are various ways in which this occurs.

Firstly, there are nociceptive receptors in the adventitial sheaths of the vessels in the wall of the synoval sac, and when the latter becomes inflamed, stretching of these receptors leads to the production of pain.

Secondly, pain occurs because chemical substances such as 5-hydroxytryptamine, prostaglandins, histamine, and polypeptide kinins released from inflamed synovial cells get carried in the synovial fluid to the adjacent articular fat pads and joint capsule, where they have an irritant effect on the nociceptive receptors in these structures.

Thirdly, the fibrosis that ultimately develops in the capsule, and even at times in the adjacent muscles, in cases in which the inflammatory process becomes chronic, causes the tissues to contract, and this again leads to stimulation of their sensory receptors, particularly with movements of the joint.

Fourthly, pain develops because the changes that take place in an osteoarthritic joint lead to strain developing in various periarticular structures including the adjacent collateral ligaments, the muscle tendons, particularly at their sites of attachment to bone, the muscles around the joint, and in cases where a faulty posture develops, in muscles some distance from it.

The outcome of all this is that exquisitely tender 'spots' develop in the articular fat pads, the capsule, and the various periarticular structures just mentioned. The precise nature of these tender 'spots' is not certain but because, as will be shown, treatment directed to counteracting abnormal neurogenic activity in them, often

abolishes the pain, it is reasonable to assume that they are the main source from which it arises, and it is for this reason that they have come to be known as trigger points.

Pain and its correlation with X-ray changes

It can therefore be seen from what has just been said that the reasons for pain developing in an osteoarthritic joint is not because of cartilage damage, or of structural alterations in the subchondrial bone's architecture, but because of changes in the soft tissues of the joint and the various periarticular structures leading to the development of trigger points. And, as previously mentioned, this explains why pain in osteoarthritis does not necessarily correlate with the extent of the radiological changes. The one exception to this is osteoarthritis of the hip when the pain in general is proportional to the extent of the joint damage seen on a radiograph (Kellgren 1961) — this will be referred to again when discussing methods of alleviating hip pain.

The practical implications of all this, therefore, are that in the assessment of osteoarthritic pain, and in deciding how best to alleviate it, more information can often be obtained from a careful examination of the soft tissues than from an inspection of radiographs.

Examination of the soft tissues

In examining an osteoarthritic joint in order to determine sources of pain in the soft tissues, it is necessary to carry out a systematic search in structures such as ligaments, tendons, fat pads, and muscles for exquisitely tender 'spots' or what Steindler (1959) in his lecture on 'The pain syndrome of the knee joint' more aptly calls trigger points. As Harkness et al (1984) so rightly state 'the importance of a careful search for, and treatment of tender spots needs stressing in the management of osteoarthritis'.

Management of osteoarthritis

As there is, as yet, no means of arresting osteoarthritis, its management in the main is directed towards the symptomatic relief of pain.

It is my belief that a trigger point approach to acupuncture has an important place in this but it should not be looked upon as a technique necessarily to be used on its own but rather one that at times should be used in conjunction with other forms of therapy including, in particular, the administration of pain-alleviating drugs. It is therefore necessary to say something about the advantages and disadvantages of these in order that their place relative to that of acupuncture can be seen in a proper perspective.

Analgesics

Simple analgesics may be helpful but the discovery that the occurrence of pain in this disorder is closely associated with the development of an inflammatory process means that the use of a non-steroidal anti-inflammatory drug is often more effective.

When considering the use of an analgesic or a non-steroidal anti-inflammatory drug, it is as well to remember that aspirin has the properties of both.

Non-steroidal anti-inflammatory drugs (NSAIDs)

It has to be kept in mind when contemplating the use of NSAIDs in osteoarthritis that most of the patients suffering from this are elderly, and that because of this their metabolism and excretion of drugs are often impaired. Moreover, because those in later life frequently need a variety of drugs for many different complaints there is always the risk of drugs interacting. NSAIDs, for example, often increase the effects of anticoagulants, and decrease those of diuretics.

NSAIDs, too, by inhibiting the synthesis of prostaglandins are liable to aggravate late-onset asthma, and in conditions such as the nephrotic syndrome, hepatocellular failure, and cardiac failure, in which glomerural filtration is prostaglandin-dependent, their use is liable to precipitate uraemia and increase oedema. Also, because of their effect on prostaglandins they are liable to cause gastrointestinal bleeding, either from an erosive gastritis or peptic ulcer, which is a particularly serious event in an elderly artereosclerotic person.

It will be remembered that it was because of benoxaprofen causing liver failure in the elderly that it had to be withdrawn. And that it was because of an appreciable incidence of aplastic anaemia and agranulocytosis developing in those treated with phenylbutazone that the use of this drug in the treatment of osteoarthritis is no longer permitted.

Although it is generally agreed that all NSAIDs have potentially dangerous side-effects, their advantages must be weighed against their disadvantages, and there is no doubt that when used judiciously this group of drugs often gives dramatic relief.

It is important to bear in mind that they should never be prescribed on a long-term basis but always intermittently and even then in the lowest possible dosage; also, there are times when the presence of other conditions or individual intolerance precludes their use; and, that since adverse reports concerning them have reached the popular press, an increasing number of the public are refusing to take them.

There is thus much to be said for examining other forms of treatment to see which, if any, are worth using, either to supplement the effects of drug therapy or as an alternative to it.

Physiotherapy

Controlled trials of different forms of physiotherapy including immersing the hands in warm wax, short-wave diathermy, infra-red irradiation, and faradism show that all of them give a certain amount of temporary relief but none are of any lasting value (Hamilton et al 1959). There are certain physical measures, however, that are of considerable help. For those with osteoarthritis of the hip or knee, it is useful to carry a walking stick held in the contralateral hand, and when the quadriceps are wasted to strengthen these with exercises. Warm baths and swimming are also of benefit for those with hip disease.

Intra-articular injections of corticosteroids

As the pain in osteoarthritis would seem to be directly related to the development of an inflammatory reaction in the synovium it might be thought that it would be helpful to inject a corticosteroid into the joint. In general, however, the results have been disappointing. Miller et al (1958) and Wright et al (1960) showed that such injections give no better results than can be obtained from injections of a placebo. Admittedly Dieppe et al (1980), using a long acting preparation, triamcinolone hexacetonide, found that the relief from pain with this was greater than with a placebo, but even so the benefit was so slight and short lasting as to lead them to conclude that this form of treatment could not be recommended for use in everyday clinical practice.

Aspiration of the effusion

The effusion developing as a result of synovitis is sometimes so large that the volume of fluid itself causes pain. In such a case simply aspirating it often affords considerable relief.

Treatment directed at trigger points in and around the joint

There is no doubt that when attempting to alleviate osteoarthritic pain by some method applied locally to the joint, by far the best is to employ some technique directed specifically at trigger points, which as stated earlier, are to be found in various structures in and around the joint, including ligaments, tendons, articular fat pads, and muscles. There are essentially three ways of doing this — either to inject hydrocortisone or a local anaesthetic into periarticular tender spots as advocated by Dixon (1965) for the relief of osteoarthritic knee joint pain; or, alternatively, to deactivate the trigger points by means of the acupuncture technique of stimulating A-delta nerve fibres in the tissues overlying them with dry needles.

When deciding which of these methods to adopt it has to be remembered that a local anaesthetic, when injected into a trigger point, does not depend for its pain-suppressing effect on its ability to anaesthetize nerve endings, and a corticosteroid does not achieve this effect solely because of its local anti-inflammatory action, but, in common with many other substances, including saline, by having a non-specific irritant effect on A-delta nerve fibres in and around trigger points, which in turn activates centrally placed pain-modulating mechanisms, in exactly the same manner as the acupuncture technique of dry needle stimulation achieves this. And certainly, from everyday clinical experience, it would seem that there is no advantage in using either a corticosteroid or a local anaesthetic over that of using the much simpler and far more straightforward technique of acupuncture. With respect to acupuncture, it is also worth bearing in mind that medical scientists in China have shown that it is capable of stimulating the production of cortisol (for a detailed discussion of this, see Ch. 15), and although this requires to be confirmed by further studies, on the present evidence, it is reasonable to suppose, that because of this, it may well have an anti-inflammatory action. If this is so, then of course it considerably increases the usefulness of this form of therapy in a condition such as osteoarthritis in which there is an appreciable articular and periarticular inflammatory response. Certainly the clinical observation that not infrequently following acupuncture there is a significant decrease in the periarticular soft tissue swelling would seem to support this idea. The following case provides a particularly striking example of this.

A housewife (62) was referred to me with a 6-month history of severe pain from an osteoarthritic first carpometacarpal joint. On examination, the tissues around the joint were noted to be considerably swollen. Nevertheless, within 3 days of deactivating trigger points with dry needles for the first time, the swelling totally disappeared, and after a further three treatment sessions there was long-term relief from pain.

It therefore follows that in alleviating osteoarthritic pain there is a good case for either injecting hydrocortisone into trigger points or for deactivating them with dry needles. The latter, in my experience, is in general to be preferred for routine use, but there are occasional circumstances when an injection of hydrocortisone is the treatment of choice. An example of this is when, as not infrequently happens, the strain of walking on an osteoarthritic knee results in the development of considerable swelling of the tissues in the region of the vastus medialis muscle just above the knee. These types of treatment, therefore, as always, are not mutually exclusive, and there are circumstances when the two used together in the same patient give better results than one alone.

NON-ARTHRITIC JOINT PAIN

Pain from a sprained joint

Trigger points in the soft tissues around a sprained joint may become activated and their deactivation with dry needles is helpful in alleviating the pain associated with this type of lesion.

Myofascial trigger point pain

Pain may develop in the region of a joint due to it being referred there from myofascial trigger points some distance away. It therefore follows that with pain in and around a joint it is not only necessary to examine the joint itself but also to exclude the presence of trigger points in the surrounding muscles.

The use of acupuncture in alleviating pain in and around certain specific joints will now be discussed.

PAIN IN AND AROUND THE KNEE JOINT

Pain in and around the knee joint may, as is well known, be referred there from hip joint disease, also from trigger point activity in muscles some distance from the joint, or from trigger point activity in the periarticular soft tissues of a normal joint, or an arthritic one.

Osteoarthritis of the knee joint

Osteoarthritis commonly involves the knee joint and when it does so it affects either the patello-femoral compartment, or the medial or lateral tibiofemoral compartments, or any combination of these.

Patellofemoral compartment

Involvement of the patellofemoral compartment is occasionally the predominant feature and when

this occurs prematurely, it is known as chondromalacia patellae. Chondromalacia patellae often starts between the ages of 15 and 30 years and usually begins on the medial aspect of the patella. The reason for this, as Wiberg (1941) has shown, is that whereas contact between the lateral facet of the patella and the femur is good at all stages of flexion, contact between the medial facet and its corresponding condyle on the femur is poor at about 90° of flexion, with, as a consequence of this, undue wear of the cartilage taking place at this site. The condition, somewhat surprisingly, sometimes gradually remits but at other times slowly progresses over the years and becomes indistinguishable from osteoarthritis.

The symptoms of the condition are pain behind the patella on walking and, in particular, on descending stairs. On examination of the joint, there is patella crepitation. A good diagnostic test is the eliciting of pain by getting the patient to contract the quadriceps whilst the patella is held firmly against the femoral condyles. Also, in favour of the diagnosis is the eliciting of pain by sliding the patella to one side or the other, with the leg extended. On palpation of the soft tissues trigger points are to be found along the sides of the patella. The commonest site for these is its upper lateral edge (Dixon 1965).

The pain in this condition which typically is intermittent in nature, is readily alleviated by deactivating these trigger points by means of inserting dry needles into the tissues overlying them. It is a procedure, however, because of the nature of the disease, that usually has to be repeated from time to time. It is only in the occasional patient, though, that the pain is so persistent as to necessitate some form of surgery being carried out.

Tibiofemoral compartments

With osteoarthritis of the tibiofemoral compartments, changes usually occur in both the medial and lateral ones but they are commonly most marked on the medial side.

Pain occurring as a result of this is associated with trigger points developing in the collateral ligaments, in tendons adjacent to them, in the articular fat pads, and in muscles near to and at times some distance from the joint; also, at times it occurs in and around the popliteal fossa.

Trigger points in the collateral ligaments

Trigger points are usually to be found in these ligaments at their upper and lower attachments (Fig. 19.1). One of the commonest sites is the anteromedial aspect of the upper part of the tibia in the area somewhat fancifully known as the pes anserinus or goose's foot (Fig. 18.7). The pes

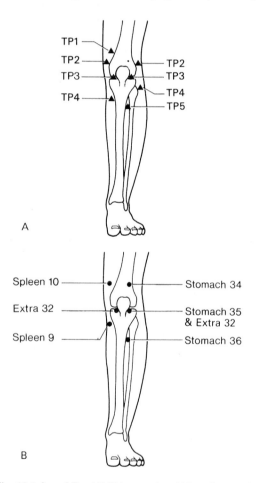

A

B

Fig. 19.1 A and B   (A) Trigger points (▲) on the anterior aspect of the knee. (1) in the vastus medialis muscle. (2) & (4) at the upper and lower insertions of the collateral ligaments. (3) in fat pads (Both these trigger points corresponding in position with traditional Chinese acupuncture points Extra 32 and, on the lateral side also with Stomach 35). (5) Trigger point corresponding in position with traditional Chinese acupuncture point Stomach 36. (B) Traditional Chinese acupuncture points (•).

anserinus is where the lower part of the medial collateral ligament, and superficial to this, the tendons of the sartorius, gracilis, and semitendinosus muscles become attached to the tibia. A bursa is present between the ligament and tendons.

Careful inspection will often reveal several trigger points in this area, and for the best results, it is necessary to deactivate each one of them with a dry needle. It is interesting to note, however, that in the traditional Chinese system, there is only one acupuncture point in this area — the so-called Spleen 9 (Fig. 16.1)

Trigger points in the medial and lateral articular fat pads

The fat pads are extrasynovial, but intracapsular, and change their shape with every movement of the knee. Trigger points in these structures are to be found on either side of the quadriceps tendon. The medial fat pad is the one most commonly affected (Fig. 19.1).

Trigger points in the vastus medialis muscle

Trigger points are often found in the vastus medialis muscle just above the knee (Fig. 19.1). In conjunction with trigger points at other sites they may be a source of pain, but on occasions without pain developing, they are the cause of the knee suddenly buckling. As Travell (1951) has pointed out, this structure is the main muscular support of the knee and when, as sometimes happens, trigger point activity in it occurs in isolation, the contraction of the muscle is in some way inhibited before pain develops, with, in consequence, the knee suddenly giving way without warning, and causing what is tantamount to a 'drop' attack.

Trigger points in the iliotibial tract

The strain imposed on the lower limb by an osteoarthritic knee joint sometimes leads to trigger points developing along the outer side of the thigh in the iliotibial tract, and below the knee between the tibia and fibula, with one often coinciding in position with the well-known

Chinese acupuncture point, Stomach 36 (Fig. 19.1).

Trigger points in the popliteal fossa

The main sites where trigger points are sometimes to be found in the popliteal fossa are in the midline and along its outer borders (Fig. 19.2). The point, at the centre of the fossa in the midline, situated in the popliteus muscle, corresponds in position with the traditional Chinese acupuncture point, Urinary Bladder 40. On the outer side points may be found, above, in the biceps femoris, and below, in the lateral head of the gastrocnemius. And, on the inner side, points may be found, above, in the vicinity of the semimembranosus and semitendinosus tendons, and

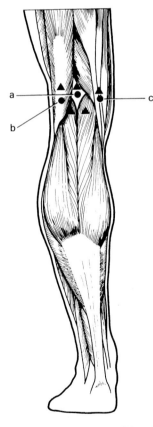

Fig. 19.2 Trigger points (▲) an traditional Chinese acupuncture points (•) in the region of the popliteal fossa. The central trigger point corresponding in position with the traditional Chinese acupuncture point Urinary Bladder 40 (a). Acupuncture points b & c are Urinary Bladder 39 and Kidney 10 respectively.

below, in the medial head of the gastrocnemius. It is interesting to note that there are two Chinese acupuncture points on the outer sides of the popliteal fossa namely, Urinary Bladder 39 on the lateral side, and Kidney 10 on the medial side (Fig. 19.2).

Factors influencing response to treatment

Whilst bearing in mind that osteoarthritic pain in the knee, certainly in the earlier stages of the disease, tends to be episodic with natural remissions, it would seem that with treatment directed at trigger points in and around the joint, it is possible to obtain, often in a quite dramatic manner, long lasting relief from pain of many months duration.

Factors, however, that may influence the response include joint instability, obesity, and unequal leg length.

Joint instability

Progressive degenerative changes in the cartilage and subchondral bone may ultimately lead to development of considerable joint instability. When this occurs, the strain imposed upon the surrounding ligaments and muscles causes trigger points in these structures to remain in a state of persistent activity. It is because of this that any relief from pain obtained by deactivating these trigger points with dry needles tends to be only short-lived. However, in spite of this, it is often possible by repeating treatment at frequent intervals to considerably improve the quality of a person's life.

A housewife (62) was referred to me for acupuncture with a 5-year history of severe pain in the right knee, which for the past year had become so bad that she could do nothing more than hobble around the house with the aid of a stick.

On examination there was evidence of marked joint instability; also, the scar of a patellectomy carried out for osteoarthritis of the patellofemoral compartment. The current X-ray showed extensive changes of this disease, affecting particularly the medial tibiofemoral compartment.

Exquisitely tender trigger points were found in and around the medial collateral ligament, with deactivation of these by dry needle stimulation giving immediate relief from pain. But, in spite of repeating this procedure on several occasions, the relief never lasted for more than 2–3 weeks. The patient would not contemplate undergoing any further surgery. However, by repeating acupuncture every 3 weeks for over 4 years now, the pain has been kept under such good control as to allow her to lead a reasonably active life including doing her own shopping and gardening. The object lesson here is that with acupuncture, provided a patient has sufficient tenacity of purpose to persevere with treatment, it is often possible to obtain long-term benefit from the cumulative effects of short-term pain relief.

Obesity

It is not uncommon for a person suffering from obesity to develop osteoarthritis of the knee joint. The relationship between the two, however, is far from clear. The rarity of the disease developing in the ankle joint, except when it has been subjected to some form of trauma, shows that excessive weight bearing is not an important aetiological factor. There is no doubt, however, that obesity aggravates the condition and this is probably because of the fact that it impedes the body's normal movements. Dixon (1965) considers the 'Fat lady's knee' to be a distinct clinical syndrome that includes medial ligament strain, excessive tenderness over the medial ligament, and tender hypertrophy of fat pads medial and posterior to the knee. In his series of cases with this syndrome, infiltration of the medial ligament and tender fat pads with a local anaesthetic produced no lasting benefit.

He found that the pain was relieved in the minority who could be persuaded to lose weight but concluded that the full syndrome of 'Fat lady's knee' is hard to help. This has not always been my experience when treating osteoarthritis of the knee in obese women with acupuncture, although for any lasting benefit to be obtained this has to be repeated several times. Unfortunately Dixon does not state how often injections of a local anaesthetic were given. If only once, as the report seems to imply, then it is no wonder that the results were disappointing. Many fat middle-aged females that have been under my care with this condition have obtained relatively long remissions from pain that has been

present for several months or years by stimulating trigger points with dry needles, 3–4 times at weekly intervals. The following case is one of the more impressive examples.

A 22 stone (139.7 kg) lady hobbled into my consulting room on a stick having persuaded her general practitioner to let her try acupuncture for severe pain of 8 years' duration in osteoarthritic knees. He told her that in view of her considerable obesity she was wasting her time. This was an opinion that at that time was shared by me, especially as on examination there was considerable swelling of the joints with a well-marked genu varus deformity. However, not to disappoint her, needles were inserted into the tissues overlying trigger points in the medial ligament and the vastus medialis muscle. After two treatments the pain was sufficiently alleviated as to allow her to give up using a stick, and after two more treatments, i.e. 1 month from starting treatment, she became virtually free from pain. And in spite of only managing to lose about 2 stone she remained like this for 12 months. At that stage further treatment had to be given but once again her response was similarly gratifying.

Short leg syndrome

It is important in examining the knee joint to take account of the length of the two legs (see p. 253) for when there is real or apparent shortening of one leg, the knee on the *contralateral* side is liable to become osteoarthritic. This occurs because the compensatory position of flexion and external rotation in which the 'longer' leg is held on walking, causes abnormal stretching of the medial ligament, and the excessive lateral mobility of the knee joint occurring as a result of this, leads to the development of destructive changes in the joint and particularly its lateral femoropatellar compartment.

Any relief from pain obtained by deactivating trigger points that develop in the soft tissues is liable to be short-lived unless the shortness of the contralateral leg is corrected by the wearing of a raised shoe.

Pain referred to the knee from some distant site

As Kellgren pointed out over 40 years ago (Ch. 4), pain in the region of the knee may occur as a result of being referred there either from the hip joint, or from tissues around the lumbar spine, or from the muscles of the thigh. Any examination of a painful knee should therefore always include an examination for trigger points in muscles or tendons at these sites. Radiographic evidence of arthritis in the knee joint is no reason for omitting this search because, as already stated, no matter how extensive the cartilage and bone changes from this may be, they are not in themselves a cause of pain.

A schoolmistress (56) was sent to me with a 5-month history of severe pain in the knees, due, according to the referral letter, to radiographically confirmed osteoarthritis in these joints.

On examination, the contours and movements of the joints were normal, and most important of all there were no trigger points in the soft tissues around them. There were, however, exquisitely tender ones in the region of both sacroiliac joints, also down the outer sides of the legs in the upper parts of the iliotibial tracts, and in muscles in the upper inner parts of the thighs.

In order to alleviate the knee pain it was necessary to deactivate all of these trigger points by inserting dry needles into the tissues overlying them, and in order to obtain lasting benefit, to repeat this procedure on five occasions at weekly intervals.

Persistent pain from a 'strained' non-osteoarthritic knee

The activation of trigger points in the soft tissues around the knee joint, in exactly the same sites as in osteoarthritis, may occur as a result of trauma. As anywhere else in the body, failure to recognize their presence and to deal with them appropriately may lead to many months of unnecessary disability.

A builder's labourer (43) fell off some scaffolding, and shortly after this the left knee became swollen and painful. The swelling quickly subsided but the pain persisted and 3 months after the accident, he was seen by an orthopaedic surgeon. He detected no abnormality either on clinical examination or on arthroscopy, and, more to placate the patient than for any other reason, arranged for him to have a course of physiotherapy. When, after a further 2 months, the pain was no better, the surgeon concluded that there could be no organic cause for it.

After the patient had been off work for 9 months, and in imminent danger of losing his job, his doctor referred him to me for assessment as to whether acupuncture might be of help.

The patient, a sensible, placid, and quite obviously, normally a very hard working type of person, told me that he was in a state of despair because, although he had full movements of the knee, it ached persistently and this was so bad at nights as to prevent him from getting any sleep.

On examination, there were two exquisitely tender trigger points immediately adjacent to the upper medial and lateral edges of the patella, and another one on the medial aspect of the tibia just below the knee. After deactivating these trigger points with dry needles on only two occasions, he lost his pain and within a very short time was able to get back to work.

PAIN IN AND AROUND THE HIP

Osteoarthritis

This disorder is occasionally the cause of pain in and around the hip in adults under the age of 40, if the joint has been damaged by some inflammatory arthritis, or subjected to strain from some congenital or acquired deformity. It, of course, becomes an increasingly common cause of pain in this region from middle age onwards. It should be noted that although osteoarthritis of the hip is usually a monarticular disorder it is not unusual for a person with unilateral hip disease to develop similar changes on the opposite side at a later date.

The pain both in so-called primary and secondary osteoarthritis of the hip joint, from the outset, usually takes the form of a severe dull ache, and once started it tends to get progressively worse. It is therefore unlike the episodic type of pain that so commonly occurs with involvement of other joints. It is felt especially in the groin, the inguinal region, over the greater trochanter, and outer side of the buttock. The pain may also be referred to the knee joint due to this and the hip joint being innervated by the obturator nerve. The strain imposed on the muscles of the back may also cause lumbar pain, and pain may also radiate down the thigh, particularly on the outer side.

The pain at first is aggravated by walking and relieved by rest, but in the later stages it is present the whole time. On clinical examination, there is pain on movement of the joint, and limitation of its movements, those particularly affected being internal rotation and extension. Atrophy of the gluteal and quadriceps muscles may be observed; and on palpation there are focal points of exquisite tenderness due to the activation of trigger points. The pain, which in the case of the hip joint is in direct proportion to the extent of joint damage seen on a radiograph (De Ceulaer & Watson Buchanan 1979) would seem to be due to several different causes.

As stated previously the cartilage does not have a nerve supply, and surprisingly, neither osteophytes (Danielsson 1964) nor bone cysts (Lawrence et al 1966) in themselves would seem to give rise to pain. However, large cysts in the femoral head may cause the latter to collapse with the production of sudden intense pain.

Pain in the hip, as in the knee, both when osteoarthritis is present and when it is not, is on occasions due to intraosseous venous stasis and intraosseous hypertension — the so-called 'intraosseous engorgement pain syndrome' (Lemperg & Arnoldi 1978). This pain which is worse towards the end of the day's activities, and persists at rest, may be alleviated by lowering the intraosseous pressure by some surgical procedure such as an osteotomy (Arnoldi et al 1971). The pain, however, that can be influenced by acupuncture is that which develops as a result of trigger points becoming activated in the periarticular tissues for the same reasons as cause this to happen in osteoarthritis of the knee joint.

Examination for trigger points

No examination to establish the cause of pain in and around the hip joint is complete without a systematic search for trigger points. There are three main sites where these trigger points are usually to be found, irrespective of whether the pain is due to osteoarthritis of the hip, or is primarily muscular in origin. In distinguishing between these two causes of pain in the region it should be remembered that with osteoarthritis there is often considerable limitation of movements of the joint, and usually, but not always, by the time that pain from this condition

develops there are characteristic abnormalities to be seen on a radiograph. There are occasions, however, in the early stages of the disease when the pain of a restrictive capsulitis develops before X-ray changes become apparent.

Location of trigger points in arthritis and non-arthritic painful disorders around the hip

Trigger points are mainly to be found at one or more of the following three sites; the groin; the upper part of thigh, close to where the femoral artery passes behind the inguinal ligament; and the greater trochanter.

Trigger points in the groin usually develop in the adductor longus muscle near to its insertion into the pubic bone (Travell 1950) (Fig. 18.1).

In addition, there is sometimes a trigger point to be found immediately below the inguinal ligament, anterior to the capsule of the joint, in the iliopsoas muscle (Fig. 17.15).

Trigger points also frequently occur in muscles in the region of the greater trochanter, and in particular in the gluteus medius and minimus close to where these muscles become attached to it. In order not to overlook any of the trigger points in this region it is necessary to palpate the tissues overlying and adjacent to the greater trochanter in a systematic manner, with special attention being paid to the gluteal muscles as they converge towards it from behind; to the various muscles immediately overlying it; and as Sola & Williams (1956) pointed out, to that part of the tensor fasciae latae situated immediately below it (Fig. 19.3).

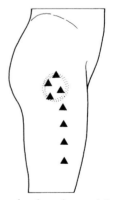

Fig. 19.3 Trigger points in and around the greater trochanter and along the tensor fasciae latae.

It should be noted that a trigger point in the gluteus medius or minimus close to the greater trochanter may not only give rise to pain in the hip region but may also cause it to be referred down the outer side of the thigh and leg (Fig. 17.11). Also, a trigger point immediately below the iliac crest in one or other of these muscles may not only give rise to pain in the hip region, but also cause it to be referred down the back of the thigh and leg (Fig. 17.12).

Deactivation of trigger points

Dry needle stimulation of activated trigger points in mild to moderate osteoarthritis of the hip gives a certain amount of relief from pain but the effect is never as dramatic or as long lasting as it is with osteoarthritis of the knee. There is therefore much to be said for combining the effects of acupuncture and drug therapy including the use of either a non-steroidal anti-inflammatory drug, or a simple analgesic, or both.

Treatment to relieve the pain of an osteoarthritic hip usually has to be given over a long period of time, and therefore one of the great advantages of using both acupuncture and a drug together is that the pain-relieving effect of the former makes it possible to keep the dose of the latter to a minimum, and thereby helps to reduce the risks of any potential side-effects from it.

Non-osteoarthritic pain

The acupuncture technique of deactivating trigger points with dry needles when pain around the hip is primarily of muscular origin is on the other hand very rewarding and often, in my experience, it is possible to bring even quite long-standing pain fairly rapidly under control.

A racehorse breeder (51) was referred to me by a gastroenterologist because of long-standing epigastric pain emanating from a myofascial trigger point just below the xiphisternum (see Ch. 20). The patient, finding that this was quite quickly relieved by acupuncture, then enquired whether similar treatment might help alleviate persistent pain in his right hip! It transpired that 18 years previously he had had a car accident, since when he had had considerable pain in

the right groin and hip region causing him to have a pronounced limp.

After having had this limp for about 10 years it got so bad that he was referred to an orthopaedic specialist who encased the lower back and hip in plaster. Apparently, apart from making his back muscles weak, this had had no effect, and he was told that although the X-ray, as yet, showed only a slight abnormality he would eventually require an operation on his hip, but that, in the meantime, he should keep the pain under control with analgesics.

On examination, there were good movements of the hip joint and the only abnormal finding was the discovery of two trigger points in the adductor longus muscle: one just below the inguinal ligament and the other at the insertion of the tendon into the pubic bone. Quite remarkably, after deactivating these trigger points with dry needles on only two occasions, the pain of 18 years standing disappeared, and when seen 2 years later it had not recurred.

This is yet another striking example of the post-traumatic persistent pain syndrome (Ch. 7) showing how trigger point activation as a result of trauma may cause pain to persist virtually indefinitely, but provided the tissues are otherwise healthy, deactivation of the trigger point, no matter how long this is delayed, quickly alleviates the pain.

Periosteal pecking

It should be noted that for pain in the hip region Mann (1974) advocates pecking the periosteum of the greater trochanter with a dry needle, and for pain in the knee region, pecking the upper medial aspect of the tibia. Stimulating periosteal nerve endings in this manner is undoubtedly a powerful form of acupuncture but a somewhat painful one, and in order to assess whether the results obtained by it are any better than those achieved by systematic deactivation of myofascial trigger points around the knee and hip as just described, it would be necessary to carry out a carefully conducted statistically controlled clinical trial.

Pain in and around the small joints of the hands

The pain from generalized osteoarthritis of the small joints of the hands is usually best controlled by the use of a non-steroidal anti-inflammatory drug, but occasionally one finger joint in particular is especially painful, and in such a case it is helpful to palpate around the joint and to insert dry needles into any particularly tender points. Pain in the first carpometacarpal joint of the thumb is usually more troublesome than in the finger joints presumably because of the important part played by the thumb in grasping objects.

Deactivation of trigger points around this joint at the base of the thumb when it is affected by osteoarthritis is only helpful in the earlier stages of the disease. It is however extremely effective in alleviating pain that sometimes persists following a sprain of the joint. Case histories illustrating this have already been given in Chapter 15.

Pain in the wrist

When a wrist is sprained, trigger points become activated in the periarticular tissues, and the deactivation of these by inserting dry needles into them is very helpful in relieving the pain associated with this condition.

Pain in the elbow

Osteoarthritis of this joint is rare unless the joint has previously been damaged by trauma or inflammation. However, when, occasionally, it does occur, the acupuncture technique of deactivating trigger points in the periarticular tissue overlying the medial and lateral epicondyles, and in the cubital fossa, is certainly helpful in relieving the pain. Much more commonly, persistent pain develops in the region of the elbow joint due to trigger point activation occurring as a result of trauma to the soft tissues. 'Tennis' elbow and 'golf' elbow with pain localized to one or other sides of the joint have already been discussed (Ch. 15). At times, however, this post-traumatic pain around the elbow is more generalized and the movements of the elbow joint, because of this, become restricted.

A man (40) was ostensibly referred to me because of persistent pain in the neck of 6 months duration. During the course of examination, however, it was noted that the left elbow was supported in a specially constructed leather splint. On enquiring about this it transpired that he had been fitted with this 10 years

previously because of persistent pain in the region of the elbow joint following an injury sustained whilst serving in the S.A.S. He said he religiously wore the splint as advised but it had done little to control the pain but he had learnt to live with it believing that nothing further could be done. All the splint seemed to have done was to make the elbow extremely stiff. An X-ray showed no significant abnormality in the joint itself. However, examination of the surrounding muscles showed there were some exquisitely tender trigger points that clearly had originally been overlooked, and after these had been deactivated with dry needles on four occasions at weekly intervals, the pain was brought under control and full movements of the joint restored.

Pain in the feet

The only joint in the foot commonly affected by osteoarthritis is the metatarsophalangeal joint of the big toe, and when this occurs as part of the generalized form of the disease is usually mild and rarely requires any special form of treatment.

Pain in the ankle

It is remarkable that considering that this joint has to bear all the weight of the body that it is rarely affected by osteoarthritis, even when subjected to repeated trauma as, for example, with footballers. When, occasionally, there is persistent pain from osteoarthritis of this joint, activated trigger points are to be found clustered around the malleoli and on the dorsum of the foot midway between these two structures. Deactivation of these by dry needle stimulation, provided this is repeated on several occasions at weekly intervals, will often cause the pain to remit for an appreciable period of time.

Trigger points at these sites also become activated when the joint is sprained (Travell & Rinzler 1952, Bonica 1953). As Bonica points out, rather than immobilizing the joint as is standard practice, it is better to get rid of the pain by deactivating the trigger points, and then encourage active movements. He advocated injecting the trigger points with a local anaesthetic, but deactivating them with a dry needle is simpler and just as effective.

CLINICAL TRIALS TO ASSESS THE VALUE OF ACUPUNCTURE IN RELIEVING OSTEOARTHRITIC PAIN

It is impossible to assess adequately the value of acupuncture in a disorder such as osteoarthritis in which, somewhat paradoxically, progressive and irreversible damage to a joint is often associated with self-limiting episodes of pain, without recourse to carefully conducted large scale clinical trials. And unfortunately up to now there has been a dearth of these.

Milligan et al (1980) compared the effectiveness of electroacupuncture and short-wave diathermy is alleviating the pain of osteoarthritis of the knee in 100 consecutive patients divided into two groups. They found at follow-up, 3 months after the completion of treatment, that pain was significantly reduced in 48.8% of patients in the acupuncture group and in 15.1% of those in the physiotherapy group.

Junnila (1982) compared the effects of acupuncture and those of piroxicam in alleviating pain associated with osteoarthritis in large joints. He found that the number of patients who experienced significant relief of pain in the acupuncture group was twice that in the piroxicam group, and noted that the additional advantage of acupuncture is its freedom from side-effects.

The difficulties associated with the carrying out of acupuncture trials in general, and in particular, the problems posed in attempting to compare its effectiveness with that of a placebo were discussed in Chapter 11. It is, however, essential to realize that such difficulties are particulary great when comparing the effectiveness of acupuncture or for that matter any other form of treatment with that of a placebo, in alleviating the pain of osteoarthritis due to the placebo treatment response in this condition often being much in excess of the normally attained 30% level.

Sidel & Abrahams (1940), for example, in comparing the effectiveness of a vaccine with that of subcutaneous saline injections in osteoarthritis found that 86% of patients treated with the latter obtained significant relief from pain. Also, Traut & Passarelli (1956) found that 59% of 182 patients with osteoarthritic pain obtained relief from this when given lactose tablets! It is therefore not possible to dissent from Evans's (1974) opinion that in order to ascertain whether any form of treatment gives better results than a placebo in the alleviation of osteoarthritic pain carefully conducted comparative trials are mandatory. This having been said, it is nevertheless essential when carrying out such trials to ensure that the properties of the treatment used in the control group are strictly limited to those of a true placebo. It would, for example, appear to have been unwise for Gaw et al (1975), in their otherwise carefully conducted trial, to assess the efficacy of acupuncture in relieving osteoarthritic pain, to have a control group in which needles were inserted into sites, 'outside of, but contiguous to, traditional acupuncture points', on the assumption that these were placebo points.

Patients in both groups responded to their respective treatments equally well, but it would be wrong to conclude from this that acupuncture in the treatment of this condition is no better than a placebo treatment for, as Mann et al (1973) so rightly observed, when discussing the subject of acupuncture in general, 'because of the lack of precise localization of acupuncture points it is difficult to conceive of nearby placebo points'. The implication of this is that the two groups in Gaw et al's study were in reality both treated with acupuncture and a trial to compare the effects of acupuncture and a true placebo in the alleviation of osteoarthritic pain has yet to be carried out!

RHEUMATOID ARTHRITIS

In considering whether or not acupuncture has a place in the management of rheumatoid arthritis it is necessary to bear in mind that the disease goes through two main stages, an early active severe inflammatory phase and a late destructive one.

Early active acute inflammatory phase

The disease has either a sudden onset with the rapid involvement of many joints or a more insidious one with a gradual spread of the pathological process until ultimately many joints are affected in a roughly symmetrical manner.

In the early active phase of the disease, irrespective of the type of onset, there is an acute inflammatory reaction affecting the synovium of the joints and tendon sheaths. In addition to synovial hypertrophy and effusions there is also considerable swelling of soft tissues as a result of the development of periarticular inflammatory oedema.

Treatment at this stage of the disease must of necessity be directed at combating the acute inflammatory reaction by means of rest, both general and local, physiotherapy, and the administration of anti-inflammatory drugs. The severity of the inflammatory reaction and the large number of joints involved would seem to me to preclude considering the use of acupuncture for pain relief at this stage.

Late destructive phase

The later stages of the disease are characterized by destructive changes in and around the joints with relatively little inflammatory reaction, although with, at times, some secondary osteoarthritic changes.

At this phase of the disease a few of the joints may remain persistently painful. In such circumstances examination of the periarticular soft tissues often reveals the presence of focal points of exquisite tenderness or what would seem to be trigger points in as much as pressure on them exacerbates the pain. In my opinion it is in attempting to relieve this type of pain that the use of acupuncture may reasonably be considered.

The insertion of dry needles into the tissues overlying these trigger points certainly often seems to be helpful, but with a disease of such complexity it is impossible to be certain about this without the objectivity of assessment provided by a large scale, well-designed clinical trial. Unfortunately up until now the only study so far completed has been a preliminary one on a limited number of patients by Man & Baragar (1974). In Man & Baragar's trial, 20 patients with seropositive rheumatoid arthritis of 5 years standing or more, and with pain confined to both knees, were divided into two groups. In the first group, one knee was treated with an intra-articular steroid injection and the other knee with acupuncture in which needles were inserted into conventional Chinese acupuncture points. In the second group, one knee was treated with intra-articular hydrocortisone and the other knee was given so-called placebo acupuncture in which needles were inserted into what were considered to be inappropriate sites. Both in those treated with acupuncture and 'placebo' acupuncture the needles were stimulated electrically.

Somewhat surprisingly, considering that these various procedures were each carried out on only one occasion, the group given acupuncture were found to obtain varying degrees of relief from pain for 1–2 months, in contrast to the 'placebo' group which only obtained transient relief for less than 1 day. It must, however, be stressed that this was only a preliminary study on a limited number of cases, and before any conclusions can be drawn as to the place of acupuncture in the relief of late stage chronic rheumatoid arthritis, much larger scale trials require to be carried out.

REFERENCES

Arnoldi C C, Lemperg R K, Linderholm H 1971 Immediate effect of osteotomy on the intramedullary pressure of the femoral head and neck in patients with degenerative osteoarthritis. Acta Orthopaedica Scandinavica 42: 357–365

Arnoldi C C, Djurhuus J C, Heerfordt J, Karte A 1980 Intraosseous phlebography, intraosseous pressure measurements and Tc-polyphosphate scintigraphy in patients with various painful conditions in the hip and knee. Acta Orthopaedic Scandinavica 51: 19–28

Bonica J J 1953 The management of pain. Lea & Febiger, Philadelphia

Collins A J, Ring F, Bacon P A, Brookshaw J D 1976 Thermography and radiology: Complementary methods for the study of inflammatory diseases. Clinical Radiology 27: 237–243

Cooper N S, Soren A, McEwen C, Rosenberger J L 1981 Diagnostic specificity of synovial lesions. Human Pathology 12: 314–328

Danielsson L G 1964 Incidence and prognosis of osteoarthrosis. Acta Orthopaedica Scandinavica, Supplement 66

De Ceulaer K, Watson Buchanan W 1979 Osteoarthrosis. Medicine 14: 693–699

Dieppe R A, Huskisson E G, Crocker P, Willoughby D A

1976 Apatite deposition disease. A new arthropathy. Lancet 1: 266–268

Dieppe P A 1978 Inflammation in osteoarthritis. Rheumatology and Rehabilitation (supplement) 59–63

Dieppe P A, Sathapatayavongs B, Jones H E, Bacon P A, Ring E F J 1980 Intra-articular steroids in osteoarthritis. Rheumatology and Rehabilitation 19: 212–217

Dixon A St. J 1965 Progress in clinical rheumatology. J A Churchill, London, p 313–329

Ehrlich G E 1975 Osteoarthritis beginning with inflammation. Journal of the American Medical Association 232: 157–159

Evans F J 1974 The placebo response in pain reduction. In: Bonica J J (ed) Advances in neurology. International Symposium on Pain. Raven Press, New York

Fassbender H G 1975 Pathology of rheumatic diseases. Springer-Verlag, Berlin (Trans. G Loewi)

Gaw A C, Chang L W, Shaw L C 1975 Efficacy of acupuncture on osteoarthritic pain. A controlled double-blind study. New England Journal of Medicine 293: 375–378

George R C, Chrisman O D 1968 The role of cartilage polysaccharides in osteoarthritis. Clinical Orthopaedics 57: 259

Goldenberg D L, Egan M S, Cohen A S 1982 Inflammatory synovitis in degenerative joint disease. Journal of Rheumatology 9: 204–209

Hamilton D E, Bywaters E G C, Please N W 1959 A controlled trial of various forms of physiotherapy in arthritis. British Medical Journal 1: 542–544

Harkness J A L, Higgs E R, Dieppe A 1984 Osteoarthritis. In: Wall P, Melzack R (eds) Textbook of pain. Churchill Livingstone, Edinburgh, p 222

Harper P, Nuki G 1980 Genetic factors in osteoarthrosis. In: The aetiopathogenesis of osteoarthrosis. Pitman Press, Bath, p 184–201

Huskisson E C, Dieppe P A, Tucker A K, Cannell L B 1979 Another look at osteoarthritis. Annals of Rheumatic Diseases 38: 423–428

Huskisson E C 1985 Osteoarthritis: Pathogenesis and management. Update Postgraduate Centre series. Update Group, London

Junnila S Y T 1982 Acupuncture superior to piroxicam in the treatment of osteoarthritis. American Journal of Acupuncture 10: 241–246

Kellgren J H 1961 Osteoarthrosis in patients and populations. British Medical Journal ii: 1–6

Kellgren J H, Lawrence J S, Bier F 1963 Genetic factors in generalized osteoarthritis. Annals of Rheumatic Diseases 22: 237–255

Lawrence J S, Bremner J M, Bier F 1966 Osteoarthrosis. Prevalence in the population and relationship between symptoms and X-ray changes. Annals of Rheumatic Diseases 25: 1–22

Lemperg R K, Arnoldi C C 1978 The significance of intraosseous pressure in normal and diseased states with special reference to the intraosseous engorgement pain syndrome. Clinical Orthopaedics and Related Research 136: 143–156

McCarty D J 1976 Calcium pyrophosphate dihydrate crystal deposition disease. Arthritis and Rheumatism 19: 295

Man Sheung-C, Baragar F D 1974 Preliminary clinical study of acupuncture in rheumatoid arthritis. Journal of Rheumatology 1 (1): 26–29

Mann F 1974 Periosteal acupuncture. In: The treatment of disease by acupuncture, 3rd edn. Heinemann Medical, London, p 193–204

Mann F, Bowsher D, Mumford J, Lipton S, Miles J 1973 Treatment of intractable pain by acupuncture. Lancet ii: 57–60

Miller J H, White J, Norton T H 1958 The value of intra-articular injections in osteoarthritis of the knee. Journal of Bone and Joint Surgery 40B: 636–643

Milligan J, Glennie-Smith K, Dowson D 1980 A comparative study between acupuncture and physiotherapy in the treatment of osteoarthritis of the knee. Paper presented at Fifteenth International Congress on Rheumatology, Paris

Radin E L, Ehrlich M M, Weiss C A, Parker H G 1976 Osteoarthritis as a state of altered pathology. In: Buchanan W W, Dick C (eds) Recent advances in rheumatology I. Churchill Livingstone, Edinburgh, p 1–18

Schumacher H R, Smolyo A P, Rose R C, Maurer K 1977 Arthritis associated with apatite crystals. Annals of Internal Medicine 87: 411–416

Schumacher H R, Gordon G, Paul H, Reginato A, Villaneuva T, Cherian V, Gibilisco P 1981 Osteoarthritis, crystal deposition and inflammation. Seminars in Arthritis and Rheumatism 11: 116–119

Sidel N, Abrahams M I 1940 Treatment of chronic arthritis. Results of vaccine therapy with saline injections used as controls. Journal of the American Medical Association 14: 1740–1742

Sola A E, Williams R L 1956 Myofascial pain syndromes. Neurology 6: 91–95

Stecher R M 1955 Heberden's nodes. A clinical description of osteoarthritis of the finger joints. Annals of Rheumatic Diseases 14: 1–10

Steindler A 1959 Lectures on the interpretation of pain. In: Orthopaedic practice. Charles C Thomas, Springfield, Illinois, U S A Lecture XV pp 555–605

Traut E F, Passarelli E W 1956 Study in the controlled therapy of degenerative arthritis. Archives of Internal Medicine 98: 181–186

Travell J 1950 The adductor longus syndrome. A case of groin pain. Its treatment by local block of trigger areas. Bulletin of the New York Academy of Medicine 26: 284–285

Travell J 1951 Pain mechanisms in connective tissues. In: Connective tissues. Transactions of the second conference, Josiah Macey Jnr Foundation, New York, p 86–125

Travell J, Rinzler S H 1952 The myofascial genesis of pain. Post-graduate Medicine 11: 425–434

Wiberg G 1941 Roentgenographic and anatomic studies of the femoropatellar joint. Acta Orthopaedica Scandinavica 12: 319

Wood P H N 1976 Osteoarthritis in the community. Clinics in Rheumatic Diseases 2: 495–507

Wright V, Chandler G N, Monson R A U, Hartfall S J 1960 Intra-articular therapy in osteoarthritis. Annals of Rheumatic Diseases 19: 257–261

Wyke B 1981 The neurology of joints. A review of general principles. Clinics in Rheumatic Diseases 7: 233–239

20. Abdominal and pelvic pain

INTRODUCTION

Pain in the abdomen and pelvis most likely to be helped by acupuncture is that which occurs as a result of the activation of trigger points in the muscles, fasciae, tendons and ligaments of the anterior and lateral abdominal wall, the lower back, the floor of the pelvis, and the upper anterior part of the thigh.

Such pain, however, is all too often erroneously assumed to be due to some intra-abdominal lesion, and as a consequence of being inappropriately treated, is often allowed to persist for much longer than is necessary. As Renaer (1984) so rightly says,

when confronted with abdominal pain complaints, most doctors will automatically think of pain originating in the abdominal viscera. Yet it would appear strange if tissues so abundantly innervated as the skin and the fasciae of the abdominal wall hardly ever caused pain.

An important reason why doctors tend to overlook the possibility of abdominal pain arising from structures encasing the internal organs is because the majority of present day textbooks on gastroenterology together with most sections on the subject in undergraduate textbooks of medicine, whilst giving detailed descriptions of diseases of the viscera and the characteristics of pain associated with these, make little or no reference to the diagnosis and treatment of pain emanating from the abdominal wall itself. This failure on the part of most authors of textbooks to emphasize the importance of distinguishing between visceral and somatic pain is not only surprising but much to be regretted for there can be no doubt that pain occurring as the result of

activation of trigger points in the abdominal wall is relatively common. One gastroenterologist, who invariably includes this possibility in his differential diagnosis whenever presented with a case of persistent abdominal pain, regularly refers to me an appreciable number of such patients for treatment with acupuncture. And it therefore came as no surprise to me to find that Ranger et al (1971), working in a large district general hospital, were able to collect a series of 100 patients with abdominal wall pain over a period of 2 years.

Despite this paucity of information concerning abdominal wall trigger point pain in most current textbooks, there have been many important contributions to the subject in various journals over the past 50 years or more. One of the earliest was contained in an address entitled *Myofibrositis as a Simulator of other Maladies*, delivered by Murray in 1929 to the Newcastle upon Tyne and Northern Counties Medical Society.

The fact that, because of the time in which Murray lived, he attributed the pain to fibrositis in no way detracts from the importance of his observations concerning what clearly today would be called myofascial trigger point pain. In the part of his address dealing with abdominal wall pain, he says 'such pain is of a dull aching character generally felt at one spot from which it tends to radiate'. He then goes on to state that pain of this type is often made worse by stretching and twisting movements of the trunk, and he stresses the importance of palpating the abdomen with the muscles both in a state of relaxation and of contraction when attempting to distinguish between visceral and somatic pain.

He describes how, by the use of this examination technique, he was able in three cases of persistent abdominal pain to demonstrate that the pain was arising from circumscribed tender areas in the muscles and that pain in the right iliac fossa previously ascribed to chronic appendicitis, pain in the right hypochondrium said to be due to biliary colic, and pain in the epigastrium attributed to a gastritis, was in each case due to what he called 'fibrositis' of the abdominal wall. He concludes by reporting that he was able to relieve this persistent pain, which in two cases had been present for several months, and in one case for 4 years, by applying an iodine and belladonna ointment to the areas of tenderness.

Other physicians who stressed the importance of distinguishing abdominal wall pain from visceral pain during the 1930s were Hunter (1933) and Telling (1935). In addition, Lewis & Kellgren (1939) carried out extremely important experimental work, in both human healthy volunteers and animals, on musculoskeletal pain that arises from the abdominal wall itself, and also that which is referred to the abdomen from muscles in the lower back (see Ch. 4).

From the 1940s onwards, several clinicians have published reports concerning the diagnosis and treatment of abdominal wall pain based on their own personal series of cases including Kelly (1942), Young (1943), Gutstein (1944), Theobald (1949), Good (1950a & b), Melnick (1954, 1957a), Long (1956), Mehta & Ranger (1971), Applegate (1972) and Bourne (1980). In addition, Travell & Simons (1983) have provided an extensive review of the whole subject in their trigger point manual.

MYOFASCIAL TRIGGER POINT ABDOMINAL WALL PAIN

Examination of the patient

In order to diagnose myofascial trigger point abdominal wall pain and to distinguish it from visceral pain, it is essential to palpate the abdomen with the muscles of the anterior wall both in a relaxed and contracted state because abdominal wall pain emanates from focal areas of exquisite tenderness, or trigger points, and the tenderness at these points is increased when the muscles are held taut and decreased when they are relaxed.

The procedure and the reason for carrying it out cannot be explained better than by quoting Long (1956) who states,

The painful area is compressed rather firmly beneath a single finger or thumb, with sufficient pressure barely to pass the threshold of pain. The patient is then asked to raise both legs straight, causing both heels to leave the examining surface by a distance of a few inches only. The resultant contraction of the anterior abdominal wall will push the examining finger away from the viscera and simultaneously increasingly compress the abdominal wall beneath the finger. If, on this manouver, the pain increases it is of abdominal wall origin; if it decreases it is of visceral origin.

Murray (1929) advocated producing tension in the abdominal muscles by getting the patient to raise the head and upper part of the body from the recumbent position. De Valera & Raftery (1976) recommend getting the patient to elevate both the feet and head. Travell & Simons (1983) advise getting the supine patient to hold a deep breath. There is little to choose between any of these methods and it is my personal practice to adopt whichever one seems to be the most suitable for a particular individual.

The muscles involved

The principal anterior abdominal wall muscles in which trigger points are liable to become activated include the two rectus abdominis muscles on either side of the midline, and the external and internal oblique muscles in the flanks (Figs 20.1 and 20.2).

Location of the trigger points

Rectus abdominis

Common sites for trigger point activation in this muscle include the epigastric region near to its insertion into the lower ribs: also in its belly, with one point half-way between the xiphisternum and the umbilicus and another point half-way between the umbilicus and the pubis; in addition to point at or near to the insertion of the muscle into the pubic bone (Fig. 20.3).

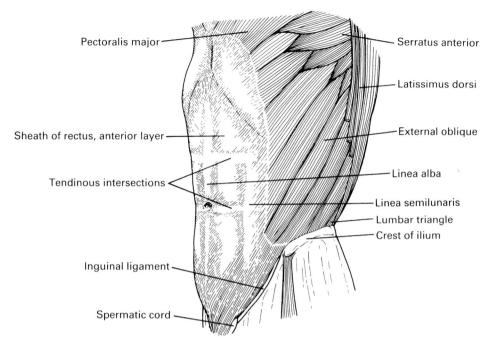

Pectoralis major

Sheath of rectus, anterior layer

Tendinous intersections

Inguinal ligament

Spermatic cord

Serratus anterior

Latissimus dorsi

External oblique

Linea alba

Linea semilunaris

Lumbar triangle

Crest of ilium

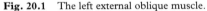

Fig. 20.1   The left external oblique muscle.

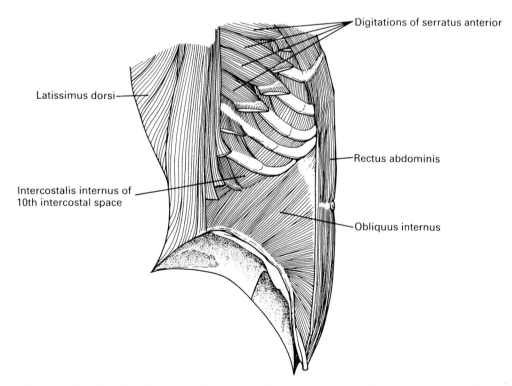

Digitations of serratus anterior

Latissimus dorsi

Intercostalis internus of 10th intercostal space

Rectus abdominis

Obliquus internus

Fig. 20.2   Muscles of the right side of the trunk. The external oblique has been removed to show the internal oblique, but its digitations from the ribs have been preserved. The sheath of the rectus abdominis has been opened and its anterior lamina removed.

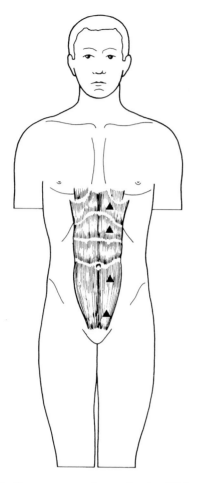

Fig. 20.3 Some common trigger point sites (▲) in the rectus abdominis muscle.

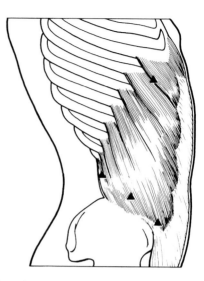

Fig. 20.4 Some commonly occurring trigger point sites (▲) in the external oblique muscle.

External and internal obliques

Common sites for trigger point activation in these muscles include the hypochondrium, the iliac crest, and close to the inguinal ligament. It may also occur anywhere along a line joining the tip of the twelfth rib above and the iliac crest below (Fig. 20.4).

Symptomatology

Activated trigger points in the anterior abdominal wall may, as trigger points anywhere else in the body, be responsible for the development of pain, but in addition, because of a somatovisceral reflex in the abdomen, they are also capable of causing other symptoms including anorexia, flatulence, nausea, vomiting, diarrhoea, colic, dysmenorrhoea and dysuria.

Melnick (1954) in a series of 56 patients with abdominal wall trigger points found the latter to be the cause of flatulence and bloating in 25% of the cases; vomiting in 11%, heartburn in 11% and diarrhoea in 4%. Theobald (1949) has reported relieving dysmenorrhoea by deactivating trigger points in the lower part of the rectus abdominis about half-way between the umbilicus and pubis, and Hoyt (1953) has reported relieving dysuria by deactivating trigger points in the lower abdominal muscles.

The pain itself often takes the form of a dull ache. Alternatively, it may, as pointed out by Ranger et al (1971) be sharp and burning in character. And it tends to be aggravated by twisting or stretching movements of the trunk. Patients sometimes complain more of discomfort than of actual pain (Kelly 1942). This is because, as Travell & Simons (1983) state, trigger points in the anterior abdominal wall, and particularly those in the rectus abdominis, are liable to cause the abdomen to become lax and distended with flatus.

It is also noticeable how often patients with upper abdominal trigger point pain complain of this being made worse by the pressure of their clothes. In addition, as pointed out by Murray (1929), epigastric trigger point pain may be aggravated by post-prandial distension of the stomach.

A farm labourer (50) had an 18-month history of epigastric pain that was always worse whenever his abdomen became distended following a meal. After he had been found to have a normal barium meal, gastroscopy, and ultrasound scan, in spite of there being persistent epigastric tenderness, he was referred to me as a possible case of abdominal wall trigger point pain. On examination, he had two well-defined exquisitely tender trigger points in the linea alba 3″ below the xiphisternum and after these had been deactivated with dry needles on two occasions, he had no further trouble.

In addition, pain from trigger points in muscles in the upper part of the abdomen may be brought on by flexing the trunk.

A market gardener (62), whose work involved much heavy lifting, suffered from attacks of severe pain in the right upper quadrant of the abdomen about 3–4 times a week, with each attack lasting about 15–20 minutes and coming on whenever his work necessitated him bending over for any length of time. At one stage it was thought he might have some type of diaphragmatic hernia. However, all investigations were negative and after he had had recurrent bouts of pain for 4 years, he was referred to me for an opinion as to whether acupuncture might help to relieve it. On examination, a single trigger point was located in the lateral border of the right rectus muscle just below the ribs that had presumably become activated by the strain of heavy lifting. The point was so exquisitely tender to touch that the patient visibly jumped when pressure was applied to it. Somewhat to my surprise in view of the long history, there were no further attacks of pain following deactivation of the trigger point with a dry needle on only one occasion.

Differential diagnosis

Pain and flatulence occurring as a result of trigger points in the right upper quadrant in either, one of the oblique muscles, or in the lateral border of the rectus muscle, is liable to be erroneously ascribed to gall bladder disease, particularly if, by chance, ultrasound scanning reveals the presence of gall stones.

Pain and tenderness in the right lower quadrant occurring as a result of trigger point activity in the lateral border of the rectus muscle is apt to be diagnosed as being due to appendicitis, particularly as the trigger point frequently occurs in the region of McBurney's point, approximately 1″–2″ from the anterior superior iliac spine along the line joining this spine and the umbilicus. Persistent right iliac fossa pain is rarely, if ever, due to chronic appendicitis but frequently occurs as a result of the activation of a trigger point.

Epigastric pain, particularly when accompanied by dyspeptic symptoms and occurring as a result of trigger point activity in the rectus abdominis, is liable to be attributed to a hiatus hernia if, by chance, the latter happens to be found on radiographic examination.

Finally, there is a risk of pain in the left lower quadrant from trigger points in the outer border of the rectus or the obliques being considered to be due to diverticulitis if, by chance, a barium enema reveals the presence of diverticulae in the lower part of the colon.

Factors responsible for the primary activation of anterior abdominal wall trigger points

The various factors responsible for the primary activation of abdominal wall myofascial trigger points include: acute trauma to the muscles, as a result, for example, of an accident or surgical operation; repeated minor trauma to, or chronic overloading of them, such as may occur during the course of certain occupational tasks and sporting activities; muscle strain occurring as a result of a faulty posture; viral infections; chronic anxiety, causing the muscles to be held persistently tense; and exposure of them to the cold or damp.

The following abstracts of case notes have been selected from my own series of patients with persistent abdominal wall trigger point pain in order to illustrate some of the commoner ways in which trigger points in the abdominal wall undergo primary activation.

Trauma

A company director (56) developed severe discomfort and tenderness of the muscles in the right hypochondrium. A cholecystogram was normal.

However, the pain persisted and after it had been present for 4 months, he was referred to me. It was significant that the pressure of a tight belt and also flexing his trunk made the pain worse, for on examination there were three well-defined exquisitely tender trigger points in the right external oblique muscle. These must have been activated as a result of trauma for it transpired that the onset of the symptoms coincided with him being knocked over by a dog. It was only necessary to deactivate these trigger points with dry needles on one occasion to relieve him of his symptoms.

A farrier (37) suffered bouts of pain in the left upper part of the abdomen. All investigations, including an ultrasound scan of the abdomen, were negative. When seen by me 14 months after the onset of the pain, it had become so incapacitating as to prevent him from working. There were several trigger points in the muscles behind the left lower ribs and these must have become activated by repeated occupational trauma for he gave a history that the pain always came on after he had spent 2–3 hours shoeing horses during which he pressed the legs of the animals tightly against the left upper part of his abdomen. He had no further pain once the trigger points had been deactivated with dry needles on two occasions, and he had made adjustments to the manner in which he worked.

A farmer (49) with a 5-year history of intermittent epigastric pain and with no abnormality on a barium meal or gastroscopy gave a history that he was always worse on the days when he strained himself closing a particularly stiff tailboard of a lorry. He also observed that his upper abdomen often felt quite sore after cattle had knocked against it on market days. Three trigger points were found in the upper part of the rectus muscle and his pain disappeared following the deactivation of these with dry needles on four occasions.

Faulty posture

A schoolboy (15) was referred to me with a 4-year history of pain in the right upper part of the abdomen. It was particularly troublesome whenever he put any weight on his right leg in the gymnasium or while playing rugby. He had been fully investigated at a pain clinic with the only abnormality discovered being a minor defect in the 8th dorsal vertebra. Because of this it was considered that the pain might be due to nerve root entrapment but an intercostal nerve block and an epidural injection had proved to be valueless.

On examination he had several exquisitely tender trigger points in the external oblique just below the costal margin and also a number in muscles around the greater trochanter. With hindsight, there can be no doubt that the trigger points in the leg were the first to become activated following a fall when aged 11, and that pain from these caused him to adopt a faulty posture, with the result that, as a secondary event, the trigger points in the abdominal wall became activated. After deactivating these trigger points with dry needles on three occasions, he had no further trouble.

A laboratory technician (31) with a 4-month history of pain in the right loin radiating anteriorly towards the groin, on being found to have no abnormality in the urogenital tract was referred to me as a possible case of musculoskeletal pain. There were numerous trigger points in muscles both posteriorly and anteriorly. It transpired that the pain always came on after she had been sitting for any length of time at a work bench and she felt herself that she had strained her muscles by sitting on a stool that was too low. The trigger points were readily deactivated and she has had no further pain since insisting on being given a higher stool.

Exposure to cold or damp

Pain in the muscles of the anterior abdominal wall not infrequently occurs as part of a condition, which, because of the nebulous nature of its underlying pathology, has over the years come to be known by a variety of names including fibrositis, myalgia, and, in more recent years, myofasciitis. Although there can now be no doubt that the condition is associated with the activation of trigger points in the abdominal wall muscles, the reason for this activation is far from certain. Exposure to cold or damp has traditionally been considered to be an important aetiological factor but there is of course no absolute proof of this.

Postoperative pain

Many patients referred to me with abdominal pain that has come on postoperatively have been found to have active trigger points either in the muscles of the lower back or the anterior abdominal wall or both. There is no doubt that the activation has occurred as a result of the muscles having been traumatized or strained during the course of some surgical procedure. In addition, postoperative pain is sometimes due to trigger points developing in surgical scars.

In all such cases the pain continues to be troublesome for a long time unless the trigger points are satisfactorily deactivated.

Secondary activation of abdominal wall trigger points

Trigger points in the anterior abdominal wall can become activated as a secondary event in response to the pain of visceral disease. It is then possible for pain from the abdominal wall trigger points to continue to be troublesome long after the visceral disease has been successfully treated. Melnick (1957b) describes a patient in whom epigastric pain, originally due to a duodenal ulcer, persisted for a long time after the ulcer had healed as a result of the activation of trigger points in the rectus muscle.

The reasons for trigger point activity occurring in association with the irritable bowel syndrome would seem to be more complex and therefore will be considered separately.

IRRITABLE BOWEL SYNDROME

The irritable bowel syndrome has been defined as 'symptoms of abdominal pain and disturbance of bowel action of more than 3 months duration without any organic cause' (Blendis 1984). It is a disease that affects not only adults but also children (Apley & Naish 1958). The pain in children is predominantly periumbilical (Stone & Barbero 1970) whereas in adults it is more often over the colon, with the commonest site being the left iliac fossa (Waller & Misiewicz 1969).

Holdstock et al (1969), from manometric studies using radiotelemetering capsules in the small intestine and proximal colon, and air-filled balloons in the sigmoid colon, have shown that attacks of pain in various chronic pain syndromes including the irritable bowel syndrome seem to be related to changes in intraluminal pressures in either the small or large intestine.

On clinical examination, there are areas of localized tenderness over one or other parts of the colon with this most often being over the descending part, but sometimes over the transverse part, and occasionally over the whole colon. On palpating the abdomen with the muscles relaxed it seems as if it is the colon that is tender, but, on getting the patient to tense the abdominal wall, it becomes obvious that often much of this tenderness is in localized areas of the abdominal wall muscles.

Kendall et al (1986) and also Hall (1986) consider that these focal areas of tenderness in the muscle occur as a result of a viscerosomatic reflex (Procacci & Zoppi 1983). This may be true but nevertheless it has to be remembered that Lewis & Kellgren (1939) showed that an injection of a 6% salt solution into the belly of the rectus muscle just below and an inch outside the navel gave rise to 'a continuous pain lasting 3 to 5 minutes of unpleasant severity and having a character not to be distinguished from that of colic'. In other words, Lewis & Kellgren, by artificially creating a trigger zone in an abdominal wall muscle, were able, by means of a somatovisceral reflex, to produce a pain not dissimilar to that which occurs with the irritable bowel syndrome.

Furthermore, it has to be remembered that such symptoms as dyspepsia (Watson et al 1976), dysuria (Fielding 1977), and dysmenorrhoea (Waller & Misiewicz 1969) are frequently present in the irritable bowel syndrome, and that, as discussed earlier, these are all symptoms that anterior abdominal wall trigger points, by virtue of a somatovisceral reflex, are capable of producing.

The question, therefore, that has to be asked is whether the pain and other symptoms in this condition are primarily due to a disorder of the gut with the focal areas of tenderness in the anterior abdominal wall musculature developing as a secondary event, or whether these tender points are actually trigger points and the prime cause of all these various symptoms? If it is the latter, then it would be reasonable to expect that deactivation of these points by one means or another would relieve the symptoms. Kendall et al, however, state that they have not been able to alleviate the pain by infiltrating them with local anaesthetic agents with or without the addition of steroids. They also have observed that these anterior abdominal wall tender points, unlike trigger points, do not seem to be constant in position but move from place to place.

These observations notwithstanding, what is certain is that many cases of the irritable bowel syndrome have been referred to me for treatment with acupuncture because, in addition to having visceral pain, they have also had pain, made worse by twisting and stretching movements of the trunk, that was clearly muscular in origin. In all these cases trigger points have invariably been found to be present at constant sites in the muscles of either the lower back or the anterior abdominal wall. In some instances this particular type of pain appears to have developed as a result of the skeletal muscles being held tense during bouts of intra-abdominal pain. In other cases it seems as if the irritable bowel syndrome and the trigger point pain have arisen independently of each other, which is hardly surprising considering that both this particular disorder of the gut (Esler & Goulston 1973) and musculoskeletal pain disorders (Crown 1978) frequently occur in people of an anxious disposition.

Myofascial trigger point pain occurring either coincidentally with, or developing as a result of, the irritable bowel syndrome is well worth treating with acupuncture, because once the trigger points have been deactivated with dry needles any residual visceral pain is so much more readily coped with.

Deactivation of abdominal wall trigger points

It is obviously possible to deactivate trigger points in the abdominal wall, as elsewhere in the body, by a variety of different methods. Murray (1929) clearly achieved this by applying an iodine and belladonna ointment to the skin overlying them. Many clinicians including Travell & Simons (1983) advocate injecting a local anaesthetic into them. Bourne (1980) favours the use of a corticosteroid local anaesthetic mixture.

Mehta & Ranger (1971), Ranger et al (1971), and also Applegate (1972), presumably because they considered the pain to be due to the entrapment of a cutaneous nerve as it passes through an anterior abdominal wall muscle, felt obliged to inject phenol into a point of maximum tenderness.

There can be no doubt that the reason why all of these methods are capable of alleviating this type of pain is because they all have one property in common, namely an irritant action on A-delta nerve fibres and with this in turn activating pain-modulating mechanisms in the central nervous system. This effect of course can be achieved far more straightforwardly simply by deactivating trigger points with acupuncture needles (Ch. 8). And with regard to this, it has been my experience that anterior abdominal wall trigger points are particularly easy to deactivate with dry needles so that even with pain of long duration it is rarely necessary to carry out this procedure more than 2–3 times.

PAIN IN THE ABDOMEN FROM TRIGGER POINTS IN THE LOWER BACK

Lewis & Kellgren (1939) were able to show that an injection of hypertonic saline into the supraspinous ligament at the level of the 9th thoracic vertebra gave rise to pain posteriorly in the region of the first lumbar vertebra, and anteriorly over the 9th costal cartilage and down towards the umbilicus. They also observed rigidity of the upper abdominal muscles on the side of the injection when this experimentally induced pain was at its height.

The following year, Kellgren (1940) published an account of several cases in which somatic pain simulated visceral pain. These included the case of a housewife who had a 1-year history of epigastric pain and nausea coming on an hour after meals, together with epigastric tenderness, but with no abnormality demonstrable on a barium meal. Examination of the back, however, revealed the presence of a mid-dorsal kyphosis of the spine and any attempt to straighten the latter caused the epigastric pain to be reproduced. In addition, there were focal areas of marked tenderness in the region of the 8th and 9th thoracic vertebrae and an injection of Novocain into these abolished the epigastric pain and tenderness. Also, the case of another housewife with a 6-month history of continuous pain in the right hypochondrium and lower angle of the scapula together with episodes of more severe pain, nausea, and flatulence. There was tenderness and rigidity of the upper abdominal muscles but a cholecystogram was normal. She also had a mid-dorsal kyphosis and it was possible to reproduce her pain by forcibly flexing and extending this part of the spine. There were tender areas in the region of the 6th and 7th thoracic interspinous ligaments and, as in the previous case, an injection of Novocain into these abolished the abdominal pain and rigidity.

These cases, reported by Kellgren nearly 50 years ago, have been quoted in order to show that it has for long been known that abdominal pain may, on occasions, occur as a result of being referred there from trigger points in the lower back, and that in all cases of abdominal pain not obviously due to some visceral disease, it is important to search for trigger points, not only in the anterior abdominal wall musculature, but also in the muscles and ligaments of the lower back.

PAIN IN THE LOWER BACK DUE TO TRIGGER POINTS IN ANTERIOR ABDOMINAL WALL MUSCLES

In my experience whenever a patient with low-back pain finds it is uncomfortable to stand up straight and also when any attempt passively to extend the spine makes the pain worse, it is often because of the activity of trigger points in the lower part of the rectus muscle at or near to its insertion into the pubic bone; or in the lower border of the external oblique muscle along its insertion into the inguinal ligament. It is therefore important in all such cases not only to look for trigger points in the lumbar muscles but also in the anterior abdominal wall.

PELVIC PAIN

Pelvic pain most likely to be amenable to treatment with acupuncture is that which occurs as a result of the activation of trigger points in muscles and ligaments in the pelvic floor and in

the adductor longus tendon near or at its attachment to the pubic bone.

CHRONIC PELVIC FLOOR MYOFASCIAL TRIGGER POINT PAIN SYNDROME

Trigger point activation in this condition occurs in various muscles and ligaments in the pelvic floor with the principal muscles involved being the levator ani, the coccygeus, the piriformis and the medial fibres of the gluteus maximus (Figs 20.5 and 20.6).

Thiele (1937) was one of the first to draw attention to this condition when he described what he called coccygodynia (pain around the coccyx) from spasm of the levator ani and coccygeus muscles occurring in conjunction with pain around the buttock and down the back of the thigh from spasm of the piriformis.

During the 1940s and 1950s, Thiele and others published papers on coccygodynia, with one of the most interesting being that of Dittrich (1951) for he appears to have been the first person to recognize that pain in this condition occurs as a result of it being referred from trigger points. In his paper he described two cases of coccygeal pain occurring as a result of it being referred to the coccyx from trigger points in adipose tissue in the sacral region. His contribution to the subject is, however, otherwise limited because he seems to have believed that trigger points in this condition only occur at this site and makes no mention of the possibility of them occurring in the muscles of the pelvic floor.

During the course of reviewing the clinical features of coccygodynia Thiele (1963) pointed out that it is only in the 20% of cases in which coccygeal pain is due to direct trauma that the coccyx is tender, and that in the other 80% of cases not due to trauma this lack of tenderness of the bone means that the pain cannot be due to disease of this structure itself or to arthritis of the sacrococcygeal joint, but rather that it must be referred to the coccyx from pelvic muscles which, for one reason or another, have gone into spasm.

Coccygodynia is not really a particularly apt name for this disorder because, as Thiele himself recognized when he first introduced the term in the 1930s, the pain is rarely confined to the

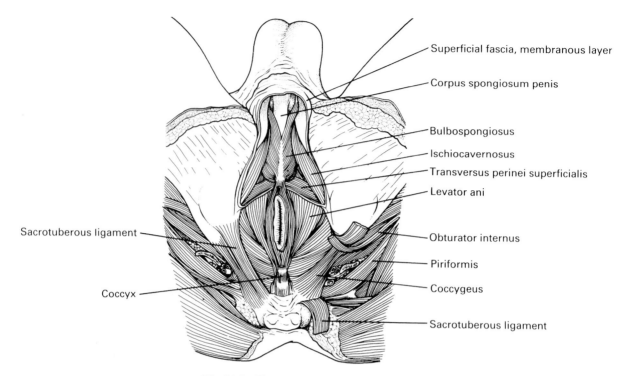

Fig. 20.5   The muscles of the male perineum.

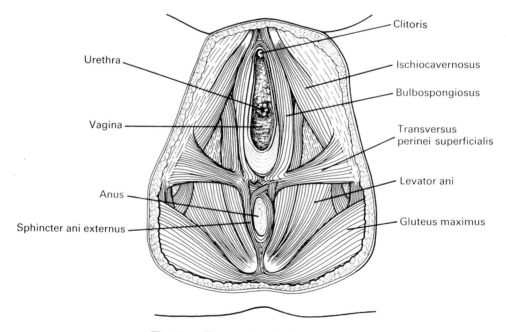

Fig. 20.6   The muscles of the female perineum.

coccyx. On the other hand, as he originally pointed out, it is a condition that is always associated with spasm of the pelvic floor muscles, and for this reason other physicians have given it a variety of other names including the levator spasm syndrome (Smith 1959) the levator syndrome (McGivney & Cleveland 1965) and the levator ani spasm syndrome (Lilius & Valtonen 1973).

However, none of these terms are entirely satisfactory as the levator ani muscle is usually only one of the muscles involved, and therefore much to be preferred is tension myalgia of the pelvic floor, a term introduced by Sinaki et al (1977). Nevertheless, even this can be improved upon for there are now good grounds for believing that the pain is referred over a fairly wide area from points of maximum tenderness or trigger points in muscles of the pelvic floor and for this reason a more appropriate term for it is the chronic pelvic floor myofascial trigger point pain syndrome.

Clinical manifestations

The condition occurs predominantly in females. It is now generally agreed that the commonest and most striking feature is pain coming on when seated. It may also be felt during the acts of sitting down and standing up. There is usually no pain on lying down or on walking about, except that sometimes sudden twisting movements of the trunk are painful. One of my patients found sitting in a chair so distressing that he was reduced to watching television or reading a book kneeling on the floor. Straining at stool may also aggravate the pain but not as often as might be thought. Sinaki et al (1977) reported it in 33% of their patients. It is also surprising that dyspareunia is rarely a problem. The pain usually takes the form of a somewhat ill-defined aching or throbbing sensation in either the anterior or posterior parts of the perineum or throughout that region. In addition the pain may spread to the buttocks, hips and backs of the thighs.

It is generally agreed that this condition mainly occurs in those of an anxious disposition, and from what some of my patients with this condition have told me, it clearly tends to occur in those who tense up the muscles of their pelvic floor at times of stress. There is usually, however, in addition some local cause for the condition developing.

On examination, exquisitely tender trigger points may be found on external examination of the perineum; in some cases, however, they can only be located by the carrying out of a rectal examination.

Patients with this condition seem to be particularly prone to trigger point activation and often give a history of trigger point pain in other parts of the body such as the neck or lower part of the back. Unfortunately this syndrome is still not as widely recognized as its important deserves, the pain all too frequently being attributed to some mechanical disorder of the spine or to some inflammatory condition such as proctitis, prostatitis, cervicitis, urethritis, or vaginitis, and, as a consequence of this, treated inappropriately. Alternatively, after the patient has been seen by a series of consultants specializing in orthopaedics, urology, gynaecology and neurology, and they each in turn having found nothing no account for the pain, it is not uncommon for the opinion of a psychiatrist to be sought.

Aetiology

Many of the physicians who over the years have published reports drawing attention to the pain being due to pelvic floor muscle spasm have considered that in many cases the spasm is secondary to some inflammatory lesion in the pelvis and have emphasized that the pain is not directly due to the latter itself. They have also stated that with many patients there is no inflammatory lesion present. And the situation would seem to be that in all cases the spasm of the pelvic floor muscles is due to the activation of trigger points in them, and that in those patients where this is not secondary to some pelvic inflammatory lesion, it is due to the muscles being subjected either to acute trauma or to repeated minor trauma or to chronic strain. The following cases exemplify how one or other of these three factors may lead to the development of this syndrome.

Acute trauma

A housewife (65) was referred to me with a 6-month history of persistent posteriorly situated perineal pain. On examination, there was a single exquisitely tender trigger point situated half-way between the coccyx and the posterior margin of the anus. The pain quickly subsided once this trigger point had been deactivated with dry needles on two occasions. There can be little doubt that this trigger point had been activated as a result of surgical trauma as the onset of the pain coincided with an operation for a rectal prolapse.

Repeated minor trauma

A businessman (58) with pain in the testicles that came on as soon as he sat down on a chair and which was relieved by standing or walking about was investigated by a general surgeon, a urologist, a neurologist, and an orthopaedic specialist. When none of these specialists could account for his pain, it was suggested to him that he should be seen by a psychiatrist. This he refused to do and after the condition had caused him considerable distress for 4 years, his general practitioner as an act of desperation referred him to me to see whether acupuncture might help.

On examination there were many exquisitely tender trigger points in the anterior perineal muscles and muscles on the inner side of the thigh near to their attachment to the public bone. Deactivation of these trigger points with dry needles gave immediate but very temporary relief and the procedure had to be repeated 12 times over the course of 5 months before the pain finally disappeared. This man had a long history of low-back pain and it would seem that the reason for him activating trigger points in the pelvic floor was because he had traumatized his perineum by sitting on the hard saddle of a rowing machine for 20 minutes twice a day for 12 years carrying out exercises designed to strengthen the muscles of his back!

Recurrent muscle strain

A housewife (48) developed a throbbing pain mainly around the rectum but spreading forwards to the anterior perineum and down the thighs. This only came on when she sat down and was relieved by standing. It was made worse, when, on sitting, she crossed her legs but was eased by opening them. Two gynaecologists and a neurologist failed to find the cause and after the pain had been present for

3 years she was referred to me to see whether acupuncture might help.

On external examination, there were many trigger points throughout the muscles of the perineum and deactivation of these with dry needles was carried out on several occasions. There was in addition much tenderness on rectal examination and she was therefore also given rectal massage. These measures, however, only gave her partial relief. She was a very tense person and there is no doubt this aggravated the situation for there was still further improvement once she had been taught autohypnosis.

The reason for her developing the condition was that she had become obsessed about completely emptying her rectum and for many years had regularly spent up to 20 minutes each day straining at stool.

Treatment

Some cases, like those quoted above, have trigger points that can readily be identified on external examination of the pelvic floor, and it is a relatively straightforward procedure to deactivate these by means of inserting dry needles into them. Response to this, however, is generally slow and in order to obtain any long-term relief it usually has to be repeated many times.

Most cases also have trigger points that are only discernible on rectal examination and with these, rectal massage, similar to that used for massaging the prostate, is very helpful (Thiele 1937, 1963).

Also deep heat, by means of diathermy, applied either per rectum or externally, is useful in helping to relax the muscles (Sinaki et al 1977). In addition, because this condition usually develops in highly anxious people and is aggravated by them nervously holding the pelvic muscles in a state of tension, relaxation techniques such as biofeedback or hypnosis should also be employed.

ADDUCTOR LONGUS SYNDROME

Pain in the groin and down the inner side of the thigh to the knee is liable to be due to a trigger point becoming activated in the adductor longus muscle (Travell 1950, Long 1956). In my experience the trigger point is most often located in the tendon of this muscle near to or at its insertion into the pubic bone (Fig. 18.1).

This activation may occur secondary to some chronic painful condition such as osteoarthritis of the hip or it may develop as the result of the muscle being subjected to trauma.

In the female this may be the cause of seemingly inexplicable vaginal pain.

A young woman developed a distressing throbbing pain in her vagina and around the urethral orifice when aged 20. It was worse after any physical activity such as dancing and sexual intercourse aggravated it. She also noticed that it was more noticeable whenever she was emotionally upset. Over the years she saw several gynaecologists but no cause for it was found and eventually she was sent to a psychiatrist. He however was unable to help and after it had been present for 14 years her general practitioner referred her to me in what he described as a faint hope that acupuncture might help!

On examination, there was an exquisitely tender trigger point in the right adductor longus tendon near to its insertion into the pubis. Pressure on this point aggravated the pain and on inserting a needle into it, she exclaimed 'that is my pain' as an electric shock-like sensation shot up into the vagina and down the inner side of her thigh.

Deactivation of the trigger point with a dry needle gave temporary relief and after the procedure had been repeated 8 times during the course of 12 weeks, the pain no longer returned.

On seeking a reason for the activation of the trigger point, it transpired that for some months prior to the onset of the pain she had been in the habit of frequently travelling very long distances seated on the pillion of a motor cycle whilst gripping tightly with her thighs for support.

In the male, trigger point activation in this muscle may be the cause of seemingly inexplicable scrotal pain. Several men referred to me with pain in this region have been found to have trigger points in this muscle; but, at the same time, it has to be remembered that trigger points at other sites may also be responsible for this pattern of pain referral.

SCROTAL PAIN

Whenever scrotal pain develops for no obvious reason the possibility of it being referred to the scrotum from trigger points elsewhere has to be considered. These trigger points may be either in the external oblique muscle just above the inguinal ligament; or in the adductor longus muscle near to its insertion into the pubic bone; or in the muscles of the pelvic floor; or, as Kellgren (1940) showed, in muscles and ligaments in the upper lumbar region in the vicinity of the 1st lumbar vertebra. The referral of pain to the scrotum from such a distant site presumably is associated with the fact that the genital branch of the genito-femoral nerve arises from the 1st and 2nd lumbar nerves (Yeates 1985).

A man (74), shortly after having undergone a prostatectomy, developed scrotal pain, which was made worse by various physical activities such as gardening and was aggravated by sitting for long periods in his car. There was no obvious cause for this pain in the testicles or neighbouring pelvic organs. And he was therefore told that with time it would disappear! However, after it had been troubling him for 3 years he expressed a wish to try the effects of acupuncture.

On examination, physical signs were confined to the lower back when there were several trigger points in various parts of the musculature including two in exquisitely tender fibrositic nodules immediately to the right of the 1st lumbar vertebra. For anatomical reasons just discussed, it would seem likely that it was from these that the pain was being referred to the scrotum.

As so often happens with trigger points, the patient was unaware of their presence, but on direct questioning he did admit that for about the same period of time he had had some aching in the lower back but had not thought it worth mentioning as the scrotal pain was so much more distressing.

Deactivation of these trigger points on 5 occasions over the course of 7 weeks brought the low-back and scrotal pain under control.

The close temporal relationship between the prostatectomy and the onset of aching in the lower back and pain in the scrotum would make it reasonable to assume that the activation of the trigger points was due to the low-back muscles having been strained during the course of the patient being lifted on or off the operating table, or to them being traumatized as a result of the patient lying for some appreciable time on the table.

REFERENCES

Apley J, Naish N 1958 Recurrent abdominal pains — a field survey of 1000 schoolchildren. Archives of Diseases in Childhood 33: 165–167

Applegate W V 1972 Abdominal cutaneous nerve entrapment syndrome. Surgery 71: 118–124

Blendis L M 1984 Abdominal pain. In: Wall P D, Melzack R (eds) Textbook of pain. Churchill Livingstone, Edinburgh, p 356

Bourne I H J 1980 Treatment of painful conditions of the abdominal wall with local injections. Practitioner 224: 921–925

Crown S 1978 Psychological aspects of low back pain. Rheumatology and Rehabilitation 17: 114–124

de Valera E, Raftery H 1976 Lower abdominal and pelvic pain in women. In: Bonica J J, Albe-Fessard D (eds) Advances in pain research and therapy, vol 1. Raven Press, New York, p 933–937

Dittrich R J 1951 Coccygodynia as referred pain. Journal of Bone and Joint Surgery 44A: 715–718

Esler M D, Goulston K 1973 Levels of anxiety in colonic disorders. New England Journal of Medicine 288: 16–20

Fielding J F 1977 The irritable bowel syndrome. Clinics in Gastroenterology 6: 607–622

Good M G 1950a The role of skeletal muscles in the pathogenesis of diseases. Acta Medica Scandinavica 138: 285–292

Good M G 1950b Pseudo-appendicitis. Acta Medica Scandinavica 138: 348–353

Gutstein R R 1944 The role of abdominal fibrositis in functional indigestion. Mississipi Valley Medical Journal 66: 114–124

Hall M W 1986 Treatment of functional abdominal pain by transcutaneous nerve stimulation (correspondence). British Medical Journal 293: 954–955

Holdstock D J, Misiewicz J J, Waller S L 1969 Observations on the mechanism of abdominal pain. Gut 10: 19–31

Hoyt H S 1953 Segmental nerve lesions as a cause of the trigonitis syndrome. Stanford Medical Bulletin 11: 61–64

Hunter C 1933 Myalgia of the abdominal wall. Canadian Medical Journal 28: 157–161

Kellgren J H 1940 Somatic simulating visceral pain. Clinical Science 4: 303–309

Kelly M 1942 Lumbago and abdominal pain. Medical Journal of Australia 1: 311–317

Kendall G, Sylvester K, Lennard-Jones J E 1986 Treatment of functional abdominal pain by transcutaneous nerve stimulation (correspondence). British Medical Journal 293: 954–955

Lewis T, Kellgren J H 1939 Observations relating to referred pain, viscero-motor reflexes and other associated phenomena. Clinical Science 4: 47–71

Lilius H G, Valtonen E J 1973 The levator ani spasm syndrome: a clinical analysis of 31 cases. Annales Chirurgiae et Gynaecologiae 62: 93–97

Long C 1956 Myofascial pain syndromes. Part III. Some syndromes of the trunk and thigh. Henry Ford Hospital Medical Bulletin 4: 102–106

McGivney J Q, Cleveland B R 1965 The levator syndrome and its treatment. Southern Medical Journal 58: 505–510

Mehta M, Ranger I 1971 Persistent abdominal pain. Anaesthesia 26(3): 330–333

Melnick J 1954 Treatment of trigger mechanisms in gastrointestinal disease. New York State Journal of Medicine 54: 1324–1330

Melnick J 1957a Symposium on mechanism and management of pain syndromes. Proceedings of the Rudolf Virchow Medical Society, City of New York 16: 135–142

Melnick J 1957b Trigger areas and refractory pain in duodenal ulcer. New York State Journal of Medicine 57: 1037–1076

Murray G R 1929 Myofibrositis as a simulator of other maladies. Lancet 1: 113–116

Procacci P, Zoppi M 1983 Pathophysiology and clinical aspects of visceral and referred pain. In: Bonica J (ed) Advances in pain research and therapy, vol 5. Raven Press, New York, p 643–656

Ranger I, Mehta M, Pennington M 1971 Abdominal wall pain due to nerve entrapment. Practitioner 206: 791–792

Renaer M 1984 Gynaecological pain. In: Wall P D, Melzack R (eds) Textbook of pain. Churchill Livingstone, Edinburgh, p 373

Sinaki M, Merritt J L, Stillwell G K 1977 Tension myalgia of the pelvic floor. Mayo Clinic Proceedings 52: 717–722

Smith W T 1959 Levator spasm syndrome. Minnesota Medicine 42: 1076–1079

Stone R T, Barbero G J 1970 Recurrent abdominal pain in childhood. Pediatrics 45: 732–738

Telling W H 1935 The clinical importance of fibrositis in general practice. British Medical Journal 1: 689–692

Theobald G H 1949 The relief and prevention of referred pain. Journal of Obstetrics and Gynaecology of the British Commonwealth 56: 447–460

Thiele G H 1937 Coccygodynia and pain in the superior gluteal region and down the back of the thigh: causation by tonic spasm of the levator ani, coccygeus and piriformis muscles and relief by massage of these muscles. Journal of the American Medical Association 109: 1271–1275

Thiele G H 1963 Coccygodynia: cause and treatment. Diseases of the Colon and Rectum 6: 422–436

Travell J 1950 The adductor longus syndrome: A cause of groin pain. Bulletin of the New York Academy of Medicine 26: 284–285

Travell J G, Simons D G 1983 Myofascial pain and dysfunction. The trigger point manual. Williams & Wilkins, Baltimore, p 660–683

Waller S L, Misiewicz J J 1969 Prognosis in the irritable bowel syndrome. Lancet II: 753–756

Watson W C, Sullivan S N, Corke M, Rush D 1976 Incidence of esophageal symptoms in patients with irritable bowel syndrome. Gut 17: 827 (abstract)

Yeates W K 1985 Pain in the scrotum. British Journal of Hospital Medicine 33(2): 101–104

Young D 1943 The effects of Novocaine injections on simulated visceral pain. Annals of Internal Medicine 19: 749–756

Index